Encyclopedia of Chemical Kinetics

Encyclopedia of Chemical Kinetics

Edited by **Sarah Gates**

FOSTER ACADEMICS

New Jersey

Published by Foster Academics,
61 Van Reypen Street,
Jersey City, NJ 07306, USA
www.fosteracademics.com

Encyclopedia of Chemical Kinetics
Edited by Sarah Gates

International Standard Book Number: 978-1-63242-133-3 (Hardback)

Printed in China.

Contents

Preface

Chemical kinetics is a branch of chemistry and is also known as reaction kinetics. It is associated with studying the rates of chemical processes and certain factors, like concentration and temperature, which affect the reaction rate. These studies help in tracing the mechanism progress with appropriate evidences at each stage. This book especially targets the students and practitioners in the field of physical science to gain comprehensive knowledge regarding reaction kinetics and its mechanism. The subjects discussed in this book and examples used to demonstrate have been driven by the principle that they are understandable to any reader with basic understanding of physical science. Even the graphs and tables used to support the content are of professional understanding. This book is a rich and valuable account of information for the reference of scientists, technologists, students and professionals engaged in this field. It has been written in a compact, self-descriptive and comprehensive manner by experts of the field.

This book unites the global concepts and researches in an organized manner for a comprehensive understanding of the subject. It is a ripe text for all researchers, students, scientists or anyone else who is interested in acquiring a better knowledge of this dynamic field.

I extend my sincere thanks to the contributors for such eloquent research chapters. Finally, I thank my family for being a source of support and help.

Editor

Part 1

Introduction to Chemical Kinetics

1

Chemical Kinetics, an Historical Introduction

Stefano Zambelli
University of Padova, Italy

1. Introduction

This Chapter would provide a methodological analysis of the historical developments of chemical kinetics from the beginnings to the achievements of Transition state theory and Kramers-Christiansen approach. Chemical kinetics is often treated as a side issue of the most important disciplines of chemical science. Students in most of the cases gain knowledge of Kinetics as part of Physical Chemistry introductory courses and find it again applied in many other contests.

Despite that, it would necessitate a fundamental and main teaching course as we will see in the course of this chapter. This didactical and academic approach could have many reasons. A general one may be the philosophical and psychological disposition to put our attention more on objects rather than concepts, matter over processes.

In Science History there are many examples of this tendency: the transmission of heat and electromagnetic waves are good examples. Phlogiston and Luminiferous Aether represents a materialization of processes that processes themselves do not need to be studied, however our mind need this primitive objectivization to grasp the concept in a simpler way.

This represents a fundamental issue of scientific method: to do Science we need to go beyond banality and perception. The development of Chemical Kinetics is deeply involved in the counterfactual approach that brought from Alchemy to Chemistry as for Physics form Aristotelic Natural Philosophy to Galilean Science.

2. Origins of chemical kinetics: The declinations of affinity

The chemical affinity principle, developed during the seventeenth century, derives from the alchemical concept of chemical wedding: similar substances will interact so we can categorize them. The real innovation at the end of 17th and during the 18th centuries was the application of that concept not only as a taxonomic principle but also for the comprehension of chemical reactivity.

The interaction of bodies is simpler when there is a similitude between them, this is the base idea of Chemical Affinities and come from ancient and medieval alchemy and naturalism doctrine. At the end of 17th century this intuitive principle become a theory, although qualitative, that justify and classify interactions between different substances.

In the same period also the observation of time become important for the determination of the nature of chemical reactions. Time of decurrence was clearly contemplated for the preparation of substances with long reactions but it was seen as an ordinary technical factor. The Opera of Alchemy, for example in the transmutations of metals, was considered as a means for the acceleration of the millenary gestation of precious metals in the bowels of Earth Mother. The underestimate of real times in the alchemists conceptions resulted so natural in an activity that already theoretically reduced geological times. The paradox was that time, a fundamental principle for alchemic theory, resulted of little importance in the alchemical praxis.

Probably the first scholar that introduced a dynamical vision of the chemical phenomena was **Wilhelm Homberg (1652-1715)**. Homberg, a German scholar, worked in Magdeburg with Von Guericke, in Italy and later in England with Boyle. He introduced the first principles of quantitative measurement for chemical action: the strength of an acid towards a series of alkali depends on the time of neutralization of the various alkali.

2.1 Tabulae affinitatum

The lists of strength of alkali and the concept of chemical affinity brought **Etienne Francois Geoffroy (1672-1731)**, a French scholar initiated to chemistry by Homberg himself, to the compilation of the *Tables of Affinity*, (or Tables of Rapports) that could be considered as the first ancestor of the periodic table. The first one was done by Geffroy (Geoffroy, 1718). You can see the Encyclopédie version in the following figure.

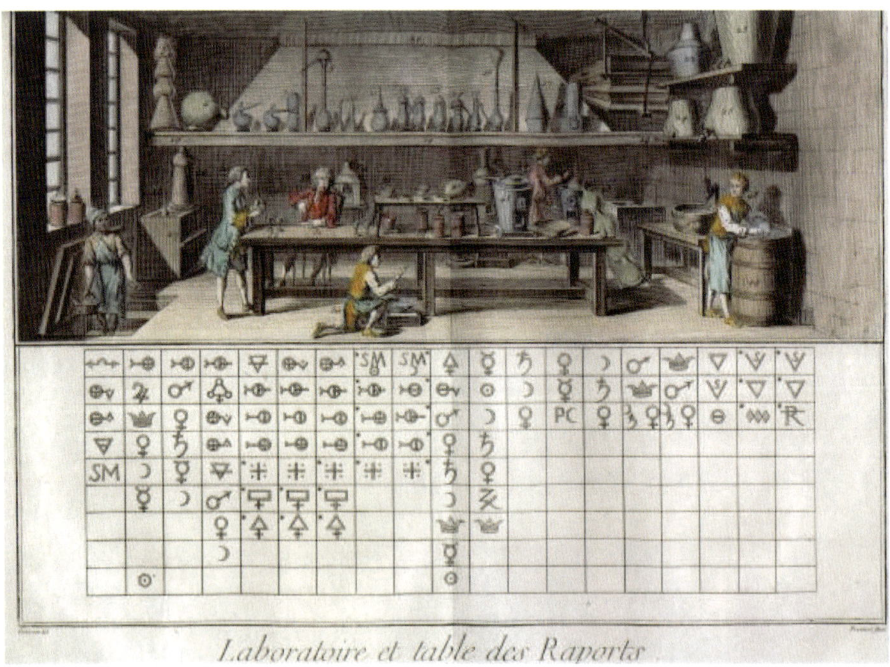

Fig. 1. Recueil de Planches, sur les Sciences, les Arts Libéraux, et les Arts Méchaniques, 1772

In the first row you can see the primary substances then going down along the columns the similar substances in order of affinity with the first one.

The development of Affinity tables was inevitably considered in the light of the main scientific discussion of the 18th century: the debate between plenistic Cartesian vision and the Newtonian distance action principle. Important chemisters of this period took parts in that debate: Boerhaave and later Buffon among Newtonian side identified affinities as a special form of gravitational attraction, Stahl on the other side negated the distance action invoking the medium of Phlogiston.

Guyton de Morveau (1737-1816), a French scholar, sustained initially phlogiston theory, but leaved it after in favor of a distance action between the different elementary particles of substances bringing the chemical affinities to a microscopic level, a similar position was taken by Berthollet and Lavoisier. De Morveau classified the kind of affinities: simple or by aggregation, composed, decomposed, double, reciprocal, intermediate, dispositional. He listed also the laws of affinity:

- Molecules have to be in fluid state to respond to affinities influence.
- Affinities acts between the elementary particles of bodies.
- Affinities between two different substances may be different from that between their composites.
- Affinity of substances acts only if it is bigger than the aggregation affinity of themselves.
- Two or more bodies united by affinity form a new body with different properties from precursors.
- Affinities action and velocity depends on temperature.

Basilar principles of Chemical Kinetics and Chemistry are going to take form. Of particular importance the last law: temperature and so ambient conditions have influence on chemical reactivity.

The position of **Torben Olof Bergman** (1735-1784), a Swedish scholar, about the influence of temperature is particularly interesting. He assumed the affinity constant at constant temperature and suggested to compile different affinity tables depending on conditions: the affinities of dry phase is different from that in liquid phase.

Bergman closed elegantly the debate on the nature of the affinities assuming a very wise position: it is not useful debating about the last nature of interacting forces between chemical particles because it will remain unknown until quantitative experiments will be done on affinities. Bergman so is the first scholar that made some hypothesis about a measure of the affinities, but their mathematical expressions and measures will be a duty for future researchers. Bergman compiled also affinity diagrams in his major opera, the **Opuscula**. They are an interesting representation of chemical reactions done with alchemical symbols: the ancestors of stoichiometric equations (although the very first one appeared even in 1615, but not systematically, in the famous **Tyrocinium Chymicum**, the first Textbook of Chemistry written by **Jean Beguin**). You can see an example in the figure 2. The diagram represents the reactions of sulfuric and hydrochloric acid with calcium carbonate and potassium hydroxide (Vitriolic and Marine for acids, Pure calcareous earth and Pure fixed vegetable alkali for the basis).

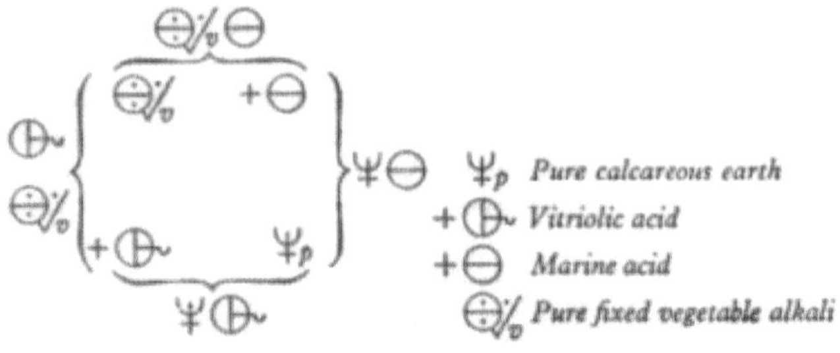

Fig. 2. This Affinity Diagram schematize two acid-base reactions

3. Chemical equilibrium conception: The law of mass action

The end of 18th Century and the first half of 19th added other essential pieces to the puzzle of Chemical Kinetics and Chemistry in general. There is a surprising absent actor in the debate on Chemical Affinities, the father of modern Chemistry: **Antoine-Laurent de Lavoisier (1743-1794)**. The Lavoisier Revolution brought quantitative measurements to Chemistry and so to Affinity Diagrams. We can see one of the first examples of stoichiometric equation from Lavoisier works in the following figure (Lavoisier 1782).

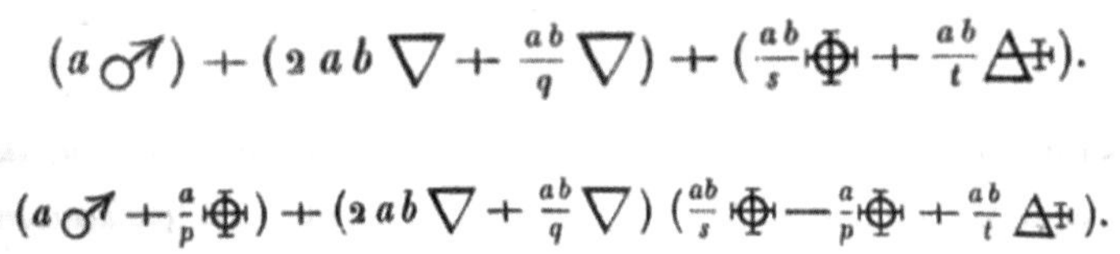

Fig. 3. Stoichimetric Equations with Lavoisier's symbols

Those symbolic equations represent one of the passages of the oxidation of iron in nitric acid where Mars symbolize iron, the nabla water, the crossed circle oxygen, the triangle and cross nitrogen oxide. In this passage iron gains the same part of oxygen that nitric acid loses, an example of the Law of Mass Conservation.

Why Lavoisier did not play a role in the debate about Affinities if he applied quantitative methods also for affinity diagrams? The causes may be many, for example the fact that he was outside main academic circles, (he was member of the French Academy of Sciences from the age of 25, but never gained an academic position). The reasons are explained by Lavoisier himself in the **Traité élémentaire de chimie**, and follow Bergan recommendations:

In this writing I followed the principle of not arguing beyond experimentations, not taking over the silence of facts. So I cannot consider those parts of Chemistry that would probably become Exact Science before the others. Scholars as Bergman, Scheele, de Morveau and many others are conducting numerous studies about Chemical Affinities and Attractions, but basic, precise and general data are lacking at the moment. Affinities theory respect to ordinary Chemistry is as Transcendent Geometry respect to Elementary one and goes over the scope of this introductory book. Mr de Morveau is writing the voice Affinity in the **Encyclopédie** *and I am worried to compete with him.*

3.1 Characterising of chemical reactions

With the development of Lavoisier's methods in the second half of the 18th Century new definitions and properties are established. A concept that for today scientists results obvious was defined: the concentration of substances. The fist timid attempts to distinguish reactivity and equilibrium was made, for example sulphuric acid was considered the most powerful because it shifted other acids from their salts, the most strong because it absorbs most water, the least active because Oleum needs water or hydrated compounds to take effect. The researches about the reactions between acids and metals are of particular interest in this period. For example many scholars did not consider more metals as primary substances thinking they was compounds with an alkaline parts (it will need nearly a Century for the comprehension of redox reactions).

In the work of **Carl Friedrich Wenzel (1740-1793)**, a dresden metallurgist, we can find the first link between reaction velocity and quantity of the reactants. He investigated the reactions between metals considering the time of dissolution of little metal cylinders inside dilute acid solutions. Using Buffon theories Wenzel considered the affinity of the acids inversely proportional to the time of dissolution but considered also the role of the solvent (water). The velocity of reaction results proportional to the affinity or the strength of the acid while inversely proportional to the resistance of the solvent. In modern terms reaction velocity is proportional to concentration. Wenzel made also interesting considerations about thermal conditions, imposing the same temperature for all the dissolutions to compare them correctly. Some scholars, Wilhelm Ostwald between the most famous, awarded Wenzel for the first qualitative definition of the *Law of Mass Action*, although the primacy is commonly given to Berthollet.

Count **Claude Louis Berthollet (1748-1822)**, member of Academy of France and founder of the Ecole Polytechnique, collaborated with Lavoisier but was more lucky than him. He had no problems during the revolution and got in the good books of Napoleonic government. He followed Bonaparte's expedition to Egypt. Visiting the Natron Lakes, Berthollet observed soda deposits on the surrounding limestone hills. He supposed a chemical reaction occurring between salt (sodium chloride) and the limestone (calcium carbonate) in the hills to produce soda (sodium carbonate) and an accompanying product, calcium chloride, which seeped away into the ground. The reaction was the reverse of the one that chemists knew under laboratory conditions, and this indicated to Berthollet that physical conditions, such as heat and pressure, and quantities of reactants could affect the course of a chemical reaction.

From these and other considerations he exposed the first qualitative form of the **Law of Mass Action** during 1803 in two famous publications: *"Essai de statique chimique"* (fig. 4) e *"Recherches sur les lois des affinités chimiques"*. The progress of a chemical reaction depends on the quantity and conditions of reacting substances. Berthollet's essays do not relate only on the velocity of the reaction but also on its equilibrium. Today these considerations may appear obvious but at the time they received fierce critics.

These theories and the embryonic conception of equilibrium was favourably considered by some important Chemists as Berzelius, Davy and Gay-Lussac, but most of the scientific community did not considered them being incompatible with Proust's and Dalton's Laws that monopolized the attention of the scientific community in the period.

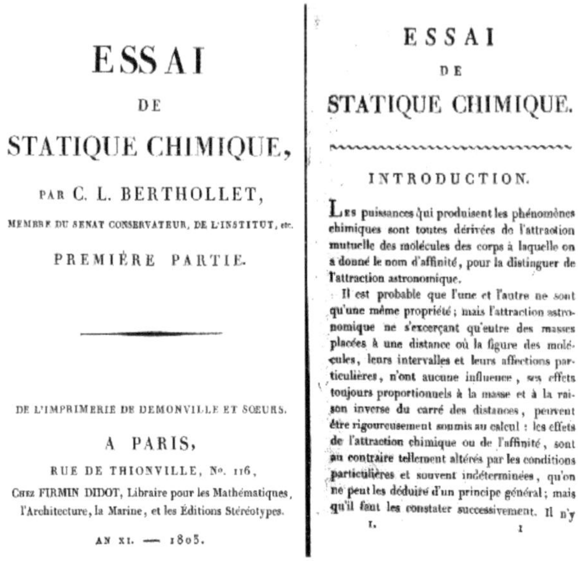

ESSAI

DE

STATIQUE CHIMIQUE,

PAR C. L. BERTHOLLET,

MEMBRE DU SENAT CONSERVATEUR, DE L'INSTITUT, etc.

PREMIÈRE PARTIE.

DE L'IMPRIMERIE DE DEMONVILLE ET SOEURS.

A PARIS,

RUE DE THIONVILLE, No. 116,

CHEZ FIRMIN DIDOT, Libraire pour les Mathématiques, l'Architecture, la Marine, et les Éditions Stéréotypes.

AN XI. — 1803.

ESSAI

DE

STATIQUE CHIMIQUE.

INTRODUCTION.

Les puissances qui produisent les phénomènes chimiques sont toutes dérivées de l'attraction mutuelle des molécules des corps à laquelle on a donné le nom d'affinité, pour la distinguer de l'attraction astronomique.

Il est probable que l'une et l'autre ne sont qu'une même propriété; mais l'attraction astronomique ne s'exerçant qu'entre des masses placées à une distance où la figure des molécules, leurs intervalles et leurs affections particulières, n'ont aucune influence, ses effets toujours proportionnels à la masse et à la raison inverse du carré des distances, peuvent être rigoureusement soumis au calcul : les effets de l'attraction chimique ou de l'affinité, sont au contraire tellement altérés par les conditions particulières et souvent indéterminées, qu'on ne peut les déduire d'un principe général; mais qu'il faut les constater successivement. Il n'y

I. 1

Fig. 4. Title and first page of Berthollet Essay

Berthollet made other significant considerations, for example the fact that for solids the Affinity remain costant. So Affinities are not absolute but become dependant on the quantities of reactants (except solids), but how those quantities was defined? In the *Essai* he defined the Affinity $A=a/E$, where a is a constant dependant on the substance and E its equivalent weight. Multiplying the mass of the substance for unit of volume w by the precedent expression he defined the A*ctive Mass* of the reactant equal to the concentration , (numbers of equivalent per unit volume: w/E).

The reasons of this rejection depended also by the fact that most of the conclusions of Berthollet and his predecessors was qualitative and not supported by adequate analytical data. To get the first quantitative observations and thermodynamic interpretations of reacting systems we have to wait the second half of 19th Century thanks to the development of analytical chemistry.

3.2 Time: A new quantitative observable

It is difficult today arguing about Chemical Kinetics without Thermodynamic but this branch of our science was established originally by simple chronological measurements of chemical processes (King 1981).

The development of quantitative relations and laws derived from the use of advanced analytical techniques but these did not give real contributions until the end of 19th Century thanks to a suitable mathematical construct.

Initially analytical observations was used to collect a multitude of data from many different systems thinking in this way to get universal laws in the optic of Natural Philosophy. It is the passage from the *many experiments* to the *good experiment* that made the true change.

The intense experimental phase around the half of 19th Century may be efficiently described by Wilhelmy and Gladstone works.

Ludwig Ferdinand Wilhelmy (1812-1864), a German physicist published in 1850 an important paper on the kinetic on the inversion of sugar with acids (Wilhelmy, 1850, Fig. 5).

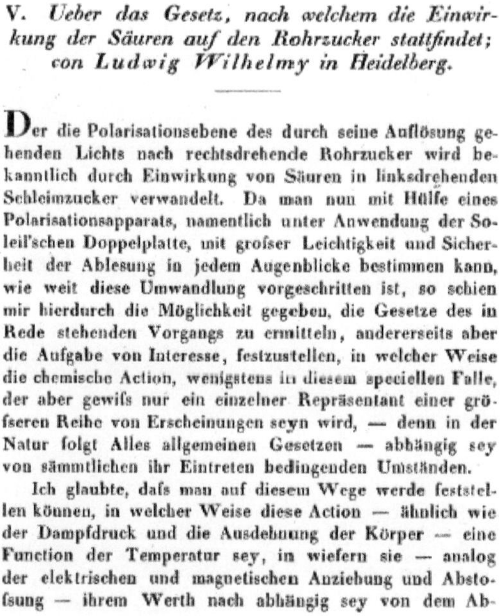

V. *Ueber das Gesetz, nach welchem die Einwirkung der Säuren auf den Rohrzucker stattfindet; von Ludwig Wilhelmy in Heidelberg.*

Der die Polarisationsebene des durch seine Auflösung gehenden Lichts nach rechtsdrehende Rohrzucker wird bekanntlich durch Einwirkung von Säuren in linksdrehenden Schleimzucker verwandelt. Da man nun mit Hülfe eines Polarisationsapparats, namentlich unter Anwendung der Soleil'schen Doppelplatte, mit grofser Leichtigkeit und Sicherheit der Ablesung in jedem Augenblicke bestimmen kann, wie weit diese Umwandlung vorgeschritten ist, so schien mir hierdurch die Möglichkeit gegeben, die Gesetze des in Rede stehenden Vorgangs zu ermitteln, andererseits aber die Aufgabe von Interesse, festzustellen, in welcher Weise die chemische Action, wenigstens in diesem speciellen Falle, der aber gewifs nur ein einzelner Repräsentant einer gröfseren Reihe von Erscheinungen seyn wird, — denn in der Natur folgt Alles allgemeinen Gesetzen — abhängig sey von sämmtlichen ihr Eintreten bedingenden Umständen.

Ich glaubte, dafs man auf diesem Wege werde feststellen können, in welcher Weise diese Action — ähnlich wie der Dampfdruck und die Ausdehnung der Körper — eine Function der Temperatur sey, in wiefern sie — analog der elektrischen und magnetischen Anziehung und Abstofsung — ihrem Werth nach abhängig sey von dem Ab-

Fig. 5. Wilhelmy paper Title page

He used a new technique, Polarimetry, for evaluating the dependence of reaction velocity on the quantity of reactants and temperature. In this paper probably appeared the first differential equation used in chemistry:

$$-\frac{dZ}{dt} = MZS \tag{1}$$

Reaction velocity is the negative derivative of the sugar quantity Z in time t, S the acid quantity and M the quantity of inverted sugar in the infinitesimal time dt. Considering an excess of acid S is constant and supposing also M constant the solution results:

$$Z = Z_0 e^{-MSt} \tag{2}$$

Wilhelmy verified that M remains almost constant in time and observed the dependance of that constant with temperature.

Wilhemly's paper results impressive for its anticipations, it was written forty years before Arrhenius work on the same topic. Unfortunately, although written in a prestigious Journal, (the *Poggendorffs Annalen der Physik und Chemie,* later *Annalen der Physik*), the paper passed unnoticed by contemporary scholars. It will be rediscovered only in 1884 by Ostwald.

Not only Polarimetry but also other techniques useful for kinetic studies was developed in this period. Colorimetric titrations was used by **John Hall Gladstone** (1827-1902), Fullerian Professor of Chemistry in London, to get precise measurements of equilibrium and to investigate the effect of salts on reaction dynamic.

We will quote the conclusions of Gladstone about the action of thiocyanate on iron salts to notice the evolution of the language and concepts on the topic (Gladstone, 1855):

1. Where two or more binary compounds are mixed under such circumstances that all the resulting bodies are free to act and react, each electro-positive element arrang-es itself in combination with each electro-negative element in certain constant proportions.
2. These proportions are independent of the manner in which the different elements were originally combined.
3. These proportions are not merely the resultant of the various strengths of affinity of the several substances for one another, but are dependent also on the mass of each of tie substances in the fixture.
4. An alteration in the mass of any one of the binary compounds present alters the amount of every one of the other binary compounds, and that in a regularly pro- gressive ratio; sudden transitions only occurring where a substance is present which is capable of combining with another in more than one proportion.
5. This equilibrium of affinities arranges itself in most cases in an inappreciably short space of time, but in certain instances the elements do not attain their final state of combination for hours, or even days.
6. The phenomena that present themselves where precipitation, volatilization, crystallization, and perhaps other actions occur, are of an opposite character, simply because one of the substances is thus removed from the field of action, and the equi-librium that was first established is thus destroyed.
7. There is consequently a fundamental error in all attempts to determine the relative strength of affinity by precipitation; in all methods of quantitative analysis founded on the colour of a solution in which colourless salts are also present; and in all conclusions as to what compounds exist in a solution drawn from such empirical rules as that " the strongest base combines with the strongest acid."

From Gladstone experiments Chemists on the field begun to use extensively optical methods verifying Berthollet's statements and two facts emerged clearly: the presence of the equilibrium conditions in contrast with Proust's Law, the hypothetical achieving of a complete reaction after an infinite time.

4. Clockwork stoichiometry

We will see that many exemplary experiments survived the second half of 19th Century and results still dominating in chemical didactics. The acid esterification of alcohols is emblematic in this sense: it is difficult nowadays to find an introductory textbook that does not explain this reaction as basic example.

In most of cases nevertheless the origin of that example is not cited. It comes from a series of experiments done by a couple of Parisian chemists around the 1860: **Pierre Eugene Marcelin Berthelot** (1827-1907) and **Leon Peon de Saint-Gilles** (1832-1863), the first one full professor of chemistry at the Ecole de Pharmacie, the second a wealthy dilettante.

Their work (Berthelot & Saint Gilles, 1862) will be extensively used by other two important couples of scholars: Guldberg and Waage, Harcourt and Esson. We will speak of them later in the chapter. In the title they referred to etherification but in the paper they speak about esterification, probably a misprint.

Arising from his interest in esterification, Berthelot studied the kinetics of reversible reactions. Working with Saint Gilles, he produced an equation for the reaction velocity depending on reactants concentrations. This was incorrect because they did not considered in the expression the inverse reaction. Other interesting considerations was the hypothesis of an exponential dependence on temperature and the fact that equilibrium position is independent from the kind of alcohols and acids used.

The conclusions of Berthelot and Sait Gilles was not particularly new compared to those of Wilhelmy. They found similar expressions and both esterification and sugar inversion are good systems for the study of kinetic and equilibrium. May be that the use of differential equations was not usual for the chemists at the time. Significantly Guldberg and Esson was mathematicians that helped later the chemists Waage and Harcourt.

The fact that chemists used mathematics so late after decades of data collections may surprise the actual reader, but we have to consider that a systematic study of mathematics was not considered in chemistry courses until after the second world war. This delay did not regarded only Chemical Kinetics but chemistry in general. We have to wait Physical Chemistry, other developments in Analytical Chemistry and a general evolution of Chemistry equipment and instruments to free chemists from very difficult and hard-working experimental praxis for the development of theoretical reflections and laws.

4.1 The law of mass action again

The first quantitative expression of the law of mass action was presented by **Cato Maximilian Guldberg** (1833-1902) and **Peter Waage** (1839-1900) two years later (Guldberg & Waage, 1864). They was Norwegian Professors of Mathematics and Chemistry at the Christiania University of Oslo and brothers in law (fig. 6).

It is interesting to consider the blessed situation of chemistry in Scandinavia coming from the necessities of mining industry and from the large number of eminent chemists like Scheele, Bergman, Berzelius, the same Guldberg and Waage, Arrhenius and Nobel later.

Scandinavian insulation and advanced knowledge promoted many autonomous researches and caused often independent contemporary discoveries with other European groups.

Despite being isolated as the use of the Laurent-Gherard notation demonstrate, (that notation was diffused more than ten years before), from 1862 and 1864 they repeated and examined experiments and results of Berthelot and Saint Gilles on esterification, Rose's work on Barium salts and that of Scherer on heterogeneous reaction between silica and soda. The study of so different processes derived from the will of the authors to get a new law, universal for all chemical processes. The style of the 1864 paper was polemical against the precedent theories of affinity that the authors considered inconclusive or erroneous.

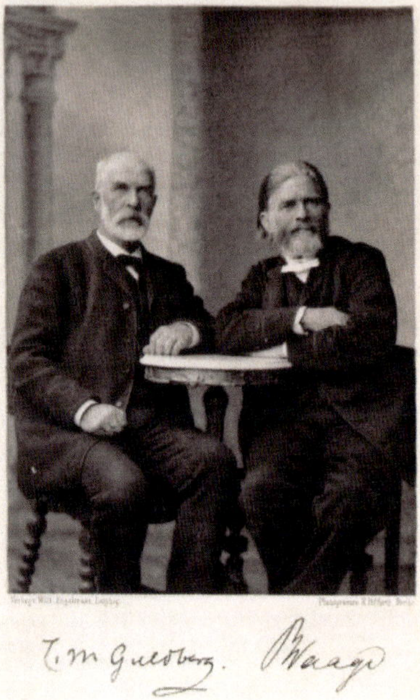

Fig. 6. Guldberg & Waage

Guldberg and Waage preferred a less speculative and more direct approach simply enunciating the formula for the definition of action of mass and volume:

$$F_{chem} = \alpha \left(\frac{M}{V}\right)^{a} \left(\frac{N}{V}\right)^{b} \quad (3)$$

Where F_{chem} represents the chemical force, M and N the quantity of the reacting substances, V the volume, α, a and b constants wich, other conditions being equal, depends only from the nature of the substances. If one begins with a general system containing four active substances pairwise interacting, (direct and opposite reactions between two reactants and two products), and considering the balance of chemical forces Guldberg and Waage obtained the expression for chemical equilibrium:

$$\alpha(p-x)^{a}(q-x)^{b} = \alpha'(p'+x)^{a'}(q'+x)^{b'} \quad (4)$$

where p, q, p', q' are the initial concentrations of reactants and products, x the amount of transformed reactants at equilibrium reaching, α, a, b, α′, a', b', constants with the previous meaning that can be calculated from the initial concentrations, the amount x and experimental data.

We can quote a passage of the 1864 paper because it resolves the apparent contradiction between affinities and equilibrium theories towards Proust's and Dalton's Laws.

That a chemical process, as so often is the case in chemistry, seems to occur in only one direction, so that either complete or no substitution takes place, arises easily from our formula. Since the active forces do not increase proportionally to the masses, but according to a power of the same, the relationship of the exponent does not have to be particularly large before the unchanged or changed amount becomes so small that it does not let itself be revealed by our usual analytical methods.

Timidly in this paper and in the following works of the two scientists there is the consciousness that the expressions derives from microscopic processes between atoms and molecules. They present a progressive clarification and distinction of the concept of chemical forces, initially considered in a Newtonian way to get the balance-equilibrium expression and in their last paper (Guldberg & Waage, 1879) assimilated to bond strength and reaction velocity, the macroscopic kinetic observable.

In this last work are present many interesting intuitions, there is an hypothesis of the microscopic interaction mechanism and from that and the stoichiometric coefficients a try to explain theoretically the exponential coefficients, previously arbitrary or purely phenomenological and there is a mild use of thermodynamic data.

Guldberg and Waage went a step further in the correct direction introducing suitable formulas for equilibrium and velocity expressions but do not have the theoretical instruments to justify and interpret it correctly. They examined a huge number of different chemical systems falling in the old trap of getting general laws from the *many experiments* rather than the *good experiment*.

5. Thermodynamics revolution

The first non systematic introduction of thermodynamics in Chemical Kinetics is due to the second couple of scientists previously cited: **Augustus George Vernon Harcourt** (1834-1919) and **William Esson** (1839-1916). Harcourt was an important chemist, member of the Royal society and president of Chemical society, Esson a mathematician and Savilian professor of Geometry. They worked at University of Oxford in a period particularly fruitful for Sciences in Britain. It is the peak of positivism and at the time different sciences, included chemistry, got clearly distinct university courses. Their activity covered a period of fifty years and represented the main passage from natural philosophy speculations to modern scientific reasoning. Influenced by Van't Hoff they will definitively abandon ambiguous terms like Affinity and Chemical Forces.

In 1864 Harcourt presented his first publications contemporary to Guldberg and Waage paper. In this work only the name of Harcourt appears but Esson asked the collaboration of a chemist around six years before to applying his mathematical methods to experimental chemistry. In 1865 it was Harcourt that asked Esson to collaborate and their partnership will continue for the rest of their lives (Harcourt & Esson 1865).

In the first part of their studies they searched chemical processes suitable for kinetics measurements. Harcourt found an initial valid system: the oxidation of oxalic acid with potassium permanganate. He supposed a two step mechanism:

1. $K_2Mn_2O_8+3MnSO_4+H_2O=K_2SO_4+2H_2SO_4+5MnO_2$
2. $MnO_2+ H_2SO_4+ H_2C_2O_4= MnSO_4+2CO_2+2H_2O$

Verifying it, like today, by the presence of the intermediate manganese oxide and by the acceleration of reaction if manganese sulphate was present at the beginning of the reaction. Examining again the data around 1866 with Esson they plotted a curve of time vs quantity of reactants verifying a logarithmic trend.

To get a better plot they needed to interrupt the reaction at will and to analyze the quantity of substances reacted at time of interruption. So they considered another reaction: the oxidation of hydroiodic acid with hydrogen peroxide in presence of definite quantities of thiosulfate and a starch indicator. They measured the time passed before the appearance of blue solutions after the consumption of thiosulfate. In this way they confirmed precisely the logarithmic trend and published their results (Harcourt & Esson, 1867).

They extended also an interesting comparison about the energetic of chemical processes. A chemical reaction is like the fall of bodies: the initial activity of reactants is converted in reaction transformation as the potential energy of a falling body in kinetic energy. Reaction velocity so does not remain constant depending on reactants activity. To get a function of velocity they need to consider an infinitesimal time interval introducing, again in analogy with Mechanics, an instantaneous reaction velocity.

The velocity of change, equal to the negative time derivative of reactants quantity, is assumed to be proportional to their original quantity y and a constant a depending on the considered system:

$$\frac{dy}{dt} = -ay \tag{5}$$

Results and methods of this system was published again and better described in other two important papers: the Bakerian Lecture (Harcourt & Esson, 1895) and the last paper written by the authors Harcourt & Esson, 1912, fig. 7).

These publications represents probably the most important works for the beginning of modern Chemical Kinetics. They introduced the today common symbol for reaction rate constant k and evaluated formally its dependence on temperature.

There is a clear conception of the microscopic nature of chemical processes, they supposed for example that rate constant nullifies at absolute zero, considering that inert atoms and molecules could not encounter and interact each other.

To describe temperature dependence of rate constant we will consider the theoretical explanation done by Esson from the experimental ratio between two rate constants at different temperatures found by Harcourt:

$$\frac{k}{k'} = \left(\frac{T}{T'}\right)^m \tag{6}$$

Where k, k' are the rate constants, T, T' the absolute temperatures and m an experimental pure number. Expressing the equation (6) in differential form m becomes a proportionality constant of infinitesimal changes of the temperatures and rate constants:

$$\frac{dk}{k} = m\frac{dT}{T} \tag{7}$$

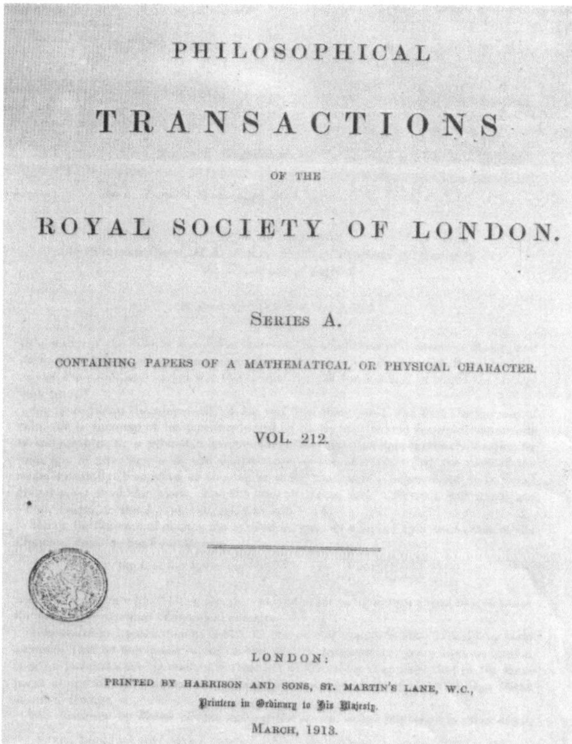
PHILOSOPHICAL

TRANSACTIONS

OF THE

ROYAL SOCIETY OF LONDON.

SERIES A.

CONTAINING PAPERS OF A MATHEMATICAL OR PHYSICAL CHARACTER.

VOL. 212.

LONDON:

PRINTED BY HARRISON AND SONS, ST. MARTIN'S LANE, W.C.,

Printers in Ordinary to His Majesty.

MARCH, 1913.

Fig. 7. Front page of the Phil. Trans. volume with the last paper of Harcourt and Esson

The value of m resulted constant for all temperatures, depending only on the chemical system considered. Considering a big excess of one reactant its chemical activity, (Esson used the term potential but we will use activity to avoid confusion with chemical potential μ), may be supposed constant during reaction course because its quantity remain nearly the same, so the variation in rate constant may be caused only by temperature variation (the precedent argumentation for equation (5) is difficult to use in this case).

In this conditions Esson talk about stable conversion of thermal energy to chemical energy with m a constant of proportionality between the different energies. Reconsidering equation (5) and integrating we can obtain an expression for chemical potential energy, (in Esson's terms), whose variation remain constant for the same variation of reactant concentration at different temperatures:

$$f(y_2) - f(y_1) = f'(y_2) - f'(y_1) = kt = k't' \tag{8}$$

Where the terms with asterisk derives from a reaction at temperature T'. From (6), (7) and (8) equations we can obtain the following expression:

$$\frac{k}{k'} = \frac{t'}{t} = \left(\frac{T}{T'}\right)^m \tag{9}$$

Contrary to rate constant the reaction times and temperatures are measurable directly, and from the equation (9) we can obtain the value of the exponent m.

Once found this relationship from the careful examination of suitable reaction systems Harcourt and Esson checked its validity for a vast number of different reactions: organic, inorganic, biological, in gas phase and so on. In all cases they obtained the value of m different from case to case but constant for different temperatures intervals.

Many experiment of Harcourt and Esson was also considered by Van't Hoff and they correlated their law with his thermodynamic hypothesis. They found confirmation also of Van't Hoff parametric formula for m:

$$m = bT^{-1} + a + cT \tag{10}$$

The dependence of m with temperature is for example $m=a$ for dissolution of metals with acids or the action of drugs in muscles, $m=cT$ for decomposition of dibromosuccinic acid, $m=bT^{-1}$ for ethyl acetate hydrolysis with sodium hydroxide. In most of the cases m results constant, but Harcourt and Esson admitted that in some cases this does not happen, contradicting their hypothesis.

For the resolution of this and other problems we have to wait Van't Hoff and Arrhenius but thermodynamics got his entrance into Chemical Kinetics thanks to Harcourt and Esson extensive work, even if it is less famous than that of Guldberg and Waage.

5.1 The birth of physical chemistry

The fundamental passage for the development of modern Chemical Kinetics was done when stages of reaction was associated to definite thermodynamic states. This passage was done by a tern of important names: **Svante August Arrhenius** (1859-1927), **Jacobus Hendricus Van't Hoff** (1852-1911) and **Wilhelm Ostwald** (1853-1932), fig. 8.

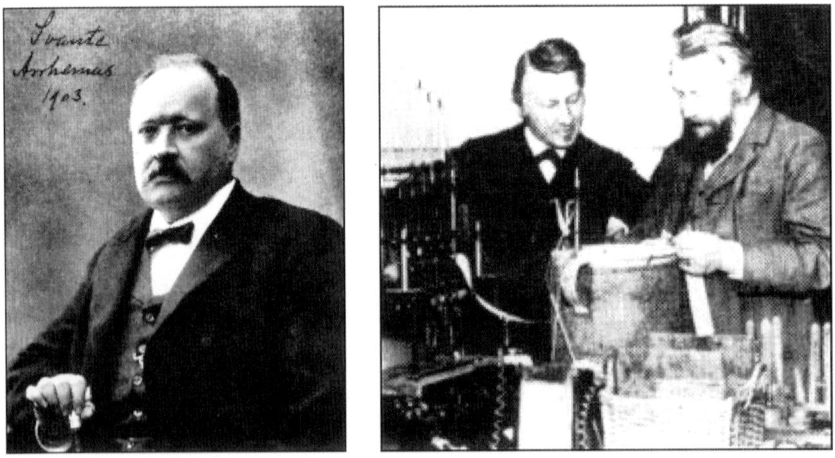

Fig. 8. From left to right: Arrhenius, Van't Hoff and Ostwald

In the first years of its construction Physical Chemistry practically corresponded to Chemical Kinetics. We will see before the contributions of Van't Hoff and Ostwald the "founders" of Physical chemistry and creators of its first journal: the *"Zeitschrift fur Physikalische Chemie"*, published for the first time in 1887 at Liepzig, fig. 9.

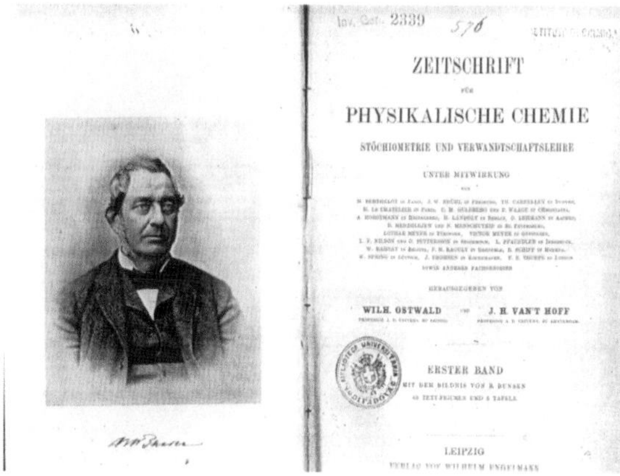

Fig. 9. Title page of the first number of the Zeitschrift

5.2 Ostwald and catalysis

Ostwald contributed directly on Chemical Kinetics less than Van't Hoff and Arrhenius, indeed he is more known for his position in the debate about atoms and for his contributions for the comprehension of Catalysis.

His main activity was done at Liepzig, where he became professor of Phisical Chemistry in 1887, after an important academic career at Riga Polytechnic where he wrote his major Opera: *"Lehrbuch der Allgemainen Chemie"*, Treatise on General Chemistry, a reference book for chemistry for many years later. In 1909 he won the Nobel Price for Chemistry thanks to his work on Catalysis. In this period he partially accepted the existence of atoms after the results of Perrin and Einstein on Brownian motion.

Even if his direct contribution on Chemical Kinetics was limited it was a field that interested him for all his academic career. His first publications regarded the verification of the Law of Mass Action on different salts hydrolysis reactions (Ostwald, 1879-1884). He later rediscovered also the work of Wilhelmy on the inversion of sugar supposing erroneously that the acids do not react directly but act as accelerator (Ostwald, 1884). That erroneous interpretation was the origin of his interest on catalytic phenomena that we will treat briefly being only partially related at the scope of the chapter.

Catalysis was discovered in the first half of 19th Century and initially was considered only as a physical action. After Berzelius studies in this field the phenomenon was considered as a chemical one and its action extended for all chemical reactions.

Liebig, a pupil of Berzelius, viewed the phenomenon in terms of the radical theory: Catalysis manifests when the forces of attraction between radicals, (activated species in modern terms), are changed due to the contact with a third body that does not combine with the original reacting species.

The explanations of Catalysis was also considered from an energetic point of view: Mitschelich, Mayer and others thought it as a sort of trigger that discharged an hidden chemical energy by physical contact.

Ostwald merged the two approaches: there is not a direct physical catalytic force or action nor a direct modification of the chemical bonds but the thermodynamic of the whole system is changed with new ways of lower free energy in the chemical transformation (Ostwald, 1902). Substantially the actual conception of the phenomena.

He pointed out that the development of the new theory of Catalysis was not possible without the development of Chemical Kinetics because it was deeply involved with the velocity of reaction (Ostwald, 1909). The correct interpretation of Catalysis was one of the first big success and confirmation of the Kinetic Theory. We are in debt with Ostwald also for the popularization of Gibbs work, not very known until the end of the 19th Century.

5.3 The link between K and *k*: Van't Hoff

Jacobus Hendricus Van't Hoff (1852-1911), was a Dutch Chemist that worked in Holland and France before joining Ostwald in Germany. He gave essential contribution to many fields of chemistry and physics: from the conception of Stereochemistry (Van't Hoff, 1875), to the thermodynamic explanations of Osmosis and solutions dynamics (Van't Hoff. 1885). For his studies on solutions he won the Nobel Prize for Chemistry in 1901.

His essential contributions to Chemical Kinetics, besides the part previously cited in the first part of this chapter, culminated in the discovery of the relation between the rate constant and the equilibrium constant (Van't Hoff, 1884). He interpreted the Chemical Equilibrium as the balance between opposite reactions so he related equilibrium constant to the ratio of the rate constants of the direct and reverse reaction. From an application of Clausius-Clapeyron equation Van't Hoff found the dependence of the equilibrium constant K from the absolute temperature T:

$$\ln K = -\frac{Q}{RT} + C \tag{11}$$

Where Q represents the isochoric heat of reaction, C an arbitrary integration constant and R the gas constant.

Equilibrium constant dependence on temperature is different for exothermic and endothermic reactions, Van't Hoff called this conclusion mobile equilibrium, a principle that Le Chatelier generalized in the same period. From the equation (11) and the relation of K with the rate constants he obtained the phenomenological equation for the dependence of the rate constant k with temperature:

$$\frac{d\ln k}{dT} = \frac{A}{T^2} + B \tag{12}$$

Where A is related to some not specified heat and B remain indeterminate. In his later works he determined experimentally the values of these constants for many reactions but did not obtain a theoretical interpretation of them.

Van't Hoff classified chemical reactions at microscopic level as mono-bi and poly molecular processes, interpreting the polymolecular processes from their stoichiometry as a sequence of mono and/or bimolecular steps. From these conclusions and the equation (12) Arrhenius will get the basis for his studies.

5.4 The Arrhenius equation

The first hypothesis on the conductibility of ions in electrolytic solutions and on the electrolyte dissociation of acid and basis of the young Swedish chemist **Svante August Arrhenius** (1859-1927) was not well accepted in his own country. He searched abroad a support for his studies and obtained it from Ostwald and Van't Hoff. He worked with them for six years between 1885 and 1891 and wrote an important paper in 1887 (Arrhenius, 1887). From thereafter his theories on ionic mobility received attention and acceptance and he won the Nobel Prize for chemistry in 1903. After the german period he returned to Sweden and studied the application of Physical chemistry to biology processes giving the basis for Biochemistry (Arrhenius, 1915).

With Ostwald and Van't Hoff he worked also on the Kinetics of electrolyte solutions and exposed his most important conclusions in a fundamental paper (Arrhenius, 1989) where he reconsidered the classical case of inversion of sugar with acids.

Arrhenius wanted to obtain the phenomenological coefficients of the precedent formulas from the number of ions in solution but found discrepancies between excepted and experimental data at high temperatures. Considering also the contributions due to more frequent collisions with the help of kinetic theory of gases applied to liquid phase he estimated a variation of 2% but the discrepancies was higher, around 15%. Moreover the acidity of the solution, or the number of H^+ ions, vary very slowly with temperature (around 0.05% for K°).

What really react therefore to justify a so big dependence with temperature? Arrhenius assumed the existence of a new specimen in the reaction: the active sugar. It is the number of molecules of active sugar that determine the velocity of reaction, they are the true reacting species. There is another subordinate equilibrium inside the reaction between sugar and active sugar that determinate its kinetic.

He reinterpreted the rate constant as the ratio between the quantities of active and total sugar and evaluated its dependence in function of the temperature:

$$\frac{d\ln k}{dT} = \frac{q}{2T^2} \tag{13}$$

It is no more necessary to define the constant B from (12) and A is now $q/2$ the half heat of activation of sugar. Arrhenius valuated also successfully the question of the activated part of the acid adding different electrolytes to solution.

The equation for the dependence of velocity of reaction with temperature results:

$$v_1 = v_0 e^{\frac{q(T_1 - T_0)}{2T_1T_0}} = v_0 e^{-q\left(\frac{1}{T_1} - \frac{1}{T_0}\right)} \tag{14}$$

Where v_1 and v_0 are the velocities at temperatures T_1 and T_0. From equations (13) and (14) he obtained directly his famous formula for the rate constant:

$$k = Ae^{-\frac{E}{RT}} \tag{15}$$

Where A is a frequency factor and E the energy of activation. The essential is the introduction of the concept of activation, but the physical explanation of the constants remained vague.

6. Genesis and development of transition state theory

Van't Hoff, Arrhenius and Ostwald put the foundation for a formal systematization of Chemical Kinetics but did not achieve a self-consistent theory. Thermodynamics alone was able to treat the reactions from a macroscopic point of view, but results insufficient to fully interpret the microscopic processes.

To get a exhaustive picture of the mechanisms from at atomic or molecular scale we will need the application of Statistical Mechanics and the development of Quantum Physics.

This is the mainly reason why we have to wait around forty years before a new for a new breakthrough in Chemical Kinetics.

Anyway this forty years are characterized by many debates and other discoveries in this field (Laidler & King 1983). First of all the Arrhenius equation, mainly welcomed, created some perplexities in the researchers that studied particular class of reactions where its use was really problematic.

Max Bodenstein (1871-1942), a German physical chemist from Heidelberg that collaborated with Walter Nernst in Gottingen and took his chair at the Berlin University after his retirement, was one of these researchers.

Bodenstein worked on gas reactions dynamics at the end of 19th Century (Bodenstein, 1899). Reactions in gas phase presents more difficulties and peculiar behaviors respect to liquid ones. Bodenstein accepted the hypothesis of activated species but supposed apparent or false equilibria between them and stable reactants especially for the particular systems he examined. Bodenstein intuited a fully new class of phenomena, what we now call non-equilibrium processes, and initially provoked some interest, but this concept was too early to get a development at the time. Theoretical basis for Transition State Theory, (hereafter called TST), needed a true equilibrium state and this approach become dominant. Other important contributions due to Bodenstein was in clarifying mechanisms of many heterogeneous and catalyzed reactions and the discovery of the mechanism of Chain Reactions around 1920, a field that we will reconsider later analyzing Christiansen work.

In this period there was a great attention about the molecularity of mechanisms and of particularly interest was a debate about unimolecular reactions. The debate was that about the so called Radiative Theory (King & Laidler, 1984), proposed mainly by **Jean Baptiste Perrin** (1870-1942), around 1917. Perrin proposed that unimolecular processes was activated only by blackbody radiation. The hypothesis, fallacious, continued for nearly ten years involving many and important figures as Einstein for example. Even being wrong Radiative Theory represents an interesting case study and boosted the research on different activation causes other than thermal collisions.

Between 1920 and 1930 many scholars like Wigner, Pelzer, Polanyi and Eyring at the Haber Laboratory of the Kaiser Wilhelm Institut of Berlin established a rigorous statistical approach to Chemical Kinetics (Polanyi & Wigner, 1928; Wigner & Pelzer, 1932). Important contributions in this sense was done also by Marcelin, that introduced the modern terminology and the Gibbs standard energy of activation, and Kramers & Christiansen (Kramers & Christiansen, 1923).

6.1 Quantum mechanical interpretation

After the achievement of the wave equation for the hydrogen molecule due to Heitler and London the Hungarian **Michael Polanyi** (1891-1976), director of the Haber Laboratory in Berlin, and his host, the young Mexican American, **Henry Eyring** (1901-1981) wanted to apply it to the quantum mechanical description of the reaction of atom exchange between ortho and para hydrogen molecules: H + H_2(orto) = H_2(para) + H.

They generalized that description for others bimolecular gas reactions between trhee atoms in a fundamental paper in 1931 (Eyiring & Polanyi 1931). The energy of the molecular and atom states during reactions was eventually exactly calculated thanks to Quantum Mechanics. They obtained the bond and activation energies plotting the energy in function of the distance between the atoms and molecules involved in the process and built the first diagrams of potential surfaces vs reaction coordinates. You can see an example in fig. 10.

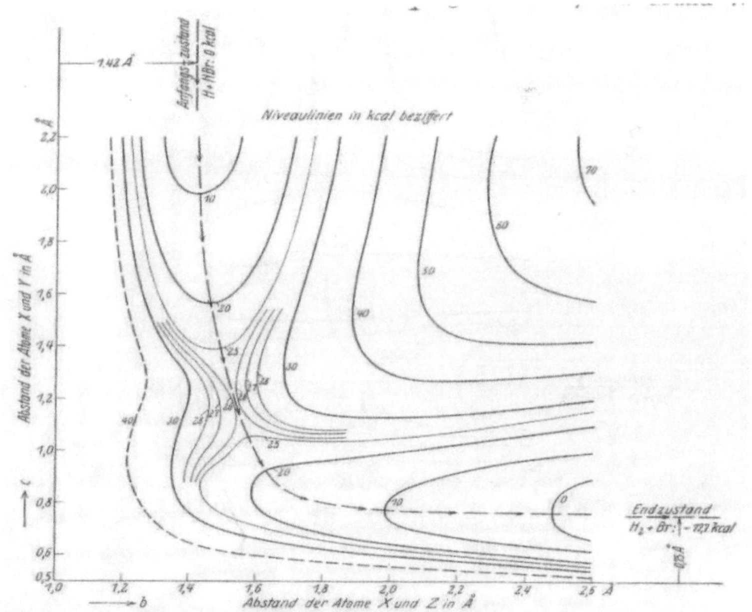

Fig. 8. „Resonanzgebirge" der Umsetzung $H + HBr \rightarrow H_2 + Br$ (Sattelgebiet) bei geradliniger Atomanordnung, aus den optischen Energiekurven von H_2 und HBr (Fig. 4) unter Vernachlässigung des COULOMBschen Anteils berechnet.

Fig. 10. Potential surface for the reaction H + HBr → H_2 + Br

6.2 TST presentation

The energetic description of all the configuration states of a chemical system was applied to Chemical Kinetics independently by the two researchers four years later, Polanyi from Manchester (Polanyi & Evans 1935) and Eyring from Princeton (Eyring 1935). The primacy is traditionally given to the most famous of the two, Eyring: the publications had some month of difference but the work was contemporary and a natural consequence of their previous joint work.

Absolute reaction rates are obtained statistically from the probability of rising of the reactants molecules from their fundamental state to the saddle of the maximum of the potential surface diagram (the activated complex). Evaluating the ratio of the partition functions of the activated and fundamental state of the reactants and the limitation of the degrees of freedom due to the particular geometry of the reaction surface (the saddle point of the activated complex reduce the degrees of freedom to one) Eyring obtained an Arrhenius type equation with a clear and definite value of the pre-exponential and exponent factors:

$$k = \left(\frac{k_b T}{h}\right) e^{-\frac{\Delta G^{\mp}}{RT}} \tag{16}$$

where $\Delta G^{\ddagger}$ is the Gibbs energy of activation, k_B is Boltzmann's constant, and h is Planck's constant. Eyring considered also the possible variations of the equation (16) due to the molecularity of the reaction.

The paper of Evans and Polanyi (Polanyi & Evans 1935) presented similar conclusions to that of Eyring but moreover tried to evaluate the interactions and energy exchanges between the reactants and the other actors of the chemical system (the solvent for example).

The investigations of Evans and Polanyi are not a simple detail, because they make evident the limits of the TST. The most known of them are the appearance of unexpected products due to particular form of the saddle surface, the tunnel effect through low energy barriers, the population of higher energy states rather than the only saddle state for high temperature reactions. A methodological limit is the vision of the process as a "big" isolated molecule where all the actors: reactants, activated complexes and products are contemporary presents and in equilibrium. This picture is valid when the main process is the establishment of the equilibrium between fundamental and activated states but results fallacious when other processes, as the interaction with solvent in diffusion controlled reactions for example become dominant. The other picture, less known, that sees the reaction as a process of diffusion will be examined in the next and last part of the chapter.

7. Genesis and development of diffusive-stochastic theories

The diffusion description, elaborated by Christiansen around 1935 (Christiansen 1936) and fully systematised in 1940 by Kramers (Kramers 1940), was an interesting and successful method complementary to transition state theory (TST). It received, however, little or no attention in chemistry circles for a long time (Zambelli 2010).

Hendrik Anthony Kramers (1894 –1952) was a Dutch physicist. He worked mainly in Germany and Denmark and was one of the most important collaborator of Bohr in the famous Copenhagen Institute of Theoretical Physics. His interest in Chemical Kinetics derived from the collaboration with **Jens Anton Christiansen** (1888–1969), later full professor of Physical Chemistry at the Copenhagen University, around 1922.

Christiansen visited the Bohr Institute after his PhD graduation for a period of nearly one year. It is possible that he already came to Copenhagen with the hope of finding some mathematical-physical assistance for his studies of chemical reactions. Christiansen's studies treated the dynamics of specific chemical reactions: in this PhD Thesis he introduced for the first time the term *chain reactions* (*ketten reaction* in Danish). His developments in this field together with that of Bodenstein previously cited resulted fundamental for the work of **Nikolay Semenov** (1896-1986) and **Cyril Norman Hinshelwood** (1897-1967) that will produce a definitive theory on chain reactions around 1950.

7.1 Christiansen's approach

Christiansen tried to apply the description and the model of chain reactions to different mechanisms (Christiansen 1922) and wrote a paper with Kramers in 1923, cited previously, about unimolecular reactions confronting the activation mechanism due to thermal collisions and radiation absorption. They treated the radiation mechanism with the fundamental Einstein's quantum theory about matter-radiation interaction (Einstein 1917). Other work of Einstein and Smoluchowski will be necessary later for Christiansen-Kramers approach. After the paper the collaboration probably ended and the two researchers will reconsider separately these arguments around fifteen years later.

Christiansen developed the model of a chemical reaction as an intra-molecular diffusion process in the half of the thirties. He published two papers in 1935 (Christiansen 1935) and 1936 (Christiansen 1936) on this research. The paper of 1936 is particularly significant. Christiansen confronted Arrhenius's theory of activated states with a little known theory (Nernst 1893) of **Walther Hermann Nernst** (1864–1941). In Nernst's theory, the reaction velocity is obtained, by analogy with Ohm's law, as the ratio between a chemical potential and a chemical resistance. Christiansen intended the chemical potential as the difference of the chemical activities of the beginning and the final states and the chemical resistance was represented by a particular integral depending on temperature and diffusion constant. The purpose of Christiansen was to demonstrate, extending Arrhenius's conception, that the methods of Nernst and Arrhenius are analogous. The generalization of Arrhenius's theory is obtained by supposing an open, possibly infinite, sequence of many consecutive steps, thus gaining an expression consistent with that of Nernst. Christiansen discretized a chemical reaction considering not only one activated state, as in Arrhenius's model, but a series of consecutive n stages which result in reciprocal virtual equilibrium. The equilibria between reactants, products and intermediates are supposed to be valid because Christiansen considered the quantity of intermediates constant during the slow stages of reaction, so the process is stationary or quasi-stationary. These are a group of assumptions similar to those made in the theory of diffusion. In fact, according to Christiansen's hypothesis, the equilibrium quantity of the activated complexes may be put in relationship to the concentrations of a diffusing substance along the sections of a column. From this diffusive description, he obtained an expression for the reciprocal reaction rate which was consistent with that obtained on a thermodynamic basis. Christiansen expressed the velocity of reaction v in the form of a diffusion equation:

$$v = -\frac{D}{\varphi}\frac{\partial c\varphi}{\partial x} \tag{17}$$

Where D and φ are the diffusion and activity coefficients, c the concentration and x a reaction coordinate. This expression implies that the transport of molecules is produced by the concentration gradient and by molecular forces (their contribution represented by the activities φ). From (17) and other assumptions about the activity coefficient Christiansen obtained another equation analogous to that of Einstein and Smoluchowski about Brownian motion:

$$v = -D\frac{\partial c}{\partial x} + \frac{D}{RT}cK \tag{18}$$

The generalization of the Arrhenius conception brings us naturally to consider the transformation of a molecule during a reaction as an intra-molecular diffusion. To demonstrate this generalization Christiansen made some fundamental assumptions. He considered the case of a simple potential barrier, a symmetrical bi-stable one as shown in Fig. 11. This case will be examined better thanks to Kramers work of 1940.

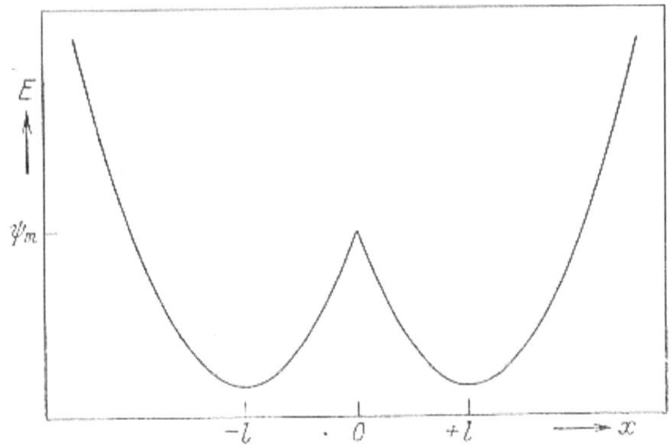

Fig. 11. Bi-stable potential barrier, the figure is taken from Christiansen's paper

7.2 The application of Klein-Kramers equation to chemical kinetics

The main biographers of Kramers, in particular Dirk ter Haar, claim that his interest in Chemical kinetics is a simple mathematical exercise of style. This may be partially true but Kramers's work would be impossible without Christiansen's previous contribution and his collaboration with **Oskar Benjamin Klein** (1894–1977) a Swedish theoretical physicist student of Arrhenius that during the years from 1917 to 1921 travelled many times back and forth between Copenhagen and Stockholm to complete his PhD thesis in which he examined the forces between ions in strong electrolyte solutions. The result was a generalized description of liquid dynamics and the formulation of what we call today the Klein-Kramers equation (Klein 1922).

Kramers paper of 1940 presents what today we call the "Kramers problem": the dynamics of a particle moving in a bi-stable external field of force, subject to the irregular forces of a surrounding medium in thermal equilibrium. The particle, originally caught in a potential well, may escape by passing over a potential barrier. Constructing a diffusion equation for the density distribution of particles in phase space it is possible to calculate the probability and the escape rate as a function of the temperature and viscosity of the medium. Kramers considered the one dimensional motion of a particle of unit mass starting from a Langevin equation of the system for the time derivative of the velocity v:

$$\frac{dv}{dt} = -\xi v + f(t) - \frac{dV(x)}{dx} \tag{19}$$

where $V(x)$ is the potential field, ξ the friction and $f(t)$ a time dependent stochastic force. Searching for the distribution law of the particle in phase space on the basis of a given distribution of the random forces he obtained the diffusion equation for the particle distribution from the statistical moments of the random force:

$$\frac{\partial P(x,x_0,v,v_0,t)}{\partial t} = -\Gamma P(x,x_0,v,v_0,t) \tag{20}$$

Where the operator Γ is defined as:

$$\Gamma = v\frac{\partial}{\partial x} - \frac{dV(x)}{dx}\frac{\partial}{\partial v} - \xi\frac{\partial}{\partial v}\left(v + k_B T\frac{\partial}{\partial v}\right) \tag{21}$$

This express the Klein-Kramers equation of the system. Kramers found solutions of equation (21) in the stationary cases in a good range of viscosity. We remark that the stationarity condition is not strictly an approximation, but rather the simplest case of a non-equilibrium state of a system. If we consider the potential surface of a chemical system and assume the role of the solvent in the viscosity coefficient Kramers approach describes efficiently the course of chemical reactions.

8. Conclusions

Kramers found the Eyring-Polanyi equation (16) as a particular case of medium-small viscosity. It may seem impressive to see that the results of TST, based on quantum mechanics, come out as a particular case of Kramers pure classical method. But there are precise limitations to the use of Kramers method.

Methodologically, even if the diffusive stochastic approach has some theoretical advantages, it is more difficult to adapt and apply to the description of chemical reactions than TST. It requires notable mathematical knowledge and physical concepts that are not so familiar in chemistry. TST on the other hand, relying on the powerful means of quantum mechanics, produces more predictive results, although we have to apply phenomenological coefficients in some cases and make some arbitrary assumptions.

Diffusion approach, although less known, and TST represents the basic theories for contemporary studies on Chemical Kinetics, a disciple that now is a part of Physical Chemistry but that before Quantum Mechanics corresponded practically to it and that contributed so deeply, as we have seen, to the whole construction of Chemical Science.

9. References

Arrhenius, S.A. (1887). Über die Dissociation der in Wasser gelösten Stoffe, *Z. Phys. Chem.*, 1, pp. 631-648, Available in English from http://www.chemteam.info/Chem-History/Arrhenius-dissociation.html

Arrhenius, S.A. (1915). *Quantitative laws in biological chemistry*, London, U.K.

Arrhenius, S.A. (1889). Uber die Reaktionsgeschwindigkeit bei der Inversion von Rohrzucker durch Säuren, *Z. Phys. Chem.*, 4, 1889, pp. 226-248

Berthelot, P.E.M. & Saint Gilles, L.P. (1862). Recherches sur les affinités de la formation et de la decomposition des ethers, *Annales de chimie et physique* (3) 65 1872, 66 1872, 68 1873, pp. 385-422, pp. 5-110, pp. 225-359, Available from http://gallica.bnf.fr/ark:/12148/bpt6k34806t/f383.image.langEN

Bodenstein, M. (1899). Gasreaktionen in der chemischen Kinetik, I, II, III, *Z. Phys. Chem.* 29, pp. 147-158, pp. 295-314, pp. 315-333

Christiansen, J.A. & Kramers, H.A. (1923). Über die Geschwindigkeit chemische Reaktionenen, *Z. Phys. Chem.* 104, pp. 451-471

Christiansen, J.A. (1922). Über das Geschwindigkeitsgesetz monomolekularer Reactionen, *Z. Phys. Chem.* 103, pp. 91-98

Christiansen, J.A. (1935). Einige Bemerkungen zur Anwendung der Bodensteinschen Methode der stationären Konzentrationen der Zwischenstoffe in der Reakionskinetik. *Z. Phys. Chem.* 28B, pp. 303-310

Christiansen, J.A. (1936). Über eine Erweiterung der Arrheniusschen Auffassung der chemischen Reaction, *Z. Phys. Chem.* 33B, pp.145-155

Einstein, A. (1917). Zur Quantentheorie der Strahlung, *Phys. Z.* 18, pp 121-128, Available in English from http://books.google.com/books?id=8KLMGqnZCDcC&pg=PA63&ots=h9g_x_ptxu&dq=%22the+formal+similarity+between+the+chromatic%%2022&sig=rrtVd32EsQTQUsYae3hRnkunW0I#v=onepage&q&f=false

Evans, M.G. & Polanyi M. (1935). Some applications of the transition state method to the calculation of reaction velocities, especially in solution, *Trans. Faraday Soc.* 31, pp. 875-893

Eyring, H. & Polanyi M. (1931). Uber einfache Gasreaktionen, *Z. Phys. Chem. B* 12, pp. 279-311

Eyring, H. (1935). The Activated Complex in Chemical Reactions, *J. Chem. Phys.* 3, pp. 107-115

Geoffroy, E.F. (1718). Table des différents rapports observés en chimie entre différentes substances, *Mémoires de l'Academie Royale des Sciences* , pp. 202-212, Available from http://gallica.bnf.fr/ark:/12148/bpt6k3519v/f330

Gladstone, J.H. (1855). On Circumstances Modifying the Action of Chemical Affinity, *Phil. Trans. Roy. Soc. London* 175, pp. 179-223, Available from http://www.jstor.org/stable/108516

Guldberg, C. M. & Waage, P. (1864). Etudes sur l'Affinité, *Forhandlinger: Videnskabs-Selskabet i Christiana*, 35, Available in English from http://www.nd.edu/~powers/ame.50531/guldberg.waage.1864.pdf

Guldberg, C.M. & Waage, P. (1879). Über Die Chemische Affinität, *Journal Prakt. Chem.*, 127, pp. 69-114

Harcourt, A. G. V. & Esson W. (1865). On the Laws of Connexion between the Conditions of a Chemical Change and Its Amount, *Phil. Trans. London 156*, 1866, pp. 193-221, Available from http://www.jstor.org/stable/108945

Harcourt, A.G.V. & Esson W. (1867). On the Laws of Connexion between the Conditions of a Chemical Change and Its Amount. II. On the Reaction of Hydric Peroxide and Hydric Iodide. *Proc. Roy Soc. 15*, 1867, pp. 262-265, Available from http://www.jstor.org/stable/112633

Harcourt, A.G.V. & Esson W. (1895). Bakerian Lecture: On the Laws of Connexion between the Conditions of a Chemical Change and Its Amount. III. Further Researches on the Reaction of Hydrogen Dioxide and Hydrogen Iodide, *Phil. Trans. London 186A*, 1895, 817-895

Harcourt, A.G.V. & Esson W. (1912). On the Variation with Temperature of the Rate of a Chemical Change, *Phil. Trans. London 212A*, 1913, 187-204

King, M.C. (1981). Experiments with time, *Ambix* 23, pp. 70-82

King, M.C. & Laidler, K.J. (1983). The Development of Transition-State Theory, *J. Phys. Chem.* 87, pp. 2657-2664, Available from http://www.qi.fcen.uba.ar/materias/qf2/TCA.pdf

King, M.C. & Laidler, K.J. (1984). Chemical kinetics and the radiation hypothesis , Archive for History of Exact Sciences 30, 1, pp. 45-86

Klein, O. (1922). Zur statistischen Theorie der Suspensionen und Lösungen, *Arkiv Mat. Astr. Fys.* 16(5), pp 1-51, Available from http://su.diva-portal.org/smash/record.jsf?pid=diva2:440187

Kramers, H.A. (1940). Brownian Motion in a Field of Force and the Diffusion Model of Chemical Reactions, *Physica* 7, pp. 284-304, Available from http://www-lpmcn.univ-lyon1.fr/~barrat/phystat-he/kramers1940.pdf

Lavoisier, A.L. (1782). Considerations sur la dissolution des metaux dans les acides, *Mémoires de l'Académie des sciences* 1782, pp. 492-527, Available from http://www.lavoisier.cnrs.fr/ice/ice_book_detail-fr-text-lavosier-Lavoisier-49-5.html

Nernst, W. (1893). Über die Beteiligung eines Lösungmittels an chemischen Reaktionen. *Z. Phys. Chem.*.11, pp 345-359

Ostwald, W. (1879-84). Chemische Affinitätsbestimmungen, *J. Prakt. Chem.*, 19, 1879, pp. 468-484; 22, 1880, pp. 251-260; 23, 1881, pp. 209-225, 517-536; 24, 1881, pp. 486-497; 29, 1884, pp. 49-52

Ostwald, W. (1884). Studien zur chemischen Dynamik. III. Die Inversion des Rohrzuckers, *J. Prakt. Chem.* 29, pp. 385-408

Ostwald, W. (1902). *Uber Katalyse*, Liepzig, 1902

Ostwald, W. (1909). *Grundriss der allgemeinen Chemie*, Liepzig, 1909

Pelzer, H. & Wigner, E. (1932). Über die Geschwindigkeitskonstante von Austauschreaktionen, *Z. Phys. Chem.* 15B, pp. 445-471

Polanyi, M. & Wigner, E. (1928). Über die Interferenz von Eigenschwingungen als Ursache von Energieschwankungen und chemischer Umsetzungen, *Z. Phys. Chem.* 139, pp. 439-452

Van't Hoff, J.H. (1875). *Chimie dans l'espace*, Rotterdam, 1875

Van't Hoff, J.H. (1884). *Etudes de dynamique chimique,* Amsterdam, 1884

Van't Hoff, J.H. (1885). L'Équilibre chimique dans les Systèmes gazeux ou dissous à I'État dilué, *Recueil des Travaux Chimiques des Pays-Bas* 4, 12, pp. 424-427

Wilhelmy, L. (1850). *Über* das Gesetz, nach welchem die Einwirkung der Säuren auf den Rohrzucker stattfindet, *Pogg. Ann.* 81, pp. 413-433, Available from http://gallica.bnf.fr/ark:/12148/bpt6k15166k/f427.table

Zambelli, S. (2010), Chemical kinetics and diffusion approach: the history of the Klein-Kramers equation, *Arch. Hist. Exact Sci.* 64, 4, pp. 395-428

Part 2

Chemical Kinetics and Mechanism

Chemical Kinetics and Inverse Modelling Problems

Victor Martinez-Luaces
Electrochemistry Engineering Multidisciplinary Research Group, University of the Republic of Uruguay, Montevideo, Uruguay

1. Introduction

Late last century and early this century, the Electrochemistry Engineering Multidisciplinary Research Group (Grupo Multidisciplinario de Ingenieria Electroquimica, in Spanish) at Montevideo, Uruguay studied the adsorption of Carbon Dioxide on Platinum surfaces (Zinola et al., 1997; Martinez-Luaces et al., 2001; Martinez-Luaces, 2001, Martinez-Luaces & Guineo, 2002; Guineo & Martinez-Luaces, 2002).

The research found three different adsorbates E_1, E_2, and E_3 and measured the surface concentrations by conventional electrochemical techniques.

The initial objective of the group was to propose a mechanism with the closest fit to the experimental curves (Zinola et al., 1997). Nevertheless, as the research progressed, the focus shifted to explain, or try to explain the double inflexion that consistently appeared in the experimental curves of surface concentration versus time for one of the adsorbates (Martinez-Luaces et al., 2001; Martinez-Luaces, 2001, Martinez-Luaces & Guineo, 2002; Guineo & Martinez-Luaces, 2002).

From a theoretical point of view, these are both inverse problems incorporating chemical and mathematical modelling at the same time. In previous papers and books, these problems were described as Inverse Modelling Problems (Martinez-Luaces, 2007, 2008, 2009a, 2009b, 2009c, 2009d).

In this paper, both inverse problems and the associated modelling are analysed from a theoretical point of view and subsequently solved. The main results will then be generalised to other Chemical Kinetics applications.

2. Theoretical framework. Inverse problems

Direct problems, according to Groestch (Groestch, 1999, 2001), can be regarded as those that provide the necessary information to follow a well-defined, stable procedure leading to a single correct solution.

Inverse problems, in contrast, are both more difficult and more interesting, largely due to their either having multiple solutions, or not being capable of being solved at all (Bunge,

2006). They frequently crop up in the practice of several professions and careers. For instance, when treating a patient for a particular illness, listing the symptoms is a simple, direct problem that has already been solved and can be looked up in any medical textbook. On the other hand, diagnosing a patient's illness from his or her symptoms is not always a straightforward task, and requires an experienced doctor.

Inverse problems have not always been properly studied, and a quote from Bunge (Bunge, 2006) is appropriate: "The fact that almost all philosophers have ignored the peculiarities of inverse problems poses another inverse problem: to guess the reasons for this huge oversight on the part of philosophers."

In principle there are two different types of inverse problems, but in order to characterise them correctly, let us begin with a schematization of direct problems, adapting a study by Groetsch (Groestch, 1999, 2001). His scheme for a direct problem is like this:

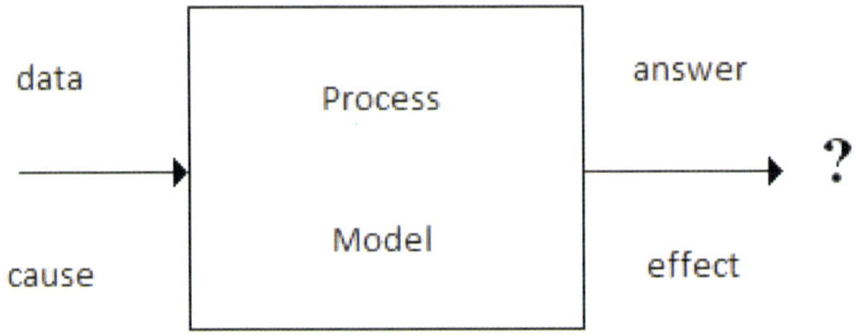

Fig. 1. Schema of direct problems

In the scheme in Figure 1, data and a given procedure are available, and the answer is sought; for instance, the reagents for a certain chemical reaction are given, and the conditions of temperature, pH, etc of the reaction are known, and we wish to know the products of the reaction.

Now we can change the schema to obtain two inverse problems. The first is the causation problem, schematized in Figure 2:

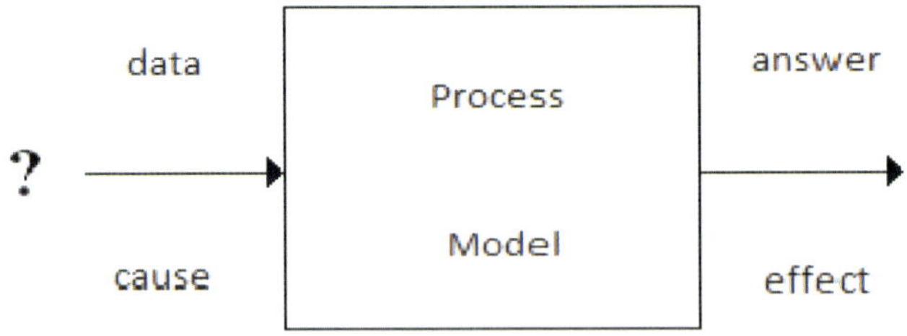

Fig. 2. Schema for causation problems

In this first type of inverse problem (causation problem), the results are known, as well as the process that produces them, but the causes are unknown. Finding the causes is the problem to be solved.

The other inverse problem generally encountered is the specification problem, schematized in Figure 3:

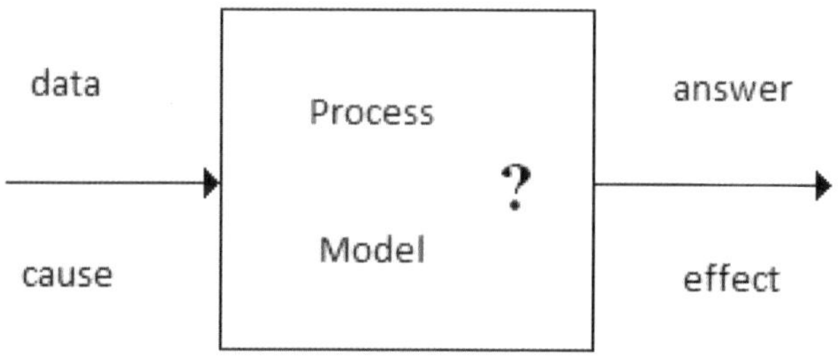

Fig. 3. Schema of specification problems

In this case, both the causes and the effects are known, and what must be determined is the process that leads from the former to the latter.

Both types of problems are common in the different branches of Chemistry. For example, in Qualitative Chemical Analysis one is frequently faced with a solution containing several unknown cations and anions. The analyst must carry out a pre-established series of reactions, and according to the results must rule out or confirm the presence or absence of the more usual cations and anions. This procedure allows the analyst, depending on the results (formation of precipitates, turbidity, colour reactions in the solution, etc.), to deduce the composition of the problem sample. Clearly, this is an example of a causation problem, because the procedure is pre-established, the results are in plain view and the objective is to know what solution composition is compatible with the results obtained (Martinez-Luaces, 2011).

In Inorganic Chemistry, on the other hand, the problem is more frequently to synthesize a given salt from simpler substances (oxides, hydroxides, anhydrides, etc.). A typical example of this is the Solvay process for obtaining sodium carbonate (Na_2CO_3) and sodium bicarbonate $(NaHCO_3)$, used in the glass, paper and soap industries among others, from sodium chloride $(NaCl)$ and carbon dioxide (CO_2) which are much more abundant and easily obtained. The problem here does not lie in identifying the reactants and/or products, but in knowing and correctly carrying out the process that will lead to the formation of the desired products, starting from cheap and easily available reagents. This is clearly a specification problem (Martinez-Luaces, 2011).

Finally, in Organic Chemistry, double inverse problems (involving causation and specification) tend to be posed simultaneously. For instance, in organic synthesis, four different ways of preparing acetone are usually presented, starting from four different reagents: ethyl acetate, acetonitrile, acetaldehyde or 2-methylpropene. Obviously the reactants are not predetermined, much less the process, and only the final product or target molecule is known (Martinez-Luaces, 2011).

3. Modelling and applications

Problem solving, modelling and applications are not synonymous, although they are obviously related. For instance, the Discussion Document preparatory to the ICMI Study 14 (Blum et al., 2002), mentions that the term "modelling" focuses in the direction that goes from the real world towards basic sciences, while the term "applications" goes in the opposite direction, that is, from science towards the real world. In addition, the term "modelling" emphasizes the process that is taking place, while the word "applications" stresses the object involved (particularly in areas of the real world that are susceptible to a given mathematical treatment). The same document uses the term "problem" in a broad sense, including, therefore, not only practical problems, but also abstract problems, or those that attempt to describe, explain, understand, or even design parts of the real world.

Obviously, solving problems and modelling are not the same thing (one can model even in the absence of a concrete problem to be solved; one would simply be giving a mathematical description of a given phenomenon), and of course, "pure" mathematics problems, which do not require any kind of modelling, can be solved.

In the light of the above, we can arrive at the following schema:

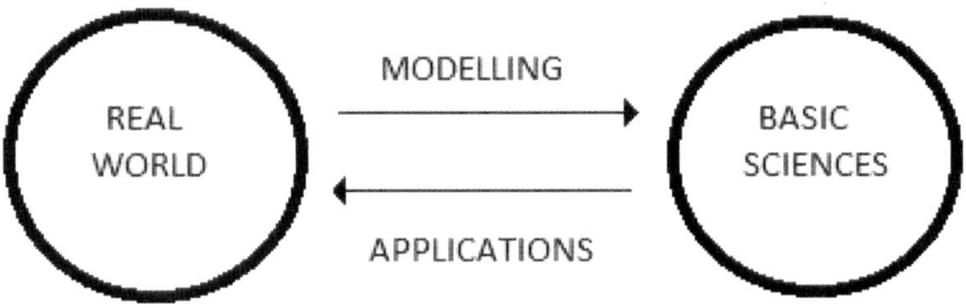

Fig. 4. Scheme of modelling and applications

Finally, it is worth mentioning that a more extensive discussion of modelling, applications and problem solving, and their teaching in university courses and secondary education in Latin America is available in previous papers (Martinez-Luaces, 2005, 2009a, 2011).

4. The first problem. The mechanism proposal

As it was mentioned before, the main objective of our research group was to study the adsorption of Carbon Dioxide on Platinum surfaces. The research found three different adsorbates E_1, E_2, and E_3 and measured the surface concentrations by conventional electrochemical techniques.

On completion of the trials of the experiment, several mechanisms were proposed and they were assessed by comparing the theoretical curves with the experimental ones. The result of this process was that the best fit was obtained by the following mechanism:

$$\begin{array}{l} E_1 \xrightarrow{k_1} E_2 \\ E_1 \xrightarrow{k_2} E_3 \\ E_2 \underset{k_{-3}}{\overset{k_3}{\rightleftarrows}} E_3 \end{array} \quad (1)$$

If $[E_1]$, $[E_2]$ and $[E_3]$ represent the adsorbates' surface concentrations and k_1, k_2, k_3 and k_{-3} the kinetic constants, then the mathematical model corresponding to this mechanism is the following:

$$\begin{cases} \dfrac{d[E_1]}{dt} = -(k_1 + k_2)[E_1] \\ \dfrac{d[E_2]}{dt} = k_1[E_1] - k_3[E_2] + k_{-3}[E_3] \\ \dfrac{d[E_3]}{dt} = k_2[E_1] + k_3[E_2] - k_{-3}[E_3] \end{cases} \tag{2}$$

or equivalently:

$$\begin{pmatrix} x \\ y \\ z \end{pmatrix}' = \begin{pmatrix} -k_1 - k_2 & 0 & 0 \\ k_1 & -k_3 & k_{-3} \\ k_2 & k_3 & -k_{-3} \end{pmatrix} \begin{pmatrix} x \\ y \\ z \end{pmatrix} \tag{3}$$

if notation is simplified.

It is interesting to observe that if the three rows of the Ordinary Differential Equations (ODE) system are added, the result is zero. This property remains true with other proposed mechanisms where only the solution will change. For example, consider the following mechanism:

$$\begin{array}{c} E_1 \underset{K_{-1}}{\overset{K_1}{\rightleftarrows}} E_2 \\ E_2 \underset{K_{-2}}{\overset{K_2}{\rightleftarrows}} E_3 \\ E_1 \underset{K_{-3}}{\overset{K_3}{\rightleftarrows}} E_3 \end{array} \tag{4}$$

where all the possible reactions between the three adsorbates are considered.

For such a mechanism, the mathematical model (i.e., the Ordinary Differential Equations system) will be as follows:

$$\begin{pmatrix} x \\ y \\ z \end{pmatrix}' = \begin{pmatrix} -k_1 - k_3 & k_{-1} & k_{-3} \\ k_1 & -k_{-1} - k_2 & k_{-2} \\ k_3 & k_2 & -k_{-2} - k_{-3} \end{pmatrix} \begin{pmatrix} x \\ y \\ z \end{pmatrix} \tag{5}$$

As in the previous case, the surface concentrations $[E_1]$, $[E_2]$ and $[E_3]$ were replaced by x, y and z in order to simplify notation.

Once again it is easy to observe that the result of adding the three rows of this new matrix is the null vector. This fact could be considered just a mathematical curiosity, though in the next section it will be the main observation to solve the second proposed problem.

5. The second problem. The double inflexion

The first proposed mechanism was the better when fitting the theoretical curves to the experimental values of surface concentration versus time. Nevertheless, one of the experimental curves consistently showed two inflexion points. Initially these inflexions were regarded as the uncertainty of the experimental measures, but each time the experiments were repeated, the results were always the same, i.e., one of the curves showed two inflexion points (Martinez-Luaces et al., 2001; Martinez-Luaces, 2001, Martinez-Luaces & Guineo, 2002; Guineo & Martinez-Luaces, 2002).

This led to other mechanisms being proposed, but none of them could explain this behaviour. As previously mentioned, all proposed mechanisms led to an O.D.E. system, for which the associated matrix had the property that the sum of all the matrix rows was zero. This observation is very useful because in all cases the matrix determinant must be zero. Finally, a null matrix determinant implies that one of the matrix eigenvalues is always zero and this determines the behaviour of the theoretical curves.

In order to explain these ideas, we shall consider a simpler chemical kinetics problem, with a simpler mechanism. For this purpose a well known process will be considered: the mutarotation of Glucose (Guerasimov, 1995; Martinez-Luaces, 2009e). In this mechanism there are only two simple uni-molecular reactions:

$$\alpha-\text{Glucose} \underset{k_{-1}}{\overset{k_1}{\rightleftarrows}} \beta-\text{Glucose} \tag{6}$$

This mechanism can be expressed mathematically through a simple ODE. In fact, if x is the concentration of β - Glucose and y that of α - Glucose, then it is easy to observe that the β - Glucose concentration can be obtained from the following ODE:

$$\frac{dx}{dt} = k_1.y - k_{-1}x \tag{7}$$

Letting a be the initial α - Glucose concentration and the corresponding initial concentration of β - Glucose being zero, then the variable y can be replaced by $a-x$ and the ODE can be written as:

$$\frac{dx}{dt} = k_1.(a-x) - k_{-1}x \tag{8}$$

Finally, very simple algebraic manipulations lead to the following linear, first order equation:

$$\frac{dx}{dt} = k_1.a - (k_1 + k_{-1}).x \tag{9}$$

The solution for this ODE is the following:

$$x(t) = \frac{k_1 a}{k_1 + k_{-1}}\left\{1 - \exp\left[-(k_1 + k_{-1})\,t\right]\right\} \tag{10}$$

This is the typical approach for studying the Glucose Mutarotation problem (Guerasimov, 1995; Martinez-Luaces, 2009e), but not the best one for this article devoted to inverse problems. In order to get a different point of view, we shall write the mechanism:

$$\alpha-\text{Glucose} \underset{k_{-1}}{\overset{k_1}{\rightleftarrows}} \beta-\text{Glucose} \tag{6}$$

in a simpler form as:

$$A \underset{k}{\overset{K}{\rightleftarrows}} B \tag{11}$$

In this case, a mathematical model, in terms of $\frac{d[A]}{dt}$ y $\frac{d[B]}{dt}$ can be written in the following form:

$$\begin{cases} \frac{d[A]}{dt} = -K[A] + k[B] \\ \frac{d[B]}{dt} = K[A] - k[B] \end{cases} \tag{12}$$

Once again, if $x=[A]$ and $y=[B]$ the ODE system can be written in matrix form, as follows:

$$\begin{pmatrix} x \\ y \end{pmatrix}' = \begin{pmatrix} -K & k \\ K & -k \end{pmatrix} \cdot \begin{pmatrix} x \\ y \end{pmatrix} \tag{13}$$

The system matrix is $M = \begin{pmatrix} -K & k \\ K & -k \end{pmatrix}$ and its eigenvalues can easily be obtained from the characteristic equation:

$$\det(M - \lambda I) = \det\begin{pmatrix} -K-\lambda & k \\ K & -k-\lambda \end{pmatrix} = 0 \tag{14}$$

This process led to a second order equation $(-K-\lambda)(-k-\lambda) - Kk = 0$ that can be written as: $\lambda^2 + (K+k)\lambda = 0$ and the eigenvalues are: $\lambda_1 = 0$ and $\lambda_2 = -(K+k)$. For these eigenvalues, the corresponding eigenvectors can be easily computed and the results are the following:

$$\vec{v}_1 = \begin{pmatrix} k \\ K \end{pmatrix} \text{ and } \vec{v}_2 = \begin{pmatrix} 1 \\ -1 \end{pmatrix}. \tag{15}$$

In this case, the system matrix is equivalent to a diagonal form (Martinez-Luaces, 2009e) and the solution of the ODE problem is the following linear combination:

$$\begin{pmatrix} x(t) \\ y(t) \end{pmatrix} = \sum_i C_i \exp(\lambda_i t)\, \vec{v}_i = C_1 \exp(\lambda_1 t)\begin{pmatrix} k \\ K \end{pmatrix} + C_2 \exp(\lambda_2 t)\begin{pmatrix} 1 \\ -1 \end{pmatrix} \tag{16}$$

and the final solution is:

$$\begin{pmatrix} x(t) \\ y(t) \end{pmatrix} = \begin{pmatrix} C_1 k + C_2 e^{-(K+k)t} \\ C_1 K - C_2 e^{-(K+k)t} \end{pmatrix} \tag{17}$$

More important than the solution itself – at least for this article – is to observe that one of the eigenvalues was zero (and the sum of both matrix rows was the null vector, as in the adsorption problem). This fact has important consequences for the asymptotic behaviour of the solutions. Moreover, as time approaches infinity:

$$\lim_{t \to +\infty} \begin{pmatrix} x(t) \\ y(t) \end{pmatrix} = \lim_{t \to +\infty} \begin{pmatrix} C_1 k + C_2 e^{-(K+k)t} \\ C_1 K - C_2 e^{-(K+k)t} \end{pmatrix} = \begin{pmatrix} C_1 k \\ C_1 K \end{pmatrix} \tag{18}$$

The qualitative result is that both concentrations tend to finite, non-zero real values, which from a chemical point of view are the equilibrium concentrations.

Similar ideas can be explored when three or even more substances are involved. In order to explain this idea, we shall consider a very simple mechanism involving three different chemical substances E_1, E_2 and E_3, like the following one:

$$E_1 \xrightarrow{k_1} E_2 \xrightarrow{k_2} E_3 \tag{19}$$

In this case, the ODE system (Martinez-Luaces, 2009e) is as follows:

$$\begin{cases} \dfrac{d[E_1]}{dt} = -k_1[E_1] \\ \dfrac{d[E_2]}{dt} = k_1[E_1] - k_2[E_2] \\ \dfrac{d[E_3]}{dt} = k_2[E_2] \end{cases} \tag{20}$$

or equivalently:

$$\begin{pmatrix} x \\ y \\ z \end{pmatrix}' = \begin{pmatrix} -k_1 & 0 & 0 \\ k_1 & -k_2 & 0 \\ 0 & k_2 & 0 \end{pmatrix} \begin{pmatrix} x \\ y \\ z \end{pmatrix} \tag{21}$$

where, as in the previous example, adding the rows the result is a null vector.

Applying the mass conservation law to the mechanism:

$$E_1 \xrightarrow{k_1} E_2 \xrightarrow{k_2} E_3 \tag{19}$$

it follows that $[E_1] + [E_2] + [E_3]$ remains constant.

Finally, if $[E_1] + [E_2] + [E_3] = C$ is differentiated with respect to t, we obtain the following equation:

$$\frac{d[E_1]}{dt} + \frac{d[E_2]}{dt} + \frac{d[E_3]}{dt} = 0 \tag{22}$$

This formula explains why the sum of all the equations of the ODE system adds up to zero. From this observation, it follows that the sum of all the rows of the system matrix will always be the null vector (Martinez-Luaces, 2007, 2009e).

For the same reasons, all the possible mechanisms involving unimolecular reactions between all the adsorbates will show the same property. As a consequence of this fact, the system matrix has a null determinant for all the proposed mechanisms. This observation can be easily proved, because if $row_1 + row_2 + row_3 = 0$, then $row_3 = -row_1 - row_2$ and since each of the rows is a linear combination of the others, it follows that $\det(A) = 0$, where A is the matrix associated with the ODE system.

Therefore, if $\det(A) = 0$, then matrix A will have a null eigenvalue, which is independent of the mechanism proposed. For each mechanism the ODE system will have three eigenvalues: $\lambda_1 \in R$, $\lambda_2 \in R$ and $\lambda_3 = 0$. This observation has important consequences in the solutions of ODE systems and their qualitative behaviour. In order to get qualitative results, three different cases will be investigated:

1. all the eigenvalues are different,
2. two eigenvalues are the same and the other is a simple one
3. there exists an unique eigenvalue with algebraic multiplicity three.

All these cases will be analysed in order to discover whether the two inflexion points can be explained by mechanisms involving only electrochemical unimolecular reactions.

5.1 First case: Three different eigenvalues ($\lambda_1 \neq \lambda_2$, $\lambda_1 \neq 0$, $\lambda_2 \neq 0$)

In this case, if $\vec{E} = (E_1, E_2, E_3)$, a well known formula - valid if all the eigenvalues are different - expresses that $\vec{E} = \sum_{i=1}^{3} c_i \exp(\lambda_i t)\, \vec{v}_i$, where c_i represents the coefficients, λ_i the eigenvalues and $\vec{v}_i$ the associated eigenvectors (Martinez-Luaces, 2009e). In fact, this formula was used to solve the mutarotation problem, as in (16). The same formula can be used for other diagonal forms with repeated eigenvalues.

Taking into account that $\lambda_1 \neq 0$, $\lambda_2 \neq 0$ and $\lambda_3 = 0$, all the surface concentrations have this form: $E_i = \alpha \exp(\lambda_1 t) + \beta \exp(\lambda_2 t) + \gamma$ and by differentiating we obtain: $\frac{d^2E_i}{dt^2} = \alpha \lambda_1^2 \exp(\lambda_1 t) + \beta \lambda_2^2 \exp(\lambda_2 t) = \exp(\lambda_1 t)\left[\alpha \lambda_1^2 + \beta \lambda_2^2 \exp(\lambda t)\right]$ where $\lambda = \lambda_2 - \lambda_1$, so $\frac{d^2E_i}{dt^2} = 0$ if and only if $\alpha \lambda_1^2 + \beta \lambda_2^2 \exp(\lambda t) = 0$, which only happens if $t = \frac{1}{\lambda} \ln\left(\frac{-\alpha \lambda_1^2}{\beta \lambda_2^2}\right)$.

Then, in this case, only one inflexion point can be explained and so, two inflexion points are not possible.

5.2 Second case: A double eigenvalue and a simple one

There are three possibilities under this case:

5.2.1 First sub-case ($\lambda_1 \neq 0$ and $\lambda_2 = \lambda_3 = 0$)

In this sub-case, the ODE system matrix A is not equivalent to a diagonal matrix D, but it is equivalent to a triangular matrix J (the Jordan canonical form). More precisely, there exists a matrix P (it is important to note that in this case not all the columns of P are eigenvectors) such that $P^{-1}AP = J$ and as a consequence, the ODE system $\dot{X} = AX$ can be easily converted in the following one $\dot{Y} = JY$ by a simple change of variables $X = PY$.

As a consequence of this fact, the new ODE system to solve is: $\begin{pmatrix} \dot{y}_1 \\ \dot{y}_2 \\ \dot{y}_3 \end{pmatrix} = \begin{pmatrix} \lambda_1 & 0 & 0 \\ 0 & 0 & 0 \\ 0 & 1 & 0 \end{pmatrix} \begin{pmatrix} y_1 \\ y_2 \\ y_3 \end{pmatrix}$ then $\dot{y}_1 = \lambda_1 y_1$, $\dot{y}_2 = 0$ and $\dot{y}_3 = y_2$. The solution of this new ODE problem is $y_1 = c_1 \exp(\lambda_1 t)$, $y_2 = c_2$ and $y_3 = c_2 t + c_3$. Finally, since $X = PY$, it follows that all the E_i are linear combinations of these functions y_1, y_2 and y_3 and so, all of them are of the form: $E_i = \alpha \exp(\lambda_1 t) + \beta t + \gamma$ and differentiating twice with respect to time, the result is: $\frac{d^2 E_i}{dt^2} = \alpha \lambda_1^2 \exp(\lambda_1 t) \neq 0 \ \forall t \in R$.

As a consequence of this fact, there are no inflexion points in this sub-case.

5.2.2 Second sub-case ($\lambda_1 = \lambda_3 = 0$ and $\lambda_2 \neq 0$)

This case is the same as the previous one, except for a change in the order of the eigenvalues, so, the main result is the same: there are no inflexion points in this sub-case.

5.2.3 Third sub-case ($\lambda_1 = \lambda_2 \neq 0$ and $\lambda_3 = 0$)

In this new sub-case, the corresponding Jordan canonical form has the following form: $J = \begin{pmatrix} \lambda & 0 & 0 \\ 1 & \lambda & 0 \\ 0 & 0 & 0 \end{pmatrix}$, where $\lambda = \lambda_1 = \lambda_2$ and the new ODE system is:

$\begin{pmatrix} \dot{y}_1 \\ \dot{y}_2 \\ \dot{y}_3 \end{pmatrix} = \begin{pmatrix} \lambda & 0 & 0 \\ 1 & \lambda & 0 \\ 0 & 0 & 0 \end{pmatrix} \begin{pmatrix} y_1 \\ y_2 \\ y_3 \end{pmatrix}$ or equivalently $\dot{y}_1 = \lambda y_1$, $\dot{y}_2 = y_1 + \lambda y_2$ and $\dot{y}_3 = 0$. Then, the solution of the first and the third ODE are $y_1 = c_1 \exp(\lambda t)$ and $y_3 = c_3$. Finally, the second ODE can be written as $\dot{y}_2 - \lambda y_2 = c_1 \exp(\lambda t)$ and the solution is $y_2 = (c_1 t + c_2)\exp(\lambda t)$.

Finally, taking into account the change of variables $X = PY$, all the surface concentrations are of the following form: $E_i = (\alpha t + \beta)\exp(\lambda t) + \gamma$. Once again, if $E_i(t)$ is differentiated twice with respect to t, the result is: $\frac{d^2 E_i}{dt^2} = \left(\lambda^2 \alpha t + \lambda^2 \beta + 2\lambda\alpha\right)\exp(\lambda t)$ As in previous cases, this expression can be zero only for a unique t value, concretely $\frac{d^2E_i}{dt^2}$ is zero only for $t=\frac{-\lambda^2\beta-2\lambda\alpha}{\lambda^2\alpha}$. Then, in this sub-case, only one inflexion point can be explained.

5.3 Third case: A unique eigenvalue ($\lambda_1=\lambda_2=\lambda_3=0$)

In this last case the Jordan canonical form is: $J=\begin{pmatrix}0&0&0\\1&0&0\\0&1&0\end{pmatrix}$ and the new ODE system is in this case: $\begin{pmatrix}\dot{y}_1\\\dot{y}_2\\\dot{y}_3\end{pmatrix}=\begin{pmatrix}0&0&0\\1&0&0\\0&1&0\end{pmatrix}\begin{pmatrix}y_1\\y_2\\y_3\end{pmatrix}$ or equivalently $\dot{y}_1=0$, $\dot{y}_2=y_1$ and $\dot{y}_3=y_2$. Then $y_1=c_1$, $y_2=c_1t+c_2$ and $y_3=c_1\frac{t^2}{2}+c_2t+c_3$ and taking into account the change of variables $X=PY$, all the surface concentrations are second order polynomials, such as: $E_i=\alpha t^2+\beta t+\gamma$. Finally, double differentiation of $E_i(t)$ with respect to t, gives: $\frac{d^2E_i}{dt^2}=2\alpha$, so in this case there are no inflexion points.

As a consequence of this analysis, two inflexion points cannot be explained by mechanisms involving electrochemical uni-molecular reactions.

Finally, as mentioned in other papers, this double inflexion is explained in terms of electrocatalytic reactions (Martinez-Luaces, 2001: Guineo & Martinez-Luaces, 2002).

6. Other qualitative results

As an example, let us consider again the following mechanism:

$$E_1 \underset{K_{-1}}{\overset{K_1}{\rightleftarrows}} E_2 \quad E_2 \underset{K_{-2}}{\overset{K_2}{\rightleftarrows}} E_3 \quad E_1 \underset{K_{-3}}{\overset{K_3}{\rightleftarrows}} E_3 \tag{4}$$

where all the possible reactions between the three adsorbates are considered.

As it was mentioned before, for such a mechanism, the mathematical model is:

$$\begin{pmatrix}\dot{x}\\\dot{y}\\\dot{z}\end{pmatrix}=\begin{pmatrix}-k_1-k_3 & k_{-1} & k_{-3}\\ k_1 & -k_{-1}-k_2 & k_{-2}\\ k_3 & k_2 & -k_{-2}-k_{-3}\end{pmatrix}\begin{pmatrix}x\\y\\z\end{pmatrix} \tag{5}$$

In this problem - as in other models, corresponding to other mechanisms - the result of the sum of all the rows is the null vector, and this fact implies the existence of a null eigenvalue.

In the previous section, this fact was utilised to prove the impossibility of two inflexion points in the surface concentration curves. Now, in this section, these facts will be used to reach other conclusions about qualitative behaviours, particularly in terms of stability of the solutions and several inverse problems related with this sequence of reactions.

6.1 Stability of the solutions

From a mathematical viewpoint when an ODE solution is altered slightly for instance, changing the initial conditions, a set of new curves may or may not show a different behaviour from the original one. From this fact, the heuristic basis for the concepts of stability and instability may be found. Moreover, a third possibility - asymptotically stable solutions - can arise when the altered solutions tend to the original one over a period of time, i.e., time nullifies any changes made to original solution (Martinez-Luaces, 2009e).

From a chemical point of view, the last option is the most desirable one, because it means that small errors due to measurements can be expected to diminish and almost disappear as reaction time proceeds.

In these cases, as in other mathematical models corresponding to ODE linear systems, stability and/or asymptotical stability strongly depend on the eigenvalues, particularly on their signs and multiplicity.

In all the unimolecular mechanisms studied there exists a null eigenvalue, and this fact implies that the solutions cannot be asymptotically stable (Martinez-Luaces, 2007, 2009e). As a consequence of chemical kinetics, small errors in the initial surface concentrations cannot be expected to vanish as the reaction tends to completion. Moreover, in the best hypothesis, we can expect these errors to be small and bounded, if the other eigenvalues are negative (i.e., this best possibility takes place only if $\lambda_1 < 0$, $\lambda_2 < 0$ and $\lambda_3 = 0$, or any other similar combination).

Let us return to the first mechanism considered in this article:

$$\begin{array}{l} E_1 \xrightarrow{k_1} E_2 \\ E_1 \xrightarrow{k_2} E_3 \\ E_2 \underset{k_{-3}}{\overset{k_3}{\rightleftarrows}} E_3 \end{array} \tag{1}$$

As mentioned before, the mathematical model corresponding to this mechanism is the following one:

$$\begin{cases} \dfrac{d[E_1]}{dt} = -(k_1 + k_2)[E_1] \\ \dfrac{d[E_2]}{dt} = k_1[E_1] - k_3[E_2] + k_{-3}[E_3] \\ \dfrac{d[E_3]}{dt} = k_2[E_1] + k_3[E_2] - k_{-3}[E_3] \end{cases} \tag{2}$$

and the corresponding ODE system matrix is:

$$A = \begin{pmatrix} -k_1 - k_2 & 0 & 0 \\ k_1 & -k_3 & k_{-3} \\ k_2 & k_3 & -k_{-3} \end{pmatrix} \tag{23}$$

In order to obtain the eigenvalues, the characteristic equation:

$$\det(A - \lambda I) = \det\begin{pmatrix} -k_1 - k_2 - \lambda & 0 & 0 \\ k_1 & -k_3 - \lambda & k_{-3} \\ k_2 & k_3 & -k_{-3} - \lambda \end{pmatrix} = 0 \tag{24}$$

must be solved.

Algebraic manipulations lead to the following equation:

$-\lambda(\lambda + k_1 + k_2)(\lambda + k_3 + k_{-3}) = 0$ and the solutions are $\lambda_1 = 0$, $\lambda_2 = -k_1 - k_2 < 0$ and $\lambda_3 = -k_3 - k_{-3} < 0$. Then, in this case two eigenvalues are negative and the other one is zero and so, solutions of the ODE system are stable, but not asymptotically.

Let us turn again to the simpler mechanism, already studied:

$$E_1 \xrightarrow{k_1} E_2 \xrightarrow{k_2} E_3 \tag{19}$$

In this case, the ODE system is as follows:

$$\begin{cases} \dfrac{d[E_1]}{dt} = -k_1[E_1] \\ \dfrac{d[E_2]}{dt} = k_1[E_1] - k_2[E_2] \\ \dfrac{d[E_3]}{dt} = k_2[E_2] \end{cases} \tag{20}$$

and the matrix system is:

$$A = \begin{pmatrix} -k_1 & 0 & 0 \\ k_1 & -k_2 & 0 \\ 0 & k_2 & 0 \end{pmatrix} \tag{25}$$

In this simpler case it is not necessary to solve the characteristic equation, i.e. $\det(A - \lambda I) = 0$, because A is a lower triangular matrix and so, the eigenvalues are the diagonal elements: $\lambda_1 = -k_1 < 0$, $\lambda_2 = -k_2 < 0$ and $\lambda_3 = 0$. Again, in this case, solutions are stable, but not asymptotically, and so, experimental errors in the initial conditions tend to remain small and bounded, but they will not tend to disappear with time.

As a final example, let us consider again the following mechanism involving all the possible reactions between the three adsorbates:

$$E_1 \underset{K_{-1}}{\overset{K_1}{\rightleftarrows}} E_2$$
$$E_2 \underset{K_{-2}}{\overset{K_2}{\rightleftarrows}} E_3 \qquad (4)$$
$$E_1 \underset{K_{-3}}{\overset{K_3}{\rightleftarrows}} E_3$$

The mathematical model for this mechanism, written in a simplified vector form is:

$$\begin{pmatrix} x \\ y \\ z \end{pmatrix}' = \begin{pmatrix} -k_1 - k_3 & k_{-1} & k_{-3} \\ k_1 & -k_{-1} - k_2 & k_{-2} \\ k_3 & k_2 & -k_{-2} - k_{-3} \end{pmatrix} \begin{pmatrix} x \\ y \\ z \end{pmatrix} \qquad (5)$$

And the characteristic equation is:

$$\det(A - \lambda I) = \det\begin{pmatrix} -k_1 - k_3 - \lambda & k_{-1} & k_{-3} \\ k_1 & -k_{-1} - k_2 - \lambda & k_{-2} \\ k_3 & k_2 & -k_{-2} - k_{-3} - \lambda \end{pmatrix} = 0 \qquad (26)$$

Once again, algebraic manipulations lead to a third order polynomial equation of this form: $-\lambda^3 - a\lambda^2 - b\lambda = 0$ that can be written as $(-\lambda)(\lambda^2 + a\lambda + b) = 0$ where $a = k_1 + k_2 + k_3 + k_{-1} + k_{-2} + k_{-3} = \sum_i k_i > 0$ and
$b = k_1k_2 + k_1k_{-2} + k_1k_{-3} + k_2k_3 + k_2k_{-3} + k_3k_{-1} + k_3k_{-2} + k_{-1}k_{-2} + k_{-1}k_{-3} > 0$.

On the other hand, since the eigenvalues are λ_1 , λ_2 and $\lambda_3 = 0$, this polynomial equation can be expressed as: $(\lambda_1 - \lambda)(\lambda_2 - \lambda)(0 - \lambda) = 0$ which can be written in the alternative form: $(-\lambda)(\lambda^2 - (\lambda_1 + \lambda_2)\lambda + \lambda_1\lambda_2) = 0$.

Finally, if $(-\lambda)(\lambda^2 + a\lambda + b) = 0$ and $(-\lambda)(\lambda^2 - (\lambda_1 + \lambda_2)\lambda + \lambda_1\lambda_2) = 0$ are different forms of the same equation, then: $\lambda_1 + \lambda_2 = -a < 0$ and $\lambda_1\lambda_2 = b > 0$. These inequalities lead to the following result: $\lambda_1 < 0$, $\lambda_2 < 0$ and $\lambda_3 = 0$, as in the other examples previously analysed and, once again, this fact means that the ODE solutions will be stable, but not asymptotically.

In all the previous examples, results can be summarised as: $\lambda_1 < 0$, $\lambda_2 < 0$ and $\lambda_3 = 0$ or any other similar combination. It is important to mention that the null eigenvalue can be obtained simply as a consequence of Lavoisier's law, as shown previously (in section 5), while the others must be obtained from the characteristic equation.

In all cases analysed solutions are just stable (a weak stability, not asymptotic stability) and as a consequence, experimental errors in the initial concentrations tend to remain bounded, but they do not tend to vanish with time.

6.2 Inverse modelling problems

Each chemical or electrochemical mechanism involving unimolecular reactions leads to a linear ODE system. This is a well known result, but what happens with the inverse question:

does any ODE linear system correspond - at least theoretically - to a given mechanism? If not, what condition must be considered to ensure that a given ODE linear system corresponds to a chemical unimolecular reaction mechanism?

In order to answer these questions we shall slightly modify the ODE system matrix corresponding to one of the mechanisms previously analysed. For instance, if we consider again the following mechanism:

$$\begin{array}{c} E_1 \underset{K_{-1}}{\overset{K_1}{\rightleftarrows}} E_2 \\ E_2 \underset{K_{-2}}{\overset{K_2}{\rightleftarrows}} E_3 \\ E_1 \underset{K_{-3}}{\overset{K_3}{\rightleftarrows}} E_3 \end{array} \tag{4}$$

and the corresponding ODE system matrix is:

$$A = \begin{pmatrix} -k_1 - k_3 & k_{-1} & k_{-3} \\ k_1 & -k_{-1} - k_2 & k_{-2} \\ k_3 & k_2 & -k_{-2} - k_{-3} \end{pmatrix} \tag{27}$$

Now, if just the first entry of this system matrix is modified, the resulting matrix will be:

$$A_\varepsilon = \begin{pmatrix} \varepsilon - k_1 - k_3 & k_{-1} & k_{-3} \\ k_1 & -k_{-1} - k_2 & k_{-2} \\ k_3 & k_2 & -k_{-2} - k_{-3} \end{pmatrix} \tag{28}$$

(it is important to note that the first entry $a_{11} = -k_1 - k_3$ was changed to a slightly different new one, $a_{11}^* = -k_1 - k_3 + \varepsilon$).

This new matrix A_ε does not correspond to a certain reaction mechanism, because if all its rows are added, the result is: $(\varepsilon, 0, 0)$ instead of the null vector as in the case of matrix A.

This observation has a dramatic consequence for the inverse modelling problem: A corresponds to a given unimolecular reaction mechanism, but A_ε cannot be associated with any of these mechanisms. As mentioned before, this is due to the mass conservation law, which in this case can be written as $[E_1]+[E_2]+[E_3]=c$. Derivation of this equation gives the following: $\frac{d[A]}{dt}+\frac{d[B]}{dt}+\frac{d[C]}{dt}=0$ and the last formula implies that adding all the matrix rows the result must be zero. This criterion can be used in order to know whether or not a given matrix corresponds to a certain mechanism (Martinez-Luaces, 2007, 2009a, 2009e).

7. Conclusions and observations

This article describes a combination of chemical and mathematical modelling applied to the adsorption of Carbon Dioxide on Platinum surfaces, but a similar procedure can be applied to any chemical or electrochemical mechanism involving unimolecular reactions. Moreover, mathematical theorems about eigenvalues, eigenvectors, diagonalization, Jordan canonical forms, etc., and chemical laws, particularly Lavoisier's law of mass conservation can be combined to solve inverse causation and stability problems.

It is well known that any given chemical mechanism involving unimolecular reactions leads to a linear ODE system, but the converse is not true. In fact, as previously shown, slightly modifying a given ODE system matrix results in a new matrix that does not correspond to any unimolecular reaction mechanism. Then, this result gives a negative answer to the inverse problem about whether a mechanism exists for every linear ODE system. At the same time, it gives a negative answer to the "inverse stability problem", i.e., a slight change in one of the coefficients produces dramatic changes in the inverse problem. Moreover, there exists a mechanism corresponding to a certain matrix A but not for the modified matrix A_ε. This is a typical conclusion of inverse problems, where existence, uniqueness and stability do not usually occur.

Finally, other issues like the qualitative behaviour of solutions (stability, instability and asymptotic stability), can be analysed using this approach. Moreover, in all the examples studied, solutions exhibited weak stability, which in terms of the electrochemical problem means that experimental errors in the initial surface concentrations tend to remain limited as the reaction proceeds to completion. Nevertheless, these experimental errors never tend to vanish, and this fact is a consequence of having a null eigenvalue. As observed earlier, all these facts can be proved combining mathematical theorems with chemical laws, so they can be easily generalised to other unimolecular reactions mechanisms.

8. References

Blum, W. et al., (2002). ICMI Study 14: applications and modelling in mathematics education - discussion document. *Educational Studies in Mathematics,* Vol. 51, No. 1-2, 149-171.

Bunge, M., (2006), Problemas directos e inversos, In: *Grupobunge. Filosofia y ciencia,* Access: May, 2011, Available from: http://grupobunge.wordpress.com/2006/07/20/119.

Groestch, C.W., (1999), *Inverse problems: activities for undergraduates,* Mathematical Association of America (Eds.), Washington D.C., U.S.A.

Groestch, C.W., (2001). Inverse problems: the other two-thirds of the story, *Quaestiones Mathematicae,* Vol. Suppl. 1, 2001, Supplement, 89-93, ISSN 1607-3606.

Guerasimov, Y.A., et al., (1995), *Physical Chemistry,* 2nd Edition, Houghton Mifflin, (Eds.) Boston, U.S.A.

Guineo Cobs, G. & Martínez Luaces, V., (2002). Electrocatalytic reactions: An interesting problem of Numerical Calculus, *Communications of the 2nd International Conference on the Teaching of Mathematics at the undergraduate level*. Crete, Greece, July 2002.

Martínez Luaces, V., (2001). Reacciones Electroquímicas y Electrocatalíticas: Un problema de Matemática Aplicada. *Actas COMAT 95-97-99*, ISBN 959 - 160097 - 6. Matanzas, Cuba.

Martínez Luaces, V., (2005). Engaging Secondary School and University Teachers in Modelling: Some Experiences in South American Countries. *International Journal of Mathematical Education in Science and Technology*, Vol 36, No. 2-3, pp. 193-194, ISSN 0020-739X.

Martínez Luaces, V., (2007). Inverse-modelling problems in Chemical Engineering courses. *Vision and change for a new century. Proceedings of Calafate Delta '07.* ISBN: 978-9974-96-348-1, El Calafate, Argentina, November 2007.

Martínez Luaces, V., (2008). Modelado inverso y Transformada de Laplace en problemas de diseño de reactores químicos. *Proceedings of EMCI XIV. Educación Matemática en Carreras de Ingeniería*, Mendoza, Argentina, May 2008.

Martínez Luaces, V., (2009a). Modelling and inverse-modelling: experiences with O.D.E. linear systems in engineering courses, *International Journal of Mathematical Education in Science and Technology*, Vol. 40, No. 2, pp. 259-268, ISSN 0020-739X.

Martínez Luaces,V., (2009b). Problemas de modelado directo e inverso con Ecuaciones Diferenciales y Transformación de Laplace. *Proceedings of EMCI XV. Educación Matemática en Carreras de Ingeniería*, Tucumán, Argentina, September 2009.

Martínez Luaces,V., (2009c). Modelling and Inverse Modelling with second order P.D.E. in Engineering courses. *Proceedings of Southern Right Delta '09.* Gordon's Bay, South Africa, November 2009.

Martínez Luaces,V., (2009d). Modelling, applications and Inverse Modelling: Innovations in Differential Equations courses. *Proceedings of Southern Right Gordon's Bay Delta '09*, Gordon's Bay, South Africa, November 2009.

Martínez Luaces, V., (2009e). *Aplicaciones y modelado: Ecuaciones Diferenciales Ordinarias, Transformación de Laplace, Ecuaciones en Derivadas Parciales.* Matser (Eds.), ISBN 978-9974-96-621-5 Montevideo, Uruguay.

Martínez Luaces, V., (2011). Problemas inversos: los casi olvidados de la Matemática Educativa. *Acta Latinoamericana de Matematica Educativa*, 24, pp. 439-447. ISBN 978-607-95306-4-8.

Martínez Luaces, V. & Guineo Cobs, G., (2002). Un problema de Electroquímica y su Modelación Matemática, *Anuario Latinoamericano de Educación Química.* Año 2002, pp. 272 - 276, ISSN 0328 - 087X.

Martínez Luaces, V., Zinola, F. & Méndez, E., (2001). Problemas Matemáticos Computacionales en el estudio de Mecanismos de Reacciones Químicas", *Actas de COMAT 95-97-99*, ISBN 959 - 160097 - 6. Cuba.

Zinola, F., Méndez, E. & Martínez Luaces, V., (1997). Modificación de estados adsorbidos de Anhídrido Carbónico reducido por labilización electroquímica en superficies facetadas de platino. *Proceedings of X Congreso Argentino de Fisicoquímica,* Tucumán, Argentina, April 1997.

3

On the Interrelations Between Kinetics and Thermodynamics as the Theories of Trajectories and States

Boris M. Kaganovich, Alexandre V. Keiko, Vitaly A. Shamansky and Maxim S. Zarodnyuk
Melentiev Energy Systems Institute, Russia

1. Introduction

Existence of close and obligatory relations between kinetics and thermodynamics is the truth well known to experts. It is clear that propositions of the science based on the most general regularities of the macroscopic world (thermodynamics) should be used in the theories of macroscopic processes running over time (chemical and macroscopic kinetics). Application of general principles in solving specific kinetic problems in the majority of cases turns out to be related to specificity of their use. Observance of one or another principle or rule can require search for original both physicochemical statement of the problem, and mathematical model, and computational method. The art of thermodynamic analysis of kinetic equations was demonstrated in (Feinberg, 1972, 1999; Horn and Jackson, 1972; Gorban, 1984; Yablonsky et al., 1991) and works by other researchers. The character of relations between the theories of trajectories and theories of states changed qualitatively in the second half of the 20th century due to rapid development of computers and numerical methods of mathematical programming (MP). It became possible to considerably simplify formalized descriptions of problems owing to the transition from their analytical solutions to iterative, stepwise search processes. Analysis of possibilities to simplify the kinetic models and unfolding the methods to implement these possibilities on the basis of equilibrium thermodynamic principles constitute the aim of the chapter.

The main idea of the research being described is the refusal to use an equation of trajectory and construction of stepwise methods to analyse processes on the basis of the model of extreme intermediate states (MEIS) that was created by B.M.Kaganovich, S.P.Filippov and E.G.Antsiferov (Antsiferov et al., 1988; Kaganovich, 1991; Kaganovich et al., 1989). The features that make MEIS different from the traditional thermodynamic models are: 1) statement of the problem to be solved (instead of search for a sole point of final equilibrium x^{eq} the entire set of thermodynamic attainability $D_t(y)$ from the given initial state y is considered and the states x^{ext} with extreme values of modeled system characteristics of interest to a researcher are found); 2) dual interpretation of the equilibrium notion, i.e. both as a state of rest and as an instant of motion in which the equality of action and counteraction is observed; and 3) dual interpretation of dynamic quantities (work ℓ, heat q, rate w, flow of substance x, etc.) both as functions of state and as functions of a trajectory. The last modifications of MEIS (Gorban et al., 2006; Kaganovich et al., 2007, 2010) include constraints on the rates of limiting stages of transformations, transfer and exchange of mass, energy and charges.

For these rates we set dependences on constants that have dimension of time (for example the total duration of chemical reaction or its certain stages). However, since it is possible to make an assumption about stationarity of motion when dividing the studied process into sufficiently small time periods the need for the use of time functions does not arise. Increasing the number of steps (segments) for choosing the solutions makes it possible to determine the trajectory of motion on the basis of these solutions with any required accuracy of calculations. The methods of affine scaling (Dikin, 1967, 2010; Dikin and Zorkaltsev, 1980) and dynamic programming (DP) (Bellman, 2003; Wentzel, 1964) are considered as numerical methods to be used to implement the MEIS capabilities.

The authors substantiated the validity of the entire methodological approach, mathematical models and computational methods on the basis of: 1) the historical analysis of developing interactions between the theories of trajectories and the theories of states; 2) the experience gained in the use of MEIS to study the processes of fuel combustion and processing, atmospheric pollution with anthropogenic emissions and motion of viscous liquids in multi-loop hydraulic systems; and 3) the establishment of mathematical relations between the applied dependences and thermodynamic principles.

Theoretical and applied efficiency of the equilibrium thermodynamic modeling in kinetic studies is illustrated by conditional and real examples: izomerization, formation of nitrogen oxides at fuel combustion, distribution of viscous liquid flows in multi-loop cirquits and optimization of schemes and parameters of these networks, analysis of mechanisms of physicochemical processes.

2. Remarks on the history of interactions between the theories of motion and the theories of rest

The authors believe that the joint development of statics and dynamics, theories of states and trajectories can be divided into five stages.

The first stage is related to the names of Galileo and Newton. Galileo was the first to consider the notions of equilibria as an obligatory component in the study of natural regularities. The principle of relativity that was discovered by Galileo revealed that the state of a body (a particle) subject to the action of forces that are in equilibrium can be described with the model of rest and the model of uniform rectilinear motion. The last formalized analysis made by D'Alamber showed that the dual interpretations can be extended to any instant of any nonuniform mechanical motion. The third law of Newton that should undoubtedly be observed in stationary and non-stationary, in reversible and irreversible processes helped greatly to better understand the relations between static and dynamic interpretations of equilibria. Newton used the equilibrium principles not only to establish the laws of nature but also to create a computational instrument intended to solve certain problems on the basis of these laws. The most important notion of infinitesimal calculus (the key Newton computational instrument) is the notion of differential - an infinitesimal linear increment in the function of state. But fixing the value of function is related to the assumption about equilibrium of the forces tending to change this value.

At the second stage of the considered historical process after Galileo and Newton a greater step in the development of equilibrium principles and their application to the analysis of trajectories and states was made by Lagrange. In (Lagrange, 1788) he gave the first systematic description of mechanics (which in the 18th century was equivalent to the description of physics) in terms of mathematics[1]. This book contains physical-mathematical explanation of the laws of nature and relations among them; the single theory of statics and dynamics, states and trajectories; choice of the methods to solve specific problems and substantiation of their physical (interpretational) and computational efficiencies; deductive derivation of partial regularities obtained by Newton in (Newton, 1999).

The initial equation chosen by Lagrange to build the structure of the Newton mechanics was the equation for equilibrium of a mechanical system

$$\sum_j c_j(x)dx_j + \sum_i \lambda_i(\varphi)d\varphi_i = 0\,, \tag{1}$$

where c, x, λ and φ are a motive force, a coordinate, an uncertain multiplier (resistance force of bonds) and bond deformation, respectively; j – index of motive forces and respective coordinates; i – index of resistances and bonds. The first sum in the left-hand side of equation (1) represents a differential of work of motive forces tending to change the system state and the second sum – a differential of work of resistance forces that hinder any changes.

Formulation of equation (1) was based on two remarkable ideas. The first of them belongs to Newton who, according to Einstein, was the first to understand that physics can describe the laws of nature only in differential form. Integral relationships are often true only in certain ranges of values of variables and are less universal than differential ones used by Lagrange. The second idea implies division of potential forces applied to system into two groups: motive forces and resistances. Tendency of the difference between the works of these forces (taking into account the signs) to zero when nearing the point x^{eq} makes it possible to find the state of final equilibrium by solving the one-criterion extreme problem:

$$\text{find} \qquad \text{extr}\left(L = \sum_j c_j(x)x_j + \sum_i \lambda_i(\varphi)\varphi_i \right), \tag{2}$$

where L – the function that was later called the function of Lagrange.

The uniqueness of criterion (2) is explained by the uniqueness of division of forces into motive and "resisting" ones. Solving problem (2) as compared to solving the closed system of equations makes it also possible to easily vary statements of the problems by changing the set of variables, adding different equalities and inequalities to the system of constraints (bonds) or excluding them. Based on (1) we reveal physical and mathematical relations between the principles of equilibrium and principles of conservation. Since all the members in this equality have the dimension of work (energy) it can be interpreted as the principle of

[1] Newton in (Newton, 1999) used mathematics exclusively as a calculation tool, i.e. as a means for solving certain problems. The laws were stated by him only in verbal formulations.

zero work, i.e. zero energy consumption (conservation) at an infinitesimal deviation of a system from equilibrium. This interpretation of (1) represents the principle of virtual work (PVW).

The identification of relations between statics and dynamics became a constituting part in the explanation of unity of the laws of mechanics in (Lagrange, 1788). Deriving the equations of trajectories from the equation of state (1) turned out to be possible owing to the assumptions made about observance of the relativity principle of Galileo and the third law of Newton and, hence, about representability of any trajectory in the form of a continuous sequence of equilibrium states. From the representability, in turn, follow the most important properties of the Lagrange motion curves: existence of the functions of states (independent of attainability path) at each point; possibility to describe the curves by autonomous differential equations that have the form $\dot{x} = f(x)$; dependence of the optimal configuration of any part of the curve upon its initial point only. These properties correspond to the extreme principles of the optimal control theory.

The single description of statics and dynamics made it also possible to extend the interpretations of the notions of state and trajectory functions. The work in an infinitesimal period of time in the vicinity of equilibrium point was interpreted by Lagrange as a function of state. Representation of the trajectory in the form of a continuous sequence of equilibrium states makes it possible to interpret the work as a virtual (possible) function of rest during the entire modeled process.

Based on the dual (dynamic and static) interpretations of equilibria and PVW (equations (1)) Lagrange formulated the integral extreme principle, i.e. the principle of the least action (PLA):

$$\delta J = \delta \int_{\tau_1}^{\tau_2} L d\tau = \delta \int_{\tau_1}^{\tau_2} (T - \Pi) d\tau = 0 , \tag{3}$$

where δ is variation of function; J - action; τ - time; T and Π - kinetic and potential energy of the system, respectively. The possibility to replace the Lagrange integrand L by the difference $(T - \Pi)$ is obvious, since the work of motive forces (the first sum in (1) and (2)) is performed by consuming kinetic energy and the work of resistance forces (the second sum) is a result of change in potential energy.

The equation of extreme trajectory that meets condition (3)

$$\frac{\partial L}{\partial x} - \frac{d}{d\tau}\left(\frac{\partial L}{\partial \dot{x}}\right) = 0 \tag{4}$$

was derived by Euler (for one point) and by Lagrange (for a system of points).

Along with many-sided and rigorous description of physical regularities the book by Lagrange (Lagrange, 1788) represents an invaluable contribution to the development of mathematical methods for analysis of states and trajectories. Specifically, the ideas of "The analytical mechanics" are related to the creation and application of the method of multipliers, mathematical programming and calculus of variations. The method of multipliers which became the primary tool for Lagrange to derive and interpret the principles of statics and dynamics of mechanical systems also became a key tool for solving the problems of search for conditional extrema. Lagrange's analysis of the method of multipliers and conditions for equilibrium of mechanical systems laid foundation to construct in the second half of the 20th century the modern mathematical theory called mathematical programming (MP). The theory deals with search for extrema and equilibria. The work of motive forces started to play the role of objective function in the problems of mathematical programming and expressions for the work of bond deformation made up the system of constraints. The above physical interpretations of these works elucidated the possibility to divide the MP problems into direct (maximization) and dual (minimization), and clarified the term "dual estimates" which is used by mathematicians as applied to the Lagrange multiplier λ. Generally speaking, the unified physical-mathematical description of classical mechanics, that was made by Lagrange on the basis of equilibrium principles, i.e. his "Analytical mechanics" can be considered to be the first general theory of equilibrium states and equilibrium trajectories.

At the third stage the equilibrium thermodynamics was created by Clausius, Helmholtz, Boltzmann and Gibbs. Since that time the equilibrium principles started to develop as applied to macroscopic systems of any physical nature. The main, second law of thermodynamics was discovered by Clausius (Clausius, 2008). He found out the existence of the state function, entropy (S), that can change in the isolated systems exclusively towards increase. The inequality that shows such monotonicity of change

$$dS \geq 0 \tag{5}$$

is one of the mathematical formulations of this law and determines irreversibility of natural processes, i.e. their compliance with "an arrow of time". They approach the point of global maximum of entropy, i.e. the state of final equilibrium x^{eq}. Thus, the second law is simultaneously the principle of both extremality and equilibrium. It can be applied to the analysis of trajectories ($dS \geq 0$) and states ($\max S$), reversible ($dS = 0$) and irreversible ($dS > 0$) processes. Motion towards point $\max S$ according to Clausius is an equilibrium motion since entropy was assumed by him as the function of state and its value can be fixed at any time instant only when respective forces are in equilibrium.

However, the practical application of the second law in the analysis of equilibrium irreversible trajectories faced great difficulties. Clausius and then Helmholtz, Boltzmann, J. Thomson, Planck and other researchers tried to harmonize the second law of thermodynamics with the principle of the least action and derive the equation that meets this principle similar to the equations (3) or (4) for dissipative macroscopic systems (in which the organized energy forms turn into a non-organized form, i.e. heat, due to friction). As is known their attempts were unsuccessful and resulted in understanding the necessity to statistically substantiate thermodynamics (Polak, 2010).

Such a substantiation was given by Boltzmann (Boltzmann, 1877), who chose the probability of attaining a state as its basic property that determines all other properties of thermodynamic system. Equilibrium transition from the least to the most probable states is at once irreversible since the reverse motion towards decrease in probabilities is immeasurably more difficult. Boltzmann's determination of a non-decreasing function (entropy) on the basis of equation

$$S = k \ln w \tag{6}$$

seems also natural, where k is the Boltzmann constant and w – thermodynamic probability (a statistical weight).

Similar to Lagrange, Boltzmann harmonized equilibrium theories of states and trajectories but in terms of probabilities. The transition from representation of entropy by a function of heat based on

$$dS = dq / T \tag{7}$$

(q is heat; T – absolute temperature) to the representation by a function of probability (6) interrelates deterministic and statistical descriptions. It also facilitates representability of heat as well as work as functions of state at infinitesimal time intervals. Indeed, according to Boltzmann the probability of a state does not depend on the path of its destination and, correspondingly, is a function of solely that state. Therefore, the entropy and heat, that are single-valued functions of probability, are logically to be considered as functions of state. Therefore, any trajectory related to both reversible and irreversible dynamics can be described by a continuous sequence of equilibrium states. In this case if variable w is used the modeled processes are interpreted as random ones, and if variable q – as deterministic ones. The mathematical macroscopic explanation of the applicability of differential equations to thermodynamic problems was given by Caratheodory (Caratheodory, 1909) and Born (Born, 1921).

The Boltzmann integro-differential kinetic equation written in terms of statistical physics became the foundation for construction of the structure of physical kinetics that included derivation of equations for transfer of matter, energy and charges, and determination of kinetic coefficients that entered into them, i.e. the coefficients of viscosity, heat conductivity, diffusion, electric conductivity, etc. Though the interpretations of physical kinetics as description of non-equilibrium processes of relaxation towards the state of equilibrium are widespread, the Boltzmann interpretations of the probability and entropy notions as functions of state allow us to consider physical kinetics as a theory of equilibrium trajectories. These trajectories as well as the trajectories of Euler–Lagrange have the properties of extremality (any infinitesimal part of a trajectory has this property) and representability in the form of a continuous sequence of states of rest. These trajectories can be used to describe the behavior of (a) isolated systems that spontaneously proceed to final equilibrium; (b) the systems for which the differences of potentials with the environment are fixed; (c) and non-homogeneous systems in which different parts have different values of the same intensive parameters.

Despite the creation of physical kinetics at the third stage of the history of interactions between statics and dynamics substantiated admissibility of equilibrium modeling of macroscopic processes of any physical nature at the forth stage the relations between macroscopic theories of motion and rest have sharply weakened. According to some scientists this was greatly due to the known discussion about the Boltzmann paradox (a seeming contradiction between the assumptions about a reversible character of interaction among separate particles and an irreversible result of these interactions aggregate). With development of the theory of dynamic systems (Arnold, 1989, Katok and Hasselblat, 2005), non-equilibrium thermodynamics' emerged from the classical thermodynamics (Prigogine, 1967; Glansdorf and Prigogine, 1971; Jou et.al., 2001), and synergetics (Haken, 1983, 2006) the equilibrium approach relating the models of states and trajectories became widely deemed to be principally unsuitable in modeling of irreversible processes, degradation and self-organization. The experience gained in equilibrium analysis of various non-equilibria and irreversibilities (for example, emission of heat by electric current, diffusion, radiation, superfluidity and superconductivity, formation of stars, phase transitions of the second kind) by the classics of physics: Kirchhoff, Maxwell, Plank, Einstein, Landau, et al. discussed in (Gorban et al., 2006; Kaganovich, 2011; Kaganovich et al., 2007, 2010) was mostly ignored.

Such an attitude to equilibrium thermodynamics - the science which revealed irreversibility of the evolution of isolated systems and asymmetry of natural processes with respect to time - is related to some circumstances that require a thorough analysis. Here we will emphasize only one of them which is the most important for understanding further text. It lies in the fact that the most important notion of thermodynamics, i.e. equilibrium, became interpreted exclusively as the state of rest (absence of any forces and flows in the thermodynamic system) and equilibrium processes - as those identical to reversible ones. These one-sided interpretations ignored the Galileo principle of relativity, the third law of Newton and the Boltzmann probabilistic interpretations of entropy that allow dynamic interpretations of equilibria and irreversible interpretations of equilibrium processes.

An incomplete one-sided definition of the main notions resulted in an erroneous assessment of equilibrium thermodynamics capabilities and some misunderstandings with respect to applicability of equilibrium modeling in different areas. A vivid misconception was the opinion that self-organization can occur only in non-equilibrium systems. The opinion was undoubtedly caused by great success of non-equilibrium thermodynamics (Glansdorff and Prigogine, 1971; Jou et al., 2001) and synergetics (Haken, 1983) in explanation of the ordering processes. These disciplines helped to reveal the mechanisms of laser radiation, the Benard phenomenon and formation of turbulent vortexes in fluid, self-organizing chemical reactions and many other phenomena. We can say that the single theory of self-organization in the inanimate nature started to take shape. However, the abovementioned results, that were obtained on the basis of the propositions of equilibrium thermodynamics and were required for integrity and versatile applicability of this theory turned out to be in no demand.

The relations between the theories of trajectories and states, kinetics and thermodynamics that were lost started to recover at the fifth stage (the last third of the 20th century) owing to the works by M.Feinberg (Feinberg, 1972, 1999; Feinberg and Hildebrant, 1997; Feinberg and Horn, 1974); F.Horn (Horn, 1964; Horn and Jackson, 1972); A.N.Gorban (Gorban, 1984, Gorban et al., 2001, 2006, 2007); G.S.Yablonsky (Yablonsky et al., 1991) and other experts in thermodynamic analysis of chemical kinetics equations that were used to assess thermodynamically attainable results of chemical processes that correspond to attainable partial or complete (final x^{eq}) equilibria.

Two remarkable ideas put forward by A.N.Gorban should be emphasized in the studies related to thermodynamic analysis of kinetics. The first of them is the idea of a thermodynamic tree (Gorban, 1984) - a one-dimension graph, whose branches are related by one-to-one correspondence to the components of arcwise connectivity (regions on the material balance polyhedron of a thermodynamic system, in which two any points can be connected by thermodynamically admissible paths), and a point of the branch reflects a set of equilibrium states on the respective component, in which the characteristic thermodynamic function has the same value. "The Gorban tree" can also be defined as a mapping of the entire thermodynamically admissible set of kinetic trajectories of the modeled system in the one-dimensional space. The presented definitions suggest high efficiency of applying the notion of a tree in geometrical explanations of relations between kinetics and thermodynamics.

The second and, apparently, the more general idea is the idea of formation of a new scientific discipline – "Model Engineering" (Gorban and Karlin, 2005; Gorban et al., 2007). The subject of the discipline is the choice of an outset statement of the solved problem which is the most suitable (optimal) both for conceptual analysis and for computations. The transfer of kinetic description into the space of thermodynamic variables became a main method for this discipline. In the method the solved problem can be represented as one-criterion problem of search for extremum of the function that has the properties of the Lyapunov functions (monotonously moving to fixed points).

3. Models of extreme intermediate states and construction of trajectories

The idea of MEIS creation first arose in analysis of synthetic liquid fuels production out of coal. The first modifications of this model were intended for estimation of the maximum yields of products in the chemical reactions (for example the maximum attainable concentration of light hydrocarbons in the process of hydrogenation of solid organic substances). The study on physical-mathematical features of MEIS that accompanied its application led to better understanding of the model capabilities and directions in its improvement. The capabilities were revealed largely owing to the specification of properties of a set of thermodynamically attainable states $D_t(y)$ from a given initial state y . Today we consider four specific features of this set to be the most important: 1) on the whole it belongs to the class of invariant manifolds in which any trajectory passing through any point of the considered manifold belongs entirely to it; 2) all the points of partial (intermediate) equilibria that belong to the manifold can be interpreted both as a state of rest (which is related to a supposition on the possibility of complete deceleration of all processes running through it) and as an instant of motion along one of the admissible trajectories; 3) dynamic variables: work, heat, flow, velocity, kinetic coefficients (including those the Onsager ones) that are applied to the description of a modeled system have the properties of the functions of states making up the set; 4) computational procedures related to the consequent monotonous change of the system's characteristic function on the set of values show one of the admissible trajectories in the space of chosen variables. The fourth feature is the sequence of the first one.

In accord with the described features the MEIS modifications gradually improved. Whereas in their first variants the admissible values of objective functions were limited only by the conditions of material and energy balances, monotonicity of entropy and thermodynamic potentials, yet in the first years of their application they started to include the constraints on possible values and limiting change of certain intensive parameters, quantities of reaction mix components and energy. The capabilities of MEIS increased sharply after the modules of macroscopic kinetics had been added to them. The modules allow one to take account of the impact the rates of the limiting stages of a modeled process have on the attainable results. The variants of formalization of constraints on macrokinetics were discussed in detail in (Gorban et al., 2006; Kaganovich, 2011; Kaganovich et al., 2007, 2010). Now a new direction in development of the models of extreme intermediate states is taking shape. It is related to their application not only in thermodynamic analysis of possible results of the processes but also in determination of the trajectories along which these results can be attained.

Setting about developing the latter direction, the authors relied on the historical experience that was briefly presented in the previous section (the experience in joint equilibrium modeling of states and trajectories), capabilities of modern computers and computational mathematics, and on their own experience acquired in the course of MEIS development and analysis of various physicochemical and technical-economic problems on its basis. The main idea in solution of the stated problem was refusal to use the equation of the sought extreme trajectory and its determination in the stepwise decision making process. During the stepwise process the assumptions about the observance of the above characteristics of $D_t(y)$ turn out to be admissible on each negligibly small section (of space or time).

To explain the suggested approach to construction of trajectories a brief description of the MEISs underlying it is necessary. Unlike the descriptions presented in (Kaganovich et al., 1993, 1995, 2007, 2010) here a new classification attribute (a form of extremality criterion which can be objective and subjective) will be added to the MEIS classification. The objective criterion is the one the system itself tends to observe under the set conditions of its change. The subjective criterion corresponds to the interest expressed by a researcher during the study[2]. An example of the objective criterion is the minimum Gibbs energy ($\min G$) of a system in which temperature T and pressure P are held constant. The examples of subjective criterion can be the maximum yield of methanol ($\max x_{CH_4O}$) at its synthesis from the mixture of CO and H_2, or the minimum formation of nitrogen oxide ($\min x_{NO}$) at coal combustion. According to the old classification features here we will consider three types of MEIS: MEIS with variable parameters, MEIS of the mechanisms of physicochemical processes and MEIS of hydraulic circuits.

At fixed T, P and initial composition of components y of the physicochemical system the MEIS with variable parameters and subjective extremality criterion (the maximum concentration of a set of useful or harmful products of the process) has the form:

find

$$\max\left(F(x) = \sum_{j\in J^{ext}} c_j x_j\right) = F\left(x^{ext}\right) \tag{8}$$

subject to

[2] The idea of such a classification was suggested to authors by the works by Yu.L.Klimontovish who used the notions of objective and subjective criteria of order (Klimontovich, 1995)

$$Ax = b\,, \tag{9}$$

$$D_t(y) = \left\{ x : \left| \begin{array}{c} x \le y, \\ \varphi_r(x_r) \le \psi_r, r \in R^{\lim}, \end{array} \right. \right\} \begin{array}{r} (10) \\ (11) \end{array}$$

$$G(x) = \sum_j G_j(x) x_j\,, \tag{12}$$

$$x_j \ge 0\,, \tag{13}$$

where $x = (x_1, \ldots, x_n)^T$ is vector of composition; $y \subset x$ - vector of initial composition; c_j - coefficient ranking the property of the j-th component x of interest to a researcher; x^{ext} - vector of composition in the desired extreme state; J^{ext} - set of indices of components with the extreme concentration of their mix to be determined; $A-(m \times n)$ - matrix of contents of the elements in the system components; b - vector of mole quantities of components of dimension m; φ_r - limiting kinetic function of the r-th component x, Ψ_r - its limiting value which depends on admissible values of variables that enter into the equation of limiting stage of the modeled process and on constants that determine its duration; $R^{\lim}$ - a set of indices of constraints on macroscopic kinetics; G and G_j - Gibbs energies of the system and its j-th component. The sign "$\le$" in expression (10) is understood in thermodynamic sense: $x \le y$, if it is possible to pass from y to x along a continuous trajectory along which $G(x)$ monotonously does not increase.

The equalities (9) and (13) represent a material balance. Expressions (10) and (11) determine the region of thermodynamic attainability from the point y. Equation (11) is used to specify constraints on macroscopic kinetics. The choice of equations for calculation of certain terms under the sign of sum in the right-hand side of equality (12) depends on the properties of the considered system.

The MEIS of a system described by the model (8)-(13) when choosing the objective extremality criterion has the form:

find

$$\left.\begin{array}{l} \min \left[G(x) = \sum_j G_j(x) x_j \right] = G\left(x^{eq}\right) \\ \\ \text{subject to} \qquad Ax = b, \\ \qquad \varphi_r(x_r) \le \Psi_r, \quad r \in R^{\lim}, \\ \qquad x_j \ge 0. \end{array}\right\} \tag{14}$$

Analysis of the model (14) shows that fulfillment of the condition of the minimum Gibbs energy (extremality criterion) is in line with the Lagrange PVW if to assume that the fundamental equation written for the state of equilibrium (Gibbs, 1876, 1878)

$$dG = -SdT + VdP + \sum_{j=1}^{n} \mu_j dx_j = 0 \tag{15}$$

(V is volume; μ - chemical potential) is an extension of equation (1) to thermodynamic systems with independent T, P and x. Following the formalism of Lagrange it can be conditionally considered that dG equals differential of the work of motive forces, whereas the terms in the right-hand side of the first equality (15) - differentials of the work of resistance forces, which in this case may have different signs.

Taking account of stationary process on the negligibly small trajectory section we can make sure that the product $G \cdot \tau$ (τ - time) is minimum, i.e. the principle of the least action is observed. Relations between the principles of conservative and dissipative systems were considered by the authors in (Kaganovich, 2011; Kaganovich et al., 2007, 2010). Below they will be additionally discussed in brief on the example of the models of hydraulic circuits.

By the analogy with parametric models it is also possible to represent the MEIS of mechanisms of physicochemical processes that are mapped on a conditional graph (Kaganovich, 2011; Kaganovich et al., 1993, 1995, 2007, 2010; Gorban et al., 2006) as those meeting the subjective and objective criteria. Each i-th branch of the conditional graph corresponds to the flows of matter, energy, charges that take part in the i-th stage of the overall process. The MEIS of the mechanism of chemical system with fixed T, P and y and subjective extremality criterion, similar to (8), is written in the form:

find

$$\max\left[F(x(\xi)) = \sum_{j \in J^{\text{ext}}} c_j x_j(\xi) \right] = F(x(\xi^{\text{ext}})) \tag{16}$$

subject to

$$x_j = y_j + \sum_j \nu_{ij} \xi_i , \quad j = 1,...,n , \quad i = 1,...,m , \tag{17}$$

$$D_t(y) = \left\{ \xi : \left| \begin{array}{ll} x(\xi) \le y, & (18) \\ \varphi_r(x(\xi)) \le \Psi_r, \quad r \in R^{\lim}, & (19) \end{array} \right. \right\}$$

$$G(x(\xi)) = \sum_j G_j(x(\xi)) x_j , \tag{20}$$

$$x_j \ge 0 , \quad 0 \le \xi_i \le 1 , \tag{21}$$

where $\xi = (\xi_1, ..., \xi_m)^T$; ξ_i is degree of completeness (coordinate) of the i-th reaction; ν_{ij} are stoichiometric coefficients. Equation (17) describes material balance of the j-th system component transformations. Inequalities (18) and (19) are similar to (10) and (11).

By the analogy with transition from model (8)-(13) to (14) it is possible to proceed from (16)-(20) to MEIS with the objective extremality criterion:

find

$$\left.\begin{array}{l}\min\left[G(x(\xi))=\sum_j G_j(x(\xi)x_j)\right]=G(x^{\mathrm{eq}}(\xi^{\mathrm{eq}}))\\ \text{subject to}\\ x_j=y_j+\sum_i v_{ij}\xi_i,\ j=1,\ \ldots,\ n,\ j=1,\ \ldots,\ m,\\ \varphi_r(x_r(\xi))\le\Psi_r,\ r\in R^{\mathrm{lim}},\\ x_j\ge 0,\ 0\le\xi_i\le 1.\end{array}\right\}\quad(22)$$

Analysis of relations between the principles of extremality of characteristic thermodynamic functions and other physical principles of extremality on the basis of models of mechanisms methodologically coincides completely with the analysis of these relations with the help of MEIS of type (8)-(13) and (14).

Possibilities to use the above presented MEIS modifications to determine both attainable results of macroscopic processes and admissible trajectories of motion towards these results are illustrated with two examples that were already used in (Kaganovich et al, 2007, 2010) to find the states x^{ext}, i.e. those meeting the subjective criteria of extremality.

The first example is a system of three isomers with constant T, P and $y=(1,0,0)$. Idealizing the problem statement, let us assume that isomers are ideal gases with standard Gibbs energies $G_1^0=-421.034$, $G_2^0=-424.620$ and $G_3^0=-420.255$ kJ/mole, the mechanism of the process that occurs in the system includes two stages: $x_1\rightarrow x_2$ and $x_2\rightarrow x_3$. Also we assume that the first stage lasts for an instant and the constant of the rate of the second k_2 equals 0.2 s^{-1}; the total duration of the chemical reactions τ_b =1.6 s. Unlike the earlier proposed MEIS (Kaganovich et al., 2007, 2010) the model with subjective criterion $\max x_3$ is replaced by the model:

find

$$\min\left[G(x)=\sum_1^3 G_j(x)x_j\right]=G(x^{\mathrm{eq}})\quad(23)$$

subject to

$$x_1+x_2+x_3=1,\quad(24)$$

$$x_3^l\le x_3^{l-1}+k_2x_2^{l-1}\tau^l,\quad(25)$$

$$x_j\ge 0,\quad(26)$$

where index l is the number of the next calculation step that corresponds to one of the stages into which τ_b is split.

When determining the attainable state of the system on the basis of model (23-26) we did not divide τ_b into separate time segments and inequality (25) was represented as

$$x_3 \le k_2 x_2^0 \tau_b ,$$

where x_2^0 is an instantaneously emerging (before formation of isomer x_3) concentration x_2. The process of transition from the state $y=(1,0,0)$ to the state $\varepsilon=(x_1^0,x_2^0)$ is shown on the triangle of material balance $A_1A_2A_3$ (Fig. 1, a) through the motion along the edge A_1A_2 from vertex A_1 $(x=y)$ towards point ε. Point ε is the equilibrium point, i.e. the point of $\min G(x)$. At this point the edge A_1A_2 touches the curve $G=G(\varepsilon)$.

For construction of the trajectory the process duration τ_b was initially divided into 5 segments. For the considered elementary example the composition of reaction mix and Gibbs energy at the final point of the process coincided with the same characteristics of x^{eq}, that were obtained from a one-stage calculation with an accuracy to the fraction of percent. Increase in the number of calculation periods did not change anyhow the calculation results.

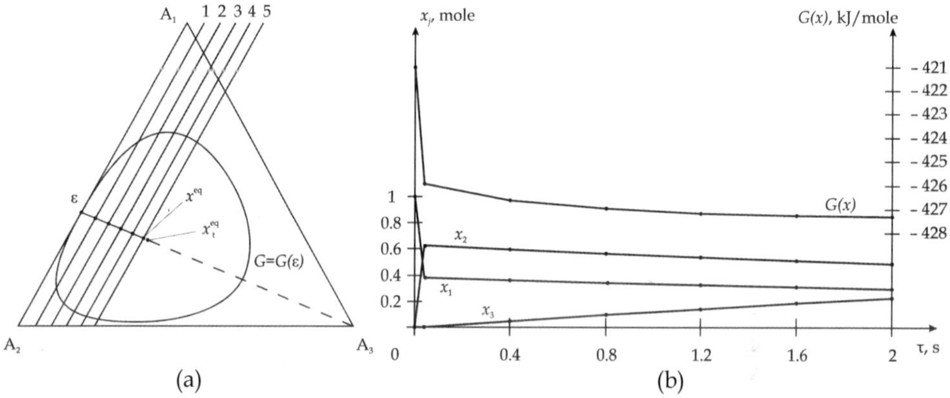

Fig. 1. Representation of the isomerization process results and trajectory on the triangle of material balance (a) and in the spaces (x,τ) and (G,τ) (b).

Lines 1-5 in Fig.1,a, that are parallel to the edge A_1A_2 are the lines of constant concentrations x_3, that are attained by the end of the first, second, third, fourth and fifth calculation periods, respectively. Intersection points of these lines with the trajectory leading from ε to point x^{eq}, for the chosen problem statement, turned out to be located on one straight line, i.e. the trajectory of motion towards equilibrium in the space of compositions (x) turned out to be rectilinear. A conditional extension of this line from x^{eq} to the purely thermodynamic (without regard to constraint (25)) equilibrium x_t^{eq} and further to the thermodynamically forbidden region of Gibbs energy rise (Fig.1 a, shown by a dashed line) leads to vertex A_3 (the point of the value x_3, equal to unity, maximum possible under the condition of material balance). The revealed linearity of the trajectory is suggested by the linearity of equality (24) and inequality (25). Physicochemical explanation of the obtained result, at least partially was already given in (Kaganovich et al, 2007, 2010). Point A_3 is a solution to the system of differential equations of chemical kinetics that was made up without regard to thermodynamic constraints for the assumed mechanism of the process with an infinitely large time interval. The revealed, though for the partial and simplest case, coincidence on the section ε - x^{eq} of the lines of "the shortest kinetic and thermodynamic distances" (the fastest change in kinetic (x_3) and thermodynamic (G) functions on set time intervals) emphasizes the unity of kinetics and thermodynamics and the unity of descriptions of natural phenomena on the basis of their principles.

The analysis of the second example - formation of nitrogen oxides at coal combustion in torch furnace at constant T and P was made on the basis of MEIS with subjective criterion of extremality:

find

$$\max x_{\mathrm{NO}} \tag{27}$$

subject to

$$Ax = b, \tag{28}$$

$$D_t(y) = \left\{ x : \begin{vmatrix} x \le y, \\ x_r \le \Psi_r,\ r \in R^{\lim}, \end{vmatrix} \right\} \qquad (29),\ (30)$$

$$G = \sum_j G_j x_j, \tag{31}$$

$$x_j \ge 0. \tag{32}$$

The condition for observance of macrokinetics requirements (30) was written as a system of inequalities (Kaganovich et al., 2007, 2010):

$$x_{\mathrm{NO}} \le 2\left[\bar{x}_{\mathrm{N}}\left(k_1 x_{OH} + k_2 y_{\mathrm{O}_2}\right)\tau_f + k_3 x_0 y_{\mathrm{N}_2}\left(\tau_b - \tau_f\right)\right], \tag{33}$$

$$x_{\mathrm{N}} \le k_{\mathrm{N}}^{\mathrm{daf}} K_f \mathrm{N}_{(\mathrm{coal})} + \left(k_3 x_0 y_{\mathrm{N}_2} + k_4 x_{\mathrm{CH}} y_{\mathrm{N}_2}\right)\tau_D, \tag{34}$$

$$x_{OH} \le (K_1 y_{H_2O})^{0.5},\quad x_O \le (K_2 y_{O_2})^{0.5}, \tag{35}$$

$$x_{\mathrm{CH}} \le k_{\mathrm{CH}}^{\mathrm{daf}} K_f \mathrm{H}_{(\mathrm{coal})}, \tag{36}$$

where τ_b, τ_f and τ_D are times of passing the reaction mixture through the furnace volume, combustion of volatiles, and diffusion of pyrolysis components from the surface of coal particle into turbulent reaction region; k_1, k_2, k_3 and k_4 - constants of reaction rates: N+OH→NO+H, N+O_2→NO+O, O+N_2→NO+N, CH+N_2→HCN+N; K_f is coefficient determining the share of volatile substances that pass from a coal particle to the gas phase during τ_D; K_1 and K_2 are equilibrium constants for reactions $H + OH \leftrightarrows H_2O$ and $O + O \leftrightarrows O_2$; $N_{(coal)}$ and $H_{(coal)}$ - amounts of nitrogen and hydrogen in coal; k_{CH}^{daf} and k_N^{daf} - coefficients depending on the composition of volatiles.

For comparison of efficiencies of thermodynamic and purely kinetic descriptions of coal combustion it should be noted that for kinetic description the whole mechanism of each stage forming the overall process (pyrolysis, combustion of volatiles and coke) and the values of kinetic coefficients of elementary stages should be known. Pyrolysis can be described based on the information about diffusion coefficients on the surface of coal particle and inside the surface layer. Measurement or theoretical description of these coefficients is very complex and unreliable because of inhomogeneity of coal particle surface and its change during combustion. A formalized representation of elementary kinetics of volatile combustion turns out unfeasible due to unavailability of exact knowledge about the composition of reaction mixture components and parameters of evaporation processes from particle surface and diffusion. The theoretical kinetic analysis of coke burning that supposes to apply the equations for molecule adsorption on the surface, surface reactions, desorption of reaction products, diffusion through pores and on particle surface is associated with insurmountable difficulties. Major portion of these processes for coke is poorly investigated. Inclusion of conditions (30), i.e. the system of inequalities (33)-(36), in MEIS requires only thermodynamic description of limiting stages. In this case the thermodynamic quantities can be determined with a sufficiently high degree of accuracy, which was shown in (Kaganovich et al., 2007, 2010).

The thermodynamic analysis of NO formation during fuel combustion is additionally improved by inclusion of trajectory construction problem in it, which is illustrated in Fig. 2,a and b. The Fig. 2 presents the calculation results for the Kansk-Achinsky coal pulverized combustion. Residence time τ_b for the reacting agent in combustion zone is taken equal to a second. Fig. 2,a shows solutions to the problem of determining attainable states: the state with maximum possible concentration of nitrogen oxide $x_{\mathrm{NO}}^{\mathrm{ext}}$ and the state of final equilibrium $x_{\mathrm{t}}^{\mathrm{eq}}$. The latter was calculated not at the complete system of conditions (29), (30) that determine the region $D_{\mathrm{t}}(y)$, but with an account of the condition for monotony (29) only. Application of the notion of equilibrium that is not related to kinetics in this case

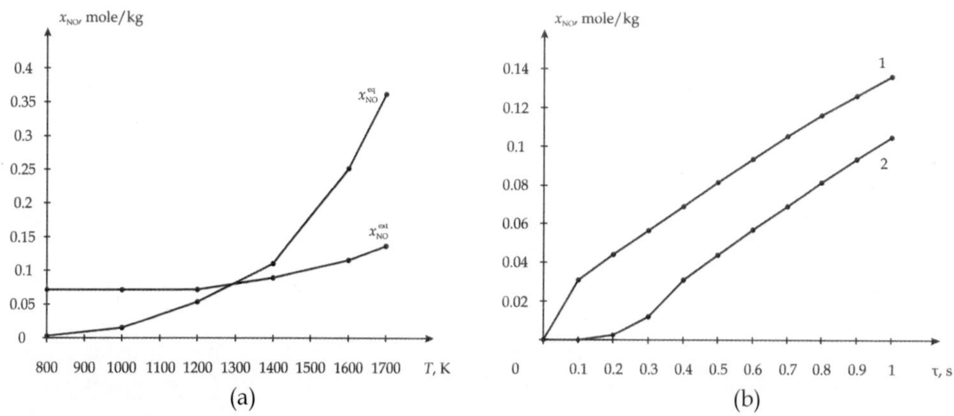

Fig. 2. Attainable equilibrium and extreme concentrations of NO as a function of temperature (a) and trajectory of attainment of $x_{\mathrm{NO}}^{\mathrm{ext}}$ (b).

proved to be interesting, since x_{NO}^{ext} at not very high temperatures (below 1200 K) were much higher than concentrations x_{NO}^{eq} even at such equilibria. The value x_{NO}^{ext}, with which we compared the value x_{NO}^{eq} determined by the stepwise computation of trajectory, was certainly found subject to the entire system of model constraints (27)-(32).

When constructing the trajectories the total process duration τ_b was divided at first into ten stages each equal to 0.1 s. As in the first example, increase in the number of stages was not needed to enhance calculation accuracy. Fig. 2,b presents two of the constructed trajectories. One of them (line 1) is determined on the basis of assumptions about ideal mixing of reagents and constant temperature (1700 K) in the whole furnace volume. The value of x_{NO} at the final point of this trajectory turned out equal to the value of the ordinate of line x_{NO}^{ext} in Fig. 2,a at point T=1700 K. The other (line 2) was constructed considering poor mixing of the initial air-fuel mixture and combustion products at the initial stages of process and temperature equality: at the first time stage – 600 K, at the second – 1200 K and at the remaining eight stages – 1700 K. The final point of this trajectory was naturally situated on the ordinate much lower than those of the first trajectory. The multistage calculation of motion in time for the second considered case illustrates the most important advantage of the stepwise process of decision making. It implies the possibility to take into account individual properties of separate time stages forming a modeled process. In the considered analysis of NO formation, for example, when passing from one step of calculations to another account can be taken of change in both the temperature and the initial composition of components that was determined at the previous step. Such a change may be caused by recirculation of flue gases, secondary blast or steam injection into the gas flow. Many other factors can also be taken into consideration. Versatile study on the change in process course in time should obviously contribute to development of justified recommendations on the process control.

Relations between the theories of states and trajectories and capabilities of equilibrium thermodynamic analysis to study reversible and irreversible kinetics can be more fully revealed by considering another type of models of extreme intermediate states, namely MEIS of hydraulic circuits (Gorban et al., 2001, 2006; Kaganovich et al., 1997, 2007, 2010). Convenience and clearness of using these models to describe the considered problems are determined by the fact that they are intended to study an essentially irreversible process, i.e. motion of a viscous fluid. Besides, they can be treated as models of the mechanism of fluid transportation from the specified source nodes of a hydraulic system to the specified consumption nodes. The major variable of the hydraulic circuit theory (Khasilev, 1957, 1964; Merenkov and Khasilev, 1985), i.e. continuous medium flow, has an obvious kinetic sense.

As opposed to the described MEIS with variable parameters and the mechanisms of physicochemical processes in this case we will try to determine the objective function of applied model for a dissipative system based on the equilibrium principle of conservative systems, i.e. the Lagrange principle of virtual works. Derivation will be given on the example of the closed (not exchanging the fluid flows with the environment) active (with sources of motive pressures) circuit. The simplest scheme of such a circuit is presented in Fig. 3,a. A common character of the chosen example is explained by the easiness of passing to other possible schemes. For example, if at the modeled network nodes there are external

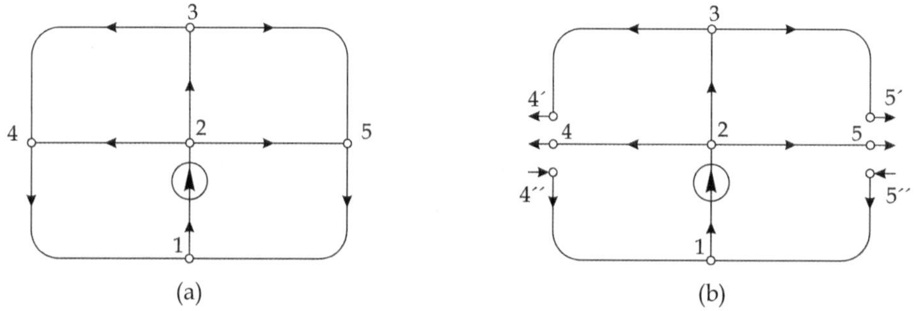

Fig. 3. Closed active circuit (a) and its transformation into a tree (b). 1–4(4´, 4´´), 5(5´, 5´´) - numbers of nodes; arrow in the circle - source of the motive pressure; arrows - specified directions of flows in branches.

sources and sinks, i.e. the circuit is open, it can be transformed to a closed scheme by adding conditional branches that connect nodes of the external sources (sinks) with the node representing environment. The motive pressures equal to the difference of pressures between the source node and environment are specified for the branches, along which the external flows move to the initial circuit. Transition to the analysis of open passive circuits (that do not contain motive pressures) is performed by removal from the initial scheme of branches with such pressures and addition of corresponding sources (sinks) to the nodes adjacent to removed branches.

Let us determine the principle of virtual works for the hydraulic circuit as follows: for every branch in any infinitesimal period of time an equilibrium of all forces (pressure, friction, gravity, etc.) acting on the fluid is observed and the work expended for infinitesimal deviation of flow on the branch from its equilibrium value is equal to zero. If only three forces are available on the i-th branch: the force caused by the difference in pressures between the initial and final cross-sections ΔP_i, the force of motive pressure (created by pump) P_i^{mov} and the force of friction, the following equation corresponds to the Lagrange principle

$$\Delta P_i dx_i + P_i^{\text{mov}} dx_i - \gamma_i x_i^{\beta} dx_i = 0, \tag{37}$$

where x_i is volumetric flow in a branch; γ_i and β are constant coefficient and exponent in the formula relating the pressure loss because of friction to the flow

$$P_i^{\text{br}} = \gamma_i x_i^{\beta}. \tag{38}$$

For the whole circuit the Lagrange equation (1) will have the form

$$dL = \sum_i P_i^{\text{mov}} dx_i - \sum_i \gamma_i x_i^{\beta} dx_i = 0, \ i = 1, \ldots, n, \tag{39}$$

where L is the Lagrange function. The term containing summands $\Delta P_i dx_i$ is not included in equation (39), since the sum ΔP_i for each closed loop and for the entire circuit is equal to zero according to the second Kirchhoff law. Products $\gamma_i x_i^{\beta} = P_i^{\text{br}}$, i.e. resistance forces of bonds, act as multipliers λ_i in (39). According to equation (39) changes of coordinates under motive forces and resistance (friction) forces are of the same sense (increase or decrease of the volumetric flow x_i) and value.

Equation (39) makes it possible to determine the objective function of MEIS and correspondingly the objective extremality criterion for stationary isothermal flow distribution of incompressible fluid in a closed active circuit. Account will be taken of the fact that because of equilibrium point stationarity the integrals corresponding to both sums in (39) take equal extreme values. For further analysis it is more convenient to make use of the latter and MEIS can be written in the form:

find

$$\text{extr}(1/T)\sum_{i=1}^{n}\gamma_i x_i^{\beta+1} \tag{40}$$

subject to

$$Ax = 0, \tag{41}$$

$$\sum_{i=1}^{n} P_i^{\text{mov}} x_i - \sum_{i=1}^{n}\gamma_i x_i^{\beta+1} = 0, \tag{42}$$

$$\sum_{i=1}^{n}\gamma_i x_i^{\beta+1} - k(T - T_{\text{env}}) = 0, \tag{43}$$

where T and T_{env} are temperatures of fluid and environment; $A = [a_{ij}]$ is $(m-1)\times n$ - matrix of independent nodes and branches incidence; m - number of nodes; k - coefficient in formula $q = k(T - T_{\text{env}})$. Equalities (41) and (42) describe material and energy balances of the circuit and equality (43) - balance of heat exchange between the circuit and environment. It is clear that multiplication of the sum in formula (40) for the objective function by multiplier $(1/T)$ that provides the function dimension and value of entropy, does not shift the extreme point along axis x at constant temperature.

The Lagrange function for problem (40)–(43) has the form:

$$L = (1/T)\sum_{i=1}^{n}\gamma_i x_i^{\beta+1} - \sum_{j=1}^{m-1}\lambda_j \sum_{i\in I_j} a_{ij}x_j + \lambda_m\left(\sum_{i=1}^{n}\gamma_i x_i^{\beta+1} - \sum_{i=1}^{n} P_i^{\text{mov}} x_i\right) + \lambda_{m+1}\left(k(T - T_{\text{env}}) - \sum_{i=1}^{n}\gamma_i x_i^{\beta+1}\right), \tag{44}$$

where I_j is subset of branches incident to node j.

It can be shown that the second partial derivatives are

$$\partial^2 L / \partial x_i^2 \le 0 \quad \text{and} \quad \partial^2 L / \partial T^2 \ge 0, \tag{45}$$

i.e. at point x^{eq} that corresponds to the steady stationary flow distribution in the circuit, the objective function has the maximum with respect to coordinates x_i and the minimum with respect to T. Hence, the second law of thermodynamics holds true in the isolated system (circuit plus environment). In this case it is derived from the principle of virtual works assumed by Lagrange as initial in the analysis of conservative systems. The minimum of T that results from (45) does not contradict the second law, since when approaching the global equilibrium point the energy dissipation (entropy production) and the difference of thermal potentials (in the considered case ($T - T_{env}$)) that directly provokes it, decrease. Therefore, in a way the second law may be called "an economy law". Energy dissipation that is not needed for complete degradation of the isolated system does not take place.

In the circuit the stationary action principle is observed. (Note that for the stationary processes the work can be multiplied by any given time without change of optimization result and for negligibly small time periods applied in our analysis the processes are always stationary). At the imposed constraints the maximum work of motive forces is done most economically. Since the fluid temperature takes a minimal value, the heat that is not caused by the work performed does not appear and the extra energy is not dissipated as well as in the case of isolated system degradation.

In the analysis of behavior of passive circuits they can be considered as "fragments" of active ones. Thus, the passive scheme that includes independent loops 2342, 2352 and 24152 can be obtained by removing from the scheme of Fig. 3,a the branch 1–2 with motive pressure and setting the source at node 2 and the sink at node 1, each being equal to the flow in the removed branch. The flow distribution for such a scheme will be determined from the model:

find

subject to

$$\left.\begin{aligned} &\operatorname{extr}(1/T)\sum_{i=1}^{n}\gamma_i x_i^{\beta+1} \\ &Ax = Q, \quad i = 1, \ldots, n. \end{aligned}\right\} \tag{46}$$

where Q is vector of independent external sources and sinks. Condition similar to (43) is excluded from model (46) upon the assumption that the temperature can be determined in calculation of the active circuit that includes a modeled one. The second derivatives of the Lagrange function

$$L = \sum_{i=1}^{n}\gamma_i x_i^{\beta+1} + \sum_{j=1}^{m-1}\lambda_j\left(Q_j - \sum_{i\in I_j} a_{ij}x_i\right)$$

of the model (46) have the form

$$\partial^2 L / \partial x_i^2 = \beta(\beta+1)\gamma_i x_i^{\beta-1} \geq 0,$$

i.e. the extremum of L is the point of minimum. Hence, it is clear that for passive circuits the least action principle and the Onsager-Prigogine theorem hold true. This is easy to explain physically, since in the passive circuits there are no work performers and exchange of flows with the environment should be fulfilled most economically.

The technique to reveal relations between different principles of extremality and equilibrium for infinitesimal time spans that is developed on the basis of thermodynamic circuit theory will be undoubtedly useful for devising methods for construction of trajectories representing continuous sequences of such spans.

4. Solution of computational problems in the analysis of trajectories

There is an appreciable groundwork for development of methods for construction and analysis of trajectories on the MEIS base. It resulted from extensive studies on the search for results of processes possible in the region of thermodynamic attainability $D_t(y)$. A key component of these studies is an extension of the experience gained in the convex analysis of ideal systems (Van der Waals and Konstamm, 1936; Zeldovich, 1938; Gorban, 1984) to modeling of real ones (Antsiferov, 1991; Kaganovich et al., 1989, 1993, 1995, 2007, 2010). They may include: an ideal (or real) gas phase, plasma, condensed substances, solutions and other components. The components of this analysis are determination of particularities of the objective function and study on the properties of set $D_t(y)$. For MEIS with variable parameters solution of the first mentioned problem proves to be non-trivial, when the sum $\sum_j c_j x_j$ in expression (8) with the constant value of y is replaced by the fractional expression $\sum_j c_j x_j / \sum_j g_j y_j$ (g is coefficient ranking worth of the j-th initial system component). The second problem contains studies on the impact of characteristic thermodynamic functions and formulations of kinetic constraints on the properties of $D_t(y)$.

The performed analysis of problems solved by using MEIS has shown the possibilities for their reduction to convex programming (CP) problems in many important cases. Such reduction is often associated with approximation of dependences among variables. There are cases of multivalued solutions to the formulated CP problems, when the linear objective function is parallel to one of the linear part of set $D_t(y)$. Naturally the problems with non-convex objective functions or non-convex attainability sets became irreducible to CP. Non-convexity of the latter can occur at setting kinetic constraints by a system of linear inequalities, part of which is specified not for the whole region $D_t(y)$, but its individual zones.

Studies on the specific features of MEIS made it possible to work out some modifications of mathematical programming methods that ensure effective application of the considered models. However, great difficulties are met even in the case when a problem solved can be reduced to a CP problem. For example, when applying MEIS of type (8)–(13) they are: 1) implicit setting of the constraints on monotony of characteristic functions (inequality (10)) and 2) large (up to 10–12 orders of magnitude) scatter in the values of sought variables, which happens in the analysis of environmental problems.

Both difficulties were successfully overcome with the help of the affine scaling method suggested by I.I. Dikin (Dikin, 1967, 2010; Dikin and Zorcaltsev, 1980). It became a key method for using models (8)–(13) and (14). The method is convenient, as it employs only interior points of the polyhedron of material balance, at which the objective function gradient can be calculated, and the motion to the extreme point always proceeds at an acute angle to this gradient taken with a reversed sign. This fact contributes to method convergence at unfavorable (with zones of minor steepness) shape of the surface, on which the extreme point is sought for. Direction of motion to this point from the point obtained in the k-th iteration is determined on the ellipsoid

$$\sum_{j=1}^{n} \frac{z_j^2}{(x_j^k)^2} \leq 1, \tag{47}$$

where $z_j = x_j^{k+1} - x_j^k$. Using the figurative comparison we can say that the affine scaling method used when descending the mountain allows determination of motion direction not by touch, as it is done, for example, in the steepest descent method, but by choosing the lowest point in the observable neighborhood. This neighborhood is represented by ellipsoid (47), whose axes are distances from x^k to the boundaries of positive orthant that determine a "visibility zone" inside the polyhedron of material balance. After the lowest point is reached in the k-th neighborhood the route of search is adjusted by means of constructing the ($k+1$)-th ellipsoid. The affine scaling method has proved high computational efficiency in the analysis of various physicochemical problems.

The mentioned difficulties were overcome in the following way. The first of them was eliminated by the two-stage technique for searching the extreme state x^{ext} that was suggested by E.G. Antsiferov (Antsiferov, 1991; Kaganovich et al., 1993, 1995, 2006). According to his idea the surface of thermodynamic function equation with point x^{ext} on it is determined at the first stage and the sought point coordinates are found on this surface at the second stage. At the first stage an auxiliary problem of linear programming is solved. As a result the maximum value (x^{mat}) of objective function (8) is determined on polyhedron (9), (13), i.e. without considering thermodynamic (10) and kinetic (11) constraints. Then the vertex of polyhedron x^{mat} is connected with the point of initial composition y, and the minimum point of characteristic function $G(x)$ is found on segment $y - x^{\text{mat}}$. At the second stage the affine scaling method is used to find x^{ext} on surface $G(x) = \text{const}$ containing this point. The chosen two-stage method is certainly approximate. However, its results have been compared with the results of the exact method of thermodynamic tree (Gorban, 1984; Gorban et al., 2006) on the examples of small dimensional systems. The latter is not implemented so far for large dimensional systems. The comparison has shown that the errors in calculations do not exceed 2-3%.

The problem of large scatter in the values of sought variables due to sharp deceleration in convergence of the computation process was solved by I.A. Shirkalin (Shirkalin, 1997) on the basis of factual transition from the affine scaling method to the general Newton method (the method of tangents) when approaching the extreme point.

Despite the long-term successful application of the affine scaling method to the MEIS-based thermodynamic analysis, extension of this analysis and primarily its extension to the studies on kinetics call for the use of dynamic programming (DP) (Bellman, 2003; Wentzel, 1964). In this context it implies not only the method of stepwise decision making, but a part of mathematical programming as the mathematical theory of equilibrium extreme states. For rigorous explanation of relations between MEIS and DP this model should be evidently treated as the basis for devising concrete methods and as part of equilibrium thermodynamics, i.e. the physical theory of equilibria and extrema. A common nature of contents of the mentioned parts is that they relate the theories of states with the theories of trajectories: DP is mathematical programming with calculus of variations and theory of optimal control; MEIS is equilibrium thermodynamics with kinetics, irreversible thermodynamics, theory of dynamic systems. For application of both MEIS and DP it is unnecessary to know (to determine) a trajectory equation and to use a time variable. The process course is clarified as a result of the stepwise (in space or time) decision making.

The relations between MEIS and DP can be better elucidated by determining connections between the ideas applied at their creation with the idea of the mentioned thermodynamic tree of A.N.Gorban. The set of thermodynamic attainability $D_t(y)$ and correspondingly all admissible macrokinetic trajectories are projected on this tree being a one-dimensional graph. Therefore, it is reasonable to apply the tree for the analysis of correctness of the results obtained on the basis of MEIS and DP. Difficulty in this application is that possible construction of a tree in (Gorban, 1984) is substantiated only for the case of convexity of set $D_t(y)$ and convexity of the characteristic thermodynamic function. But it is believed that new computational approaches will eliminate this difficulty.

The known computational advantages of the DP method are:

- possibility for comprehensive consideration of the solved problem specificity, its many aspects and multiple scale nature, particularities of decision making at individual stages;
- applicability to searching for a global extremum of non-convex, unsmoothed functions with the break points (including functions of discrete variables);
- admissibility of using complex algorithms with application of logical expressions and tables in the computation process;
- automatic determination of several optimal variants, which is very convenient for versatile analysis of the obtained solutions in terms of physicochemical, technical, economic and ecological requirements.

Neither the affine scaling method nor the other MP methods possess the majority of the noted DP advantages.

Unfortunately, until now the MEIS-based dynamic programming method has found application only in the analysis of problems of technical and economic optimization (optimal synthesis) of circuits. This particular application, however, allowed a valuable experience to be accumulated in solving the most important DP problem, namely the search for extremum of the non-additive function. We will exemplify complexities and effectiveness of applying dynamic programming by the scheme in Fig. 3,a that was already used in the MEIS-based analysis of hydraulic circuits.

Suppose it is necessary to determine the most economical variant of fluid transportation from the pumping station on branch 1–2 to consumption nodes 3, 4 and 5, i.e. find the minimum of function $F(x,d)$, where $x=(x_1,...,x_n)^T$ and $d=(d_1,...,d_n)^T$ are vectors of volumetric flow and parameters (e.g. pipe diameters on network branches); x_i and d_i – their components. MEIS of optimal flow distribution and the method of multiloop optimization that were applied for solving the stated problem were discussed in (Sumarokov, 1976; Kaganovich, 2011; Kaganovich et al., 1995, 2007, 2010; Gorban et al., 2001, 2006). The common algorithm of applying these model and method assumes division of the optimization process into five stages.

1. Setting the closed (without external sources and sinks) redundant scheme including all possible directions in locating individual branches (pipelaying).
2. Fixing parameters for each branch (e.g. maximum admissible diameters of pipes at preliminarily planned flows).
3. Determination of flow distribution on the basis of model (40)–(43) for the given scheme and parameters. As a result of this stage the interaction between flows in the scheme branches that cause non-additivity of function $F(x,d)$ is fixed, since the flow distribution is the result of this interaction. So far as the scheme is closed, there is no interaction involving constant pressures or flows at nodes of external sources or sinks. Thermal interaction of the circuit described by equation (43) as a whole with the environment remains, but does not influences additivity of the minimized function.
4. Transformation with the fixed interaction (distribution of flows among the branches) of the closed scheme (Fig. 3,a) to the tree (Fig. 3,b), specifying conditional external sources and sinks at break nodes (4, 4´, 4´´, 5, 5´, 5´´). They make it possible to preserve material balances in the network that were determined at the previous stage.
5. Choice of the optimal (corresponding to the minimum of additive function $F(x,d)$) parameters of the tree branches by the DP method. The process of stepwise search for solutions on the basis of this method is described by the functional equations

$$\left.\begin{aligned} F_j &= \min(F_{j+1} + F_{j,j+1}), \\ F_{j-1} &= \min(F_j + F_{j-1,j}), \end{aligned}\right\} \tag{48}$$

where numbers $j+1$, j, $j-1$, etc. decrease from the end nodes (5, 5´, 5´´) to the node 1 of fluid flow arrival to pumping station. It is clear that at the node, where flows are joining the minimum values of function F are summed up. Thus,

$$F_2 = \min(F_3 + F_{2,3}) + \min(F_4 + F_{2,4}) + \min(F_5 + F_{2,5}).$$

Summation is made for each of the zones, into which the admissible range of change in variables is divided and the objective function depends on these variables. (The range, for example, can be related to admissible pressures at the corresponding node that in turn depend on the chosen diameters d_i).

Procedures 3–5 are repeated iteratively. The branches with negligibly small flows are excluded from the considered scheme. (For the scheme to remain close, in the iterations of flow distribution calculation removal can be simulated by setting negligible values of d_i). The calculation process terminates, when the difference in values for $F(x,d)$ becomes lower than the given negligible value at transition from one iteration to another.

Convergence of the multiloop optimization method that is based on iterative application of dynamic programming has a strict physical explanation. The stationary flow distribution that is determined at the third stage corresponds to equilibrium optimal interaction between the flows in branches (the scheme closeness, as was noted above, stipulates the uniqueness of this interaction inside the network) and to the extreme network interaction with the environment (see Section 3). In this case in the isolated system (network plus environment) the maximum value of entropy is achieved and in the circuit the maximum work of motive pressure source is done at minimum possible fluid temperature, i.e. at minimum heat release and transfer to the environment and the minimum energy dissipation (entropy production). Optimization of network parameters by the DP method is related with sequential transition from the equilibrium extreme state of an ideal (with non-interacting components) additive system at node $j+1$ to the same state at node j. Optimization of network parameters by the DP method results in minimum dissipation of "economic energy" - money and minimum production of "economic entropy". Monotony of change in entropy production during iterative calculations of interaction between the system components for the given scheme and parameters at the fixed interaction ensures convergence of the computation process.

The results obtained in the thermodynamic analysis of circuits on the basis of dynamic programming give grounds to hope that the experience gained during this analysis will be extensively used in modeling the mechanisms of physicochemical processes on the graphs. Indeed, calculation of current or flow distribution in the circuit can be considered as determination of the mechanism of transporting charges or a substance from nodes - "suppliers" to nodes - "consumers". Unfortunately, up to now experience in thermodynamic modeling of circuits in the analysis of mechanisms was extended only to the studies of chemical reactions represented by open schemes of the form:

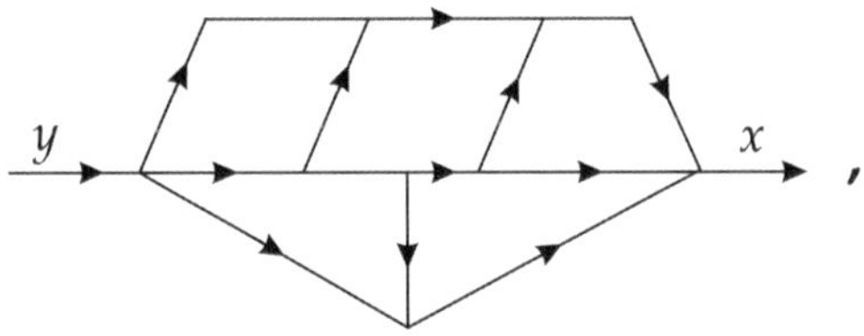

in which y and x denote vectors of the composition of initial reagents and reaction products, respectively (Kaganovich et al., 1993, 1995, 2007, 2010; Gorban et al., 2006). Transition from open schemes to closed ones that allow the iterative determination of interactions between the modeled system components and its representation as an ideal one can cause severe difficulties for complex mechanisms with processes of diverse types (transformation, exchange and transfer of substance, energy and charges). Thus, if the open electric or hydraulic circuit is transformed to the closed one by a rather easy procedure of connecting the nodes of external sources and sinks by conditional branches with the conditional node representing environment and by placement of sources of single-type motive forces on the branches connecting sources with the environment, the scheme of mechanism with stages of different physical nature will be transformed by means of including conditional branches with different (by nature) motive forces in the closed scheme. In general it is not by far a trivial problem.

Certainly, solving this problem deserves further studies. If they are successful, the dynamic programming method can prove to be an important tool for the analysis of mechanisms. DP application seems to be most effective to search for a mechanism satisfying some subjective criterion of extremality. Such application can be exemplified by the considered algorithm of optimal circuit synthesis that can be treated as a procedure of simultaneous determination of economic and physical components of the whole mechanism of pipeline system construction. In the context of physicochemical problems the optimality criteria may be the maximum yield of useful products of the modeled process or its minimum harmful impact on the environment.

MEIS with variable parameters and subjective extremality criteria of type (8)–(13) may turn out even more convenient objects for DP applications than MEIS represented by schemes in the form of graphs. This is due to the fact that the stepwise optimization on the basis of these models (e.g. determination of concentrations for the specified set of substances) can be performed without dividing the model into interacting parts. This fact ensures additivity of the objective function. Certainly it does not mean that construction of DP algorithms for MEIS (8)–(13) is an easy process. Dividing the computation process into individual steps and taking an account of specific features of these steps are still rather difficult due to a lack of formalized techniques to perform those processes.

Construction of trajectories by the DP method proves to be even more complex, when the models of type (14) with objective criteria of extremality are applied. In this case the objective function is a characteristic thermodynamic function of the system and for non-ideal systems its representation as a non-additive function of components becomes inevitable. Experience accumulated in circuit modeling is undoubtedly highly useful to solve the arising problem. Its use, however, will necessitate the search for new original methodological procedures. The search for trajectories in the case of successful intra step optimization is much easier, because it does not require inadditivity to be accounted for.

The idea of DP and relations similar to (48) have actually been used in analysis of trajectory construction examples as applied to the processes of isomerization an nitrogen oxides formation, which are considered in the section 3. Though, the possibility to simultaneously search for several "optimal" variants and to choose the best one among them subject to peculiarities of the problem solved. Development of algorithms for such a search is to be the aim of further studies.

5. Conclusion

Estimation of the results achieved until now in joint analysis of kinetics and thermodynamics, trajectories and states makes it possible to assert that the directions of further studies are laid down to a certain extent and some ideas of solving basic problems of these studies are suggested.

However, the made groundwork in studying physical-mathematical properties of the models of extreme intermediate states and in their application enables one to highly estimate the forthcoming achievements in solution of discussed problems and to prove the necessity for continuation and expansion of the scope of kinetic-thermodynamic studies.

This is so, because MEISs form the basis for analysis of states and trajectories in macroscopic systems, and they are intended for determination of (a) the results (useful or harmful) attainable on admissible motion trajectories of modeled systems and (b) control technique for their obtaining (preventing).

Rapid progress in computer technology that contributes to enhancement of competitiveness for simple algorithms that require multiple increase in computations and at the same time immeasurably decrease the labor input in creation of software and preparation of initial information gives a weighty support in the required proofs. The algorithms constructed on the basis of simple and universal prerequisites of equilibrium thermodynamics are obviously simple. They are used for stepwise description of trajectories that does not require derivation of "underivable" equations. The preparation process of initial experimental and theoretical data needed for their application becomes sharply easier. In this case the characteristics of rest states, whose sequences are applied to describe steps in decision making, are measured and calculated rather easier than characteristics of motion.

Development of the kinetic-thermodynamic direction in the analysis of macroscopic systems must essentially enrich both the applied and fundamental components of this analysis.

Improvement of the applied component is achieved first of all by increasing the versatility of studies of the most diverse technical and natural systems, which will allow the quality solution of numerous problems: updating of production processes, saving of resources, environmental protection.

Contribution to the fundamental science will influence development of macrscopic kinetics, classical equilibrium thermodynamics, and joint application of these disciplines to study the macroworld. The capabilities of kinetic analysis will be surely expanded considerably, if traditional kinetic methods that are reduced to the analysis of trajectory equations are supplemented by novel numerical methods. The latter are to be based on consideration of continuous sequences of stationary processes in infinitesimal time intervals. The problems of searching for the trajectories, being included into the subject of equilibrium thermodynamics, would make deserved the definition of this discipline as a closed theory that allows the study of any macroscopic systems and processes on the basis of equilibrium principles. Like the equilibrium analytical mechanics of Lagrange the thermodynamics may be called the unified theory of statics and dynamics. Joint application of kinetic and thermodynamic models further increases the noted potential advantages of the discussed directions of studies.

Certainly, the expected progress in development of kinetic-thermodynamic analysis cannot render worthless the current theories of evolution, the trajectories of development: the theory of dynamic systems, irreversible thermodynamics, synergy due to their great contribution to explanation of self-organization and degradation phenomena in animate and inanimate nature. When solving complex problems the researcher must have a set of models and methods and know how to choose among this set the elements, which correspond in the best way to specific properties of the considered problem. In the analysis of chemical kinetics problems the equilibrium thermodynamic models should obligatorily be included in the research instruments, because these models make it possible to study the entire region of thermodynamic attainability and to search for admissible trajectories of the modeled system motion in it.

6. Acknowledgment

The authors acknowledge Russian Foundation of Basic Research for the support (grants No. 12-08-00729 and No. 12-08-00496)

7. References

Antsiferov, E.G. (1991). *Application of mathematical programming methods to the analysis of thermodynamic systems: Abstract of doctoral thesis,* Computing Centre of AS USSR, Moscow (in Russian).

Antsiferov, E.G., Kaganovich, B.M, Yablonskii, G.S. (1988). Thermodynamic Limitations in Searching for Regions of Optimal Performance of Complex Chemical Reactions (Exemplified by Conversion of Hydrocarbons). *Reaction Kinetics and Catalysis Letters,* Vol.37, No.1, pp. 57-61, ISSN 0133-1736.

Arnold, V.I. (1989). *Mathematical Methods of Classical Mechanics,* Springer, ISBN 0-387-96890-3, New York

Bellman, R.E. (2003). *Dynamic Programming,* Courier Dover Publications, ISBN 0-486-42809-5, New York.

Boltzmann, L. (1877). Über die Beziehung zwishen dem zweiten Hauptsatze der Mechanischen Wärmetheorie und der Wahrscheinlichkeitsrechnung respective den Sätzen über das Wärmegleichgewicht. *Wiener Berichte,* Bd.76, pp. 373-435.

Born, M. (1921). Kritische Betrachtungen zur traditionellen Darstellung der Thermodynamik, *Physikalische Zeitschrift,* Bd.22, pp. 218-224, 249-254, 282-286.

Caratheodory, C. (1909). Untersuchungen über die Grundlagen der Thermodynamik. *Mathematische Annalen,* Bd.67, pp. 355–390.

Clausius, R. (2008). *The Mechanical Theory of Heat,* Bibliobazaar, ISBN 978-05-5-499584-7, Charleston.

Dikin, I.I. (1967). Iterative Solution of Linear and Quadratic Programming Problems. *Proceedings of the USSR Academy of Sciences,* Vol.174, No.4, pp. 747-748, ISSN 0869-5652 (in Russian).

Dikin, I.I. (2010). *Affine Scaling Method in Linear and Nonlinear Programming,* KRASAND, ISBN 978-5-396-00035-3, Moscow (in Russian).

Dikin, I.I., Zorkaltsev, V.I. (1980). *Iterative Solution of Mathematical Programming Problems (Algorithms of Affine Scaling Method),* Nauka, Novosibirsk (in Russian).

Feinberg, M. (1972). On chemical kinetics of a certain class. *Archive for Rational Mechanics and Analysis,* Vol.46, No1, pp. 1-41, ISSN 0003-9527.

Feinberg, M. (1999). Recent results in optimal reactor synthesis via attainable region theory. *Chemical Engineering Science,* Vol.54, No.7, pp. 2535-2543, ISSN 0009-2509

Feinberg, M., Hildebrand, D. (1997). Optimal reactor design from a geometric viewpoint –1. Universal properties of the attainable region. *Chemical Engineering Science,* Vol.52, No.10, pp. 1637–1665, ISSN 0009-2509

Feinberg, M., Horn, F. (1974). Dynamics of open chemical systems and the algebraic structure of the underlying reaction network. *Chemical Engineering Science*, Vol.29, pp. 775–787, ISSN 0009-2509

Gibbs, J.W. (1876, 1878). On the equilibrium of heterogeneous substances. *Transactions of the Connecticut Academy*, 1876, No.3, pp. 108-248; 1878 No.3, pp. 343-524.

Glansdorff, P., Prigogine, I.R. (1971). *Thermodynamic Theory of Structure, Stability and Fluctuations*, Wiley, ISBN 0-471-30280-5, New York.

Gorban, A.N. (1984). *Equilibrium Encircling: Equations of Chemical Kinetics and their Thermodynamic Analysis*, Nauka, Novosibirsk (in Russian).

Gorban, A.N., Kaganovich, B.M., Filippov, S.P, Keiko, A.V., Shamansky, V.A., Shirkalin, I.A. (2006). *Thermodynamic Equilibria and Extrema. Analysis of Attainability Regions and Partial Equilibria*, Springer, ISBN 978-0387-28575-7, New York.

Gorban, A.N., Kaganovich, B.M., Filippov, S.P. (2001). *Thermodynamic Equilibria and Extrema. Analysis of Attainability Regions and Partial Equilibria in Physicochemical and Technical Systems*, Nauka, ISBN 5-02-031702-0, Novosibirsk (in Russian).

Gorban, A.N., Karlin, I.V. (2005). Invariant manifolds for physical and chemical kinetics. *Lecture Notes in Physics*, Vol.660, Springer, ISBN 3-540-22684-2, ISSN 0075-8450, Berlin, Heidelberg, New York.

Gorban, A.N., Kazantis, N., Keverkidis, I.G., Öttinger, H.C., Theodoropoulos, C. (2007). *Model Reduction and Coarse-Graining Approaches for Multiscale Phenomena*. Springer, ISBN 978-3-540-35885-5, Berlin, Heidelberg, New York.

Haken, H. (1983). *Advanced Synergetics. Instability Hierarchies of Self-Organizing Systems and Devices*, Springer-Verlag, ISBN 3-540-12162-5, Berlin, Heidelberg, New York, Tokyo.

Haken, H. (2006). *Information and Self-Organization*, Springer, ISBN 978-3-540-33021-2, ISSN 0172-7389, Berlin, Heidelberg.

Horn, F. (1964). Attainable Regions in Chemical Reaction Technique. *The Third European Symposium on Chemical Reaction Engineering / Pergamon Press*, London, pp. 1-10.

Horn, F., Jackson, R. (1972). General mass action kinetics. *Archive for Rational Mechanics and Analysis*, Vol.47, No.2, pp. 81–116, ISSN 0009-2509

Jou, D., Casas-Vazques, J., Lebon, G (2001). *Extended Irreversible Thermodynamics*, Springer, ISBN 978-90-481-3073-3, New York, Dordrecht, Heidelberg, London.

Kaganovich, B.M. (1991). *Study on energy technologies on the basis of methods of thermodynamics and circuit theory; Doctoral thesis*, (SEI AS USSR), Irkutsk (in Russian).

Kaganovich, B.M. (2011). *Equilibrium Thermodynamics of Irreversible Processes*, MESI SB RAS, ISBN 978-5-93908-098-9, Irkutsk (in Russian).

Kaganovich, B.M., Filippov, S.P. (1995). *Equilibrium Thermodynamics and Mathematical Programming*, Nauka, ISBN 5-02-030848-X, Novosibirsk (in Russian).

Kaganovich, B.M., Filippov, S.P., Antsiferov, E.G. (1989). *Efficiency of Energy Technologies: Thermodynamics, Economy, Forecasts*. Nauka, ISBN 5-02-028740-7, Novosibirsk (in Russian).

Kaganovich, B.M., Filippov, S.P., Antsiferov, E.G. (1993). *Modeling of Thermodynamic Processes*, Nauka, ISBN 5-02-030314-3, Novosibirsk (in Russian).

Kaganovich, B.M., Keiko, A.V., Shamansky, V.A. (2007). *Equilibrium Thermodynamic Modeling of Dissipative Macroscopic Systems*, MESI SB RAS, ISBN 978-5-93908-057-6, Irkutsk (in Russian).

Kaganovich, B.M., Keiko, A.V., Shamansky, V.A. (2010). Equilibrium Thermodynamic Modeling of Dissipative Macroscopic Systems. *Advances in Chemical Engineering*, Vol.39, *Thermodynamics and Kinetics of Complex Systems*, Elsevier, ISBN 978-0-12-374459-3, ISSN 0065-2377, pp. 1-74.

Kaganovich, B.M., Keiko, A.V., Shamansky, V.A., Shirkalin, I.A., Zarodnyuk, M.S. (2010). *Thermodynamic Model Engineering. Motion Models Reduction to Rest Models*, Nauka, ISBN 978-5-02-023321-8, Novosibirsk (in Russian).

Kaganovich, B.M., Keiko, A.V., Shamansky, V.A., Zarodnyuk, M.S. (2010). *Analysis of Mathematical Communications between Equilibrium Thermodynamics and Trajectory Theories*, MESI SB RAS, ISBN 978-5-93908-078-3, Irkutsk (in Russian).

Katok, A.B. Hasselblatt, B. (1997). *Introduction to the Modern Theory of Dynamical Systems*, Cambridge University Press, ISBN 0-521-57557-5, Cambridge.

Khasilev, V.Ya. (1957). Generalized Relationships for Technical And Economic Calculations of Heat Supply And Other Networks. *Teploenergetika*, No.1, pp. 28–32 (in Russian).

Khasilev, V.Ya. (1964). Elements of the Hydraulic Circuits Theory. *Izvestiya AN SSSR. Energetika i transport*, No.1, pp. 69–88 (in Russian).

Klimontovich, Yu.L., (1995). *Statistical Theory of Open Systems*. Kluwer Academic Publishers, ISBN 0-7923-3242-3, Amsterdam.

Lagrange, J., (1997). *Analytical Mechanics*, Kluwer Academic Publishers, ISBN 0-792-34349-2, Dordrecht.

Merenkov, A.P., Khasilev, V.Ya. (1985), *Theory of Hydraulic Circuits*. Nauka, Moscow (in Russian).

Newton, I. (1999). The Principia: Mathematical Principles of Natural Philosophy. University of California Press, ISBN 0-520-08817-4, Berkeley.

Polak, L.S. (2010). *Variational Principles of Mechanics: Their Development and Application to Physics*, LIBROKOM, ISBN 978-5-397-01138-9, Moscow (in Russian).

Prigogine, I.R. (1967). *Introduction to Thermodynamics of Irreversible Processes*, John Wiley, ISBN 0-470-69928-0, New York.

Shirkalin, I.A. (1997). *Solution of Convex Programming Problem with Large Scatter of Variable Values*, SEI AS USSR, Irkutsk (in Russian).

Sumarokov, S.V. (1976). The method of solving multiextreme network problem. *Ekonomika i matematicheskiye metody*, Vol.12, No.5, pp. 1016-1018 (in Russian).

Van der Waals, J.D., Konstamm, P.A. (1936). *Course of Thermostatics: Part 1. General Thermostatics, Part 2. Binary Mixtures*, ONTI. Moscow (in Russian).

Wentzel, E.S. (1964). *Elements of Dynamic Programming*. Nauka, Moscow (in Russian).

Yablonsky, G.S., Bykov, V.I., Gorban, A.N., Elokhin, V.I. (1991). *Kinetic Models of Catalytic Reactions*. Comprehensive Chemical Kinetics, Vol.32, Elsevier, ISBN 0-444-41631-5, Amsterdam.

Zeldovich, Ja. B. (1938). Proof of the unique solution to equation of the mass action law. *Russian Journal of Physical Chemistry A*, Vol.11, No.5, pp. 658–687, ISSN 0044-4537 (in Russian).

4

Vibrational and Chemical Kinetics in Non-Equilibrium Gas Flows

E.V. Kustova and E.A. Nagnibeda
Saint Petersburg State University
Russia

1. Introduction

In this chapter, we consider the vibrational and chemical kinetics in reacting gas flows under the conditions of strong deviations from thermodynamic equilibrium. Such conditions occur, for example, near surfaces of nonexpendable space vehicles in their reentry into the Earth and Mars atmospheres, in experiments carried out in high-enthalpy facilities, in supersonic gas flows in nozzles and jets, in chemical technology processes. In many cases, the characteristic times of vibrational relaxation and chemical reactions appear to be comparable with the characteristic time for the variation of basic gas-dynamic parameters of a flow. Therefore, the equations of gas dynamics and non-equilibrium kinetics should be considered jointly. Consequently, the set of governing equations for macroscopic parameters includes not only the conservation equations for the momentum and total energy, but also the equations for chemical reactions and vibrational energy relaxation. The latter equations contain the rates of energy transitions and chemical reactions which are needed in order to solve the equations of non-equilibrium gas flows.

Originally, non-equilibrium chemical reactions were studied in thermally equilibrium gas mixtures which were assumed to be spatially homogeneous Kondratiev & Nikitin (1974). Later on, different models for vibrational–chemical coupling were proposed on the basis of the kinetic theory methods. One of the first works in this area is that by I. Prigogine Prigogine & Xhrouet (1949), followed by studies Present (1960), and Ludwig & Heil (1960). The effect of non-equilibrium distributions on the chemical reaction rate coefficients was considered in Shizgal & Karplus (1970). Later on, this effect was studied using various distributions of reacting gas molecules over the internal energy (see, for instance, Refs. Belouaggadia & Brun (1997); Knab (1996))). Most of these models are based on thermally-equilibrium distributions or non-equilibrium Boltzmann distributions over the vibrational energy of the reagents. More rigorous models of non-equilibrium kinetics in a flow take into account the non-Boltzmann quasi-stationary distributions or the state-to-state vibrational and chemical kinetics Kustova et al. (1999); Nagnibeda & Kustova (2009). The influence of state-to-state and multi-temperature distributions on reaction rates in particular flows are studied in Kustova & Nagnibeda (2000); Kustova et al. (2003). Recently the comparison of kinetic models for transport properties in reacting gas flows has been discussed in Kustova & Nagnibeda (2011).

In the present contribution, we propose mathematical description for the chemical kinetics in gas flows on the basis of the Chapman–Enskog method, generalized for strongly non-equilibrium reacting gas mixtures.

First, we consider the one-temperature model for the non-equilibrium chemical kinetics in thermally equilibrium gas flows or deviating weakly from thermal equilibrium state. Then, the models for vibrational–chemical coupling in gas flows are derived from the kinetic theory taking into account state-to-state and multi-temperature vibrational distributions.

The influence of non-equilibrium distributions, gas compressibility and space inhomogeneity on the reaction rates for different processes is discussed.

2. One-temperature model for non-equilibrium kinetics

2.1 Kinetic equations. Distribution functions

We consider strong non-equilibrium chemical kinetics in a flow under the following conditions for relaxation times

$$\tau_{el} < \tau_{int} \ll \tau_{react} \sim \theta. \tag{1}$$

Here τ_{el}, τ_{int}, τ_{react} and θ are mean times for relaxation of translation and internal degrees of freedom, chemical reactions and gas dynamic parameters changing respectively. The kinetic equations for the distribution functions have the form Nagnibeda & Kustova (2009):

$$\frac{\partial f_{cij}}{\partial t} + \mathbf{u}_c \cdot \nabla f_{cij} = \frac{1}{\varepsilon} J_{cij}^{rap} + J_{cij}^{sl}, \tag{2}$$

$\varepsilon = \tau_{rap}/\tau_{sl} \sim \tau_{rap}/\theta \ll 1$ is the small parameter, J_{cij}^{rap} and J_{cij}^{sl} are the collision integral operators for rapid and slow processes, c, i, j denote chemical species, vibrational and rotational levels respectively, $\mathbf{r}$, $\mathbf{u}$, t are coordinates, molecular velocities and time. Under condition (2), integral operators of rapid processes describe elastic collisions and collisions with rotational and vibrational energies change and can be written in the form

$$J_{cij}^{rap} = J_{cij}^{el} + J_{cij}^{rot} + J_{cij}^{vibr} = J_{cij}^{el} + J_{cij}^{int}, \tag{3}$$

The operator of slow processes $J_{cij}^{sl} = J_{cij}^{react}$ includes the integrals of reactive collisions and describes exchange reactions

$$A_c(\mathbf{u}_c, i, j) + A_d(\mathbf{u}_d, k, l) \rightleftharpoons A_{c'}(\mathbf{u}_{c'}, i', j') + A_{d'}(\mathbf{u}_{d'}, k', l'), \tag{4}$$

and dissociation-recombination reactions

$$A_c(\mathbf{u}_c, i, j) + A_d(\mathbf{u}_d, k, l) \rightleftharpoons A_{c'}(\mathbf{u}_{c'}) + A_{f'}(\mathbf{u}_{f'}) + A_d(\mathbf{u}'_d, k, l), \tag{5}$$

c', f' are the atomic species forming as reaction products; $\mathbf{u}_{c'}$, $\mathbf{u}_{f'}$, $\mathbf{u}'_d$ are the particle velocities after the collision. For the simplicity we consider dissociation of only diatomic molecules, therefore products of dissociation are only atoms. In addition to this, it is commonly supposed that the dissociation cross section does not depend on the internal state of a partner in the reaction, and this state does not vary as a result of dissociation and recombination.

The collision operator J_{cij}^{react} represents the sum of two terms, J_{cij}^{ex} and J_{cij}^{diss}. Expressions for these operators are given, for instance, in Alexeev et al. (1994); Ern & Giovangigli (1998);

Kuščer (1991); Ludwig & Heil (1960); Nagnibeda & Kustova (2009); Rydalevskaya (1977):

$$J_{cij}^{ex} = \sum_{dc'd'} \sum_{ki'k'} \sum_{lj'l'} \int \left[f_{c'i'j'} f_{d'k'l'} \frac{s_{ij}^{c} s_{kl}^{d}}{s_{i'j'}^{c'} s_{k'l'}^{d'}} \left(\frac{m_c m_d}{m_{c'} m_{d'}} \right)^3 - f_{cij} f_{dkl} \right] g \sigma_{cd,ijkl}^{c'd',i'j'k'l'} d^2\Omega d\mathbf{u}_d, \tag{6}$$

$$J_{cij}^{diss} = \sum_{d} \sum_{k} \sum_{l} \int \left[f'_{dkl} f_{c'} f_{f'} h^3 s_{ij}^{c} \left(\frac{m_c}{m_{c'} m_{f'}} \right)^3 - f_{cij} f_{dkl} \right] g \sigma_{cij,d}^{diss} d\mathbf{u}_d d\mathbf{u}_{c'} d\mathbf{u}_{f'} d\mathbf{u}'_d. \tag{7}$$

In Eq. (6), $\sigma_{cd,ijkl}^{c'd',i'j'k'l'}$ is the differential cross section of the exchange reaction, and the distribution functions after the collision are denoted $f_{c'i'j'} = f_{c'i'j'}(\mathbf{r}, \mathbf{u}_{c'}, t)$, $f_{d'k'l'} = f_{d'k'l'}(\mathbf{r}, \mathbf{u}_{d'}, t)$; in Eq. (7), $\sigma_{cij,d}^{diss}(\mathbf{u}_c, \mathbf{u}_d, \mathbf{u}_{c'}, \mathbf{u}_{f'}, \mathbf{u}'_d)$ is the formal cross section of dissociation, $f_{c'} = f_{c'}(\mathbf{r}, \mathbf{u}_{c'}, t)$, $f_{f'} = f_{f'}(\mathbf{r}, \mathbf{u}_{f'}, t)$ are the distribution functions of atomic dissociation products; $f'_{dkl} = f_{dkl}(\mathbf{r}, \mathbf{u}'_d, t)$, h is the Plank constant, m_c is the mass of a molecule c, s_{ij}^c is the statistical weight of the internal states i and j of a component c, g is the relative velocity, Ω is the solid angle in which a molecule appear after a collision.

Expressions (6), (7) are written taking into account the principle of microscopic reversibility for reactive collisions considered in Alexeev et al. (1994); Ern & Giovangigli (1998); Kuščer (1991); Ludwig & Heil (1960); Rydalevskaya (1977):

$$s_{i'j'}^{c'} s_{k'l'}^{d'} m_{c'}^2 m_{d'}^2 g'^2 \sigma_{c'd',i'j'k'l'}^{cd,ijkl}(\mathbf{g}', \Omega) = s_{ij}^{c} s_{kl}^{d} m_c^2 m_d^2 g^2 \sigma_{cd,ijkl}^{c'd',i'j'k'l'}(\mathbf{g}, \Omega'), \tag{8}$$

$$\frac{m_{c'}^3 m_{f'}^3}{h^3} \sigma_{c'f'd}^{rec,cij}(\mathbf{u}_{c'}, \mathbf{u}_{f'}, \mathbf{u}'_d, \mathbf{u}_c, \mathbf{u}_d) = s_{ij}^{c} m_c^3 g \sigma_{cij,d}^{diss}(\mathbf{u}_c, \mathbf{u}_d, \mathbf{u}_{c'}, \mathbf{u}_{f'}, \mathbf{u}'_d), \tag{9}$$

$\sigma_{c'f'd}^{rec,cij}$ is the probability density for a triple collision resulting in dissociation.

In the frame of the method proposed in Kustova & Nagnibeda (1998); Nagnibeda & Kustova (2009) for the solution of Eqs. (2), the distribution functions are expanded in a power series of the small parameter ε. The peculiarity of the modified Chapman-Enskog method is that the distribution functions and macroscopic parameters are determined by the collision invariants of the most frequent collisions. Under condition (1), the set of collision invariants contains the invariants of any collision (momentum and total energy) and the additional invariants of rapid processes. In our case, these additional invariants are any variables independent of the velocity and internal energy and depending arbitrary on chemical species c because chemical reactions are supposed to be frozen in rapid processes This set of collision invariants provides the following set of macroscopic parameters for a closed flow description: number densities of species $n_c(\mathbf{r}, t)$ $(c = 1, ..., L)$, gas velocity $\mathbf{v}(\mathbf{r}, t)$ and temperature $T(\mathbf{r}, t)$.

2.2 Governing equations. Reaction rates

Closed set of equations of the flow are derived from the kinetic equations (2). Integrating these equations over velocities and summing over the internal energy levels we obtain equations of chemical kinetics in the flow. Multiplying kinetic equations by the collision invariants of any collision, integrating over the velocity and summing over the internal energy levels, we obtain the conservation equations for the momentum and total energy. Finally the set of governing equations for macroscopic parameters $n_c(\mathbf{r}, t)$, $\mathbf{v}(\mathbf{r}, t)$, $T(\mathbf{r}, t)$ takes the form:

$$\frac{dn_c}{dt} + n_c \nabla \cdot \mathbf{v} + \nabla \cdot (n_c \mathbf{V}_c) = R_c^{react}, \quad c = 1,..,L, \tag{10}$$

$$\rho \frac{d\mathbf{v}}{dt} + \nabla \cdot \boldsymbol{P} = 0, \tag{11}$$

$$\rho \frac{dU}{dt} + \nabla \cdot \mathbf{q} + \boldsymbol{P} : \nabla \mathbf{v} = 0. \tag{12}$$

Here U is the total energy per unit mass which is the function of temperature and species number densities, $\boldsymbol{P}$ is the pressure tensor, $\mathbf{q}$ is the total heat flux, $\mathbf{V}_i$ are the diffusion velocities.

The production terms in Eqs. (10) take the form

$$R_c^{ex} = \sum_{dc'd'} \left(n_{c'} n_{d'} k_{c'c}^{d'd} - n_c n_d k_{cc'}^{dd'} \right), \tag{13}$$

$$R_c^{diss} = \sum_d n_d \left(n_{c'} n_{f'} k_{rec,c}^d - n_c k_{c,diss}^d \right). \tag{14}$$

Production terms (13) (14) contain the rate coefficients of exchange chemical reactions $k_{cc'}^{dd'}$, dissociation $k_{c,diss}^d$, and recombination $k_{rec,c}^d$ Nagnibeda & Kustova (2009).

For practical calculations it is more suitable to use component mass fractions $\alpha_c = \rho_c/\rho$ instead of number densities n_c (ρ is the total mass density, ρ_c is the component c mass density). In this case, the set of macroscopic parameters includes $\alpha_c(\mathbf{r},t)$ $(c = 1,...,L)$, $\mathbf{v}(\mathbf{r},t)$, $T(\mathbf{r},t)$. The equations of chemical kinetics take the form:

$$\rho \frac{d\alpha_c}{dt} = -\nabla \cdot (\rho_c \mathbf{V}_c) + \sum_r \dot{\xi}_r \nu_{rc} M_c, \quad c = 1,..,L \tag{15}$$

here M_c is the component molar mass, $\dot{\xi}_r$ is the chemical reaction rate for reaction r ($r = 1,...,R$, R is the number of reactions in a mixture), $\nu_{rc} = \nu_{rc}^{(p)} - \nu_{rc}^{(r)}$ is global stoichiometric coefficient, $\nu_{rc}^{(r)}, \nu_{rc}^{(p)}$ are the stoichiometric coefficients of reactants and products.

The source terms are defined by expressions:

$$\sum_r \dot{\xi}_r \nu_{rc} M_c = m_c \sum_{ij} \int J_{cij}^{sl} d\mathbf{u}_c = m_c \sum_{ij} \int (J_{cij}^{ex} + J_{cij}^{diss}) d\mathbf{u}_c. \tag{16}$$

Let us introduce the rate coefficients of forward and backward reactions $k_{f,r}$, $k_{b,r}$. For exchange reaction (4) ($r = ex$), and recombination-dissociation reaction (5) ($r = diss$) they have the form:

$$\nu_{ex,c} k_{f,ex} = -\mathcal{N}_A \sum_{jlj'l'} \sum_{iki'k'} \int \frac{f_{cij} f_{dkl}}{n_c n_d} g\, \sigma_{cd,ijkl}^{c'd',i'j'k'l'} \, d^2\Omega \, d\mathbf{u}_d \, d\mathbf{u}_c, \tag{17}$$

$$\nu_{ex,c} k_{b,ex} = -\mathcal{N}_A \sum_{jlj'l'} \sum_{iki'k'} \int \frac{f_{c'i'j'} f_{d'k'l'}}{n_{c'} n_{d'}} g'\, \sigma_{c'd',i'j'k'l'}^{cd,ijkl} \, d^2\Omega \, d\mathbf{u}_{d'} \, d\mathbf{u}_{c'}, \tag{18}$$

$$\nu_{diss,c}\, k_{f,diss} = -\mathcal{N}_A \sum_{jl}\sum_{ik} \int \frac{f_{cij} f_{dkl}}{n_c n_d}\, g\, \sigma^{diss}_{cij,d}\, d\mathbf{u}_c\, d\mathbf{u}_d\, d\mathbf{u}_{c'}\, d\mathbf{u}_{f'}\, d\mathbf{u}'_{d'}, \tag{19}$$

$$\nu_{diss,c}\, k_{b,diss} = -\mathcal{N}_A^2 \sum_{jl}\sum_{ik} \int \frac{f_{c'} f_{f'} f'_{dkl}}{n_{c'} n_{f'} n_d}\, \sigma^{rec,cij}_{c'f'd}\, d\mathbf{u}_{c'}\, d\mathbf{u}_{f'}\, d\mathbf{u}'_d\, d\mathbf{u}_c\, d\mathbf{u}_d. \tag{20}$$

Rate coefficients (17)–(20) are connected with those appearing in equations (13), (14) by the relations:

$$k_{f,r} = -\frac{\mathcal{N}_A}{\nu_{rc}} k_{cc'}^{dd'}, \qquad k_{b,r} = -\frac{\mathcal{N}_A}{\nu_{rc}} k_{c'c}^{d'd} \tag{21}$$

for exchange reactions, and

$$k_{f,r} = -\frac{\mathcal{N}_A}{\nu_{rc}} k^d_{c,diss}, \qquad k_{b,r} = -\frac{\mathcal{N}_A^2}{\nu_{rc}} k^d_{rec,c} \tag{22}$$

for dissociation and recombination reactions, $\mathcal{N}_A$ is the Avogadro number.

Using equations (16), (17)–(20), we can write the expression for the reaction rate $\dot{\xi}_r$ in the conventional form:

$$\dot{\xi}_r = k_{f,r} \prod_{c=1}^{L} \left(\frac{\rho_c}{M_c}\right)^{\nu_{rc}^{(r)}} - k_{b,r} \prod_{c=1}^{L} \left(\frac{\rho_c}{M_c}\right)^{\nu_{rc}^{(p)}}. \tag{23}$$

One can notice that the general expressions for the rate coefficients depend on the cross-section of corresponding reactions as well as on the distribution functions, and, consequently, on the approximation of the Chapman–Enskog method.

2.3 Zero-order reaction-rate coefficients

The zero-order solution of Eqs. (2) for molecular species has the form of the Maxwell-Boltzmann distributions

$$f^{(0)}_{cij} = \left(\frac{m_c}{2\pi kT}\right)^{3/2} \frac{n_c}{Z^{int}_c(T)} s^c_{ij} \exp\left(-\frac{m_c c_c^2}{2kT} - \frac{\varepsilon^c_{ij}}{kT}\right), \tag{24}$$

with the internal partition function Z^{int}_c given by

$$Z^{int}_c(T) = \sum_{ij} s^c_{ij} \exp\left(-\frac{\varepsilon^c_{ij}}{kT}\right).$$

Here ε^c_{ij} is the internal energy of a molecule at the ith vibrational and jth rotational levels, k is the Boltzmann constant, $\mathbf{c}_c = \mathbf{u}_c - \mathbf{v}$ is the peculiar velocity. The zero-order distribution function for atomic species reads

$$f^{(0)}_c = \left(\frac{m_c}{2\pi kT}\right)^{3/2} n_c \exp\left(-\frac{m_c c_c^2}{2kT}\right). \tag{25}$$

The zero order transport terms in the flow equations take the form $\mathbf{V}^{(0)}_c = 0$, $\boldsymbol{P}^{(0)} = p\boldsymbol{I}$, $\mathbf{q}^{(0)} = 0$, the pressure is $p = nkT$, n is the total number density. Thus, in the zero-order

(Euler) approximation, the governing equations describe non-equilibrium chemical kinetics in a thermally equilibrium inviscid non-conducting gas mixture:

$$\rho \frac{d\alpha_c}{dt} = \sum_r \dot{\xi}_r^{(0)} \nu_{rc} M_c, \qquad c = 1,..,L, \tag{26}$$

$$\rho \frac{d\mathbf{v}}{dt} = -\nabla p, \tag{27}$$

$$\rho \frac{dU}{dt} = -p \, \nabla \cdot \mathbf{v}. \tag{28}$$

The right-hand side in Eqs. (26) contain the zero-order reaction rates:

$$\dot{\xi}_r^{(0)} = k_{f,r}^{(0)} \prod_{c=1}^{L} \left(\frac{\rho_c}{M_c}\right)^{\nu_{rc}^{(r)}} - k_{b,r}^{(0)} \prod_{c=1}^{L} \left(\frac{\rho_c}{M_c}\right)^{\nu_{rc}^{(p)}}. \tag{29}$$

Here $k_{f,r}^{(0)}, k_{b,r}^{(0)}$ are the thermal-equilibrium reaction-rate coefficients. For the exchange reaction (4), when the partner A_d is a molecule, $k_{f,ex}^{(0)}, k_{b,ex}^{(0)}$ are given by:

$$\nu_{ex,c} k_{f,ex}^{(0)}(T) = -\frac{\mathcal{N}_A}{Z_c^{int}(T) Z_d^{int}(T)} \left(\frac{m_{cd}}{2\pi kT}\right)^{3/2} \sum_{iki'k'} \sum_{jlj'l'} \int \exp\left(-\frac{m_{cd} g^2}{2kT}\right) \times$$

$$s_{ij}^c s_{kl}^d \exp\left(-\frac{\varepsilon_{ij}^c + \varepsilon_{kl}^d}{kT}\right) g^3 \sigma_{cd,ijkl}^{c'd',i'j'k'l'}(g,\Omega) \, dg \, d^2\Omega, \tag{30}$$

$$\nu_{ex,c} k_{b,ex}^{(0)}(T) = -\frac{\mathcal{N}_A}{Z_{c'}^{int}(T) Z_{d'}^{int}(T)} \left(\frac{m_{c'd'}}{2\pi kT}\right)^{3/2} \sum_{iki'k'} \sum_{jlj'l'} \int \exp\left(-\frac{m_{c'd'} g'^2}{2kT}\right) \times$$

$$s_{i'j'}^{c'} s_{k'l'}^{d'} \exp\left(-\frac{\varepsilon_{i'j'}^{c'} + \varepsilon_{k'l'}^{d'}}{kT}\right) g'^3 \sigma_{c'd',i'j'k'l'}^{cd,ijkl}(g',\Omega) \, dg' \, d^2\Omega, \tag{31}$$

and if A_d is an atom,

$$\nu_{ex,c} k_{f,ex}^{(0)}(T) = -\frac{\mathcal{N}_A}{Z_c^{int}(T)} \left(\frac{m_{cd}}{2\pi kT}\right)^{3/2} \sum_{ii'} \sum_{jj'} \int \exp\left(-\frac{m_{cd} g^2}{2kT}\right) \times$$

$$s_{ij}^c \exp\left(-\frac{\varepsilon_{ij}^c}{kT}\right) g^3 \sigma_{cd,ij}^{c'd',i'j'}(g,\Omega) \, dg \, d^2\Omega. \tag{32}$$

$$\nu_{ex,c} k_{b,ex}^{(0)}(T) = -\frac{\mathcal{N}_A}{Z_{c'}^{int}(T)} \left(\frac{m_{c'd'}}{2\pi kT}\right)^{3/2} \sum_{ii'} \sum_{jj'} \int \exp\left(-\frac{m_{c'd'} g'^2}{2kT}\right) \times$$

$$s_{i'j'}^{c'} \exp\left(-\frac{\varepsilon_{i'j'}^{c'}}{kT}\right) g'^3 \sigma_{c'd',i'j'}^{cd,ij}(g',\Omega) \, dg' \, d^2\Omega. \tag{33}$$

For the dissociation reaction (5), the zero-order forward-rate coefficient is obtained in the form

$$\nu_{diss,c}\, k^{(0)}_{f,diss}(T) = -\frac{4\pi \mathcal{N}_A}{Z^{int}_c(T)} \left(\frac{m_{cd}}{2\pi kT}\right)^{3/2} \sum_{ij} \int \exp\left(-\frac{m_{cd} g^2}{2kT}\right) \times$$

$$s^c_{ij} \exp\left(-\frac{\varepsilon^c_{ij}}{kT}\right) g^3 \sigma^{diss}_{cij,d}(g, \mathbf{u}_{c'}, \mathbf{u}_{f'}, \mathbf{u}'_d)\, dg\, d\mathbf{u}_{c'}\, d\mathbf{u}_{f'}\, d\mathbf{u}'_d. \tag{34}$$

The zero-order recombination (backward for dissociation) rate coefficient reads

$$\nu_{diss,c}\, k^{(0)}_{b,diss}(T) = -\mathcal{N}_A^2 \frac{\left(m_{c'} m_{f'} m_d\right)^{3/2}}{(2\pi kT)^{9/2}} \sum_{ij} \int \exp\left(-\frac{m_{c'} c^2_{c'}}{2kT} - \frac{m_{f'} c^2_{f'}}{2kT} - \frac{m_d c'^2_d}{2kT}\right) \times$$

$$\sigma^{rec,cij}_{c'f'd}(\mathbf{u}_c, \mathbf{u}_d, \mathbf{u}_{c'}, \mathbf{u}_{f'}, \mathbf{u}'_d)\, d\mathbf{u}_c\, d\mathbf{u}_d\, d\mathbf{u}_{c'}\, d\mathbf{u}_{f'}\, d\mathbf{u}'_d. \tag{35}$$

Thus, if the cross-sections of the corresponding reactions are known, the zero-order rate coefficients can easily be calculated. However, for practical applications, phenomenological models such as the Arrhenius one are commonly used.

Using the detailed balance principle (8)–(9), one can obtain the ratios of forward and backward reaction rate coefficients:

$$K^{(0)}_{ex}(T) = \frac{k^{(0)}_{b,ex}(T)}{k^{(0)}_{f,ex}(T)} = \left(\frac{m_c m_d}{m_{c'} m_{d'}}\right)^{3/2} \frac{Z^{int}_c(T) Z^{int}_d(T)}{Z^{int}_{c'}(T) Z^{int}_{d'}(T)} \exp\left(\frac{D_c + D_d - D_{c'} - D_{d'}}{kT}\right), \tag{36}$$

$$K^{(0)}_{diss}(T) = \frac{k^{(0)}_{b,diss}}{k^{(0)}_{f,diss}} = \mathcal{N}_A \left(\frac{m_c}{m_{c'} m_{f'}}\right)^{3/2} h^3 (2\pi kT)^{-3/2} Z^{int}_c(T) \exp\left(\frac{D_c}{kT}\right), \tag{37}$$

D_c is the dissociation energy of molecule c, $D_c + D_d - D_{c'} - D_{d'}$ is heat effect of an exchange reaction. Formulas (36), (37) express the chemical-equilibrium constants well known from thermodynamics and hold only for Maxwell-Boltzmann distributions over velocity and internal energy.

2.4 First order reaction rate coefficients. Chemical kinetics in viscous gases

First-order distribution functions are obtained in Nagnibeda & Kustova (2009) in the form

$$f^{(1)}_{cij} = f^{(0)}_{cij} \left(-\frac{1}{n}\mathbf{A}_{cij} \cdot \nabla \ln T - \frac{1}{n} \sum_d \mathbf{D}^d_{cij} \cdot \mathbf{d}_d - \frac{1}{n}\mathbf{B}_{cij} : \nabla \mathbf{v} - \frac{1}{n} F_{cij} \nabla \cdot \mathbf{v} - \frac{1}{n} G_{cij}\right). \tag{38}$$

Functions $\mathbf{A}_{cij}$, $\mathbf{B}_{cij}$, $\mathbf{D}^d_{cij}$, F_{cij} and G_{cij} satisfy the linear integral equations with the linearized operators of elastic collisions and inelastic ones with internal energy transitions.

Let us consider the first-order transport terms in equations Eqs. (10)–(12). For the viscous stress tensor we obtain

$$\boldsymbol{P} = (p - p_{rel})\boldsymbol{I} - 2\eta \mathbf{S} - \zeta \nabla \cdot \mathbf{v} \boldsymbol{I}. \tag{39}$$

Here, p_{rel} is the relaxation pressure, η and ζ are the coefficients of shear and bulk viscosity. In the one-temperature approach, the additional terms connected to the bulk viscosity and relaxation pressure appear in the diagonal terms of the stress tensor due to rapid inelastic internal energy transitions. The existence of the relaxation pressure is caused also by slow processes of chemical reactions proceeding on the gas-dynamic time scale.

The transport coefficients in the expression (39) can be written in terms of functions $\mathbf{B}_{cij}$, F_{cij}, and G_{cij}:

$$\eta = \frac{kT}{10}\left[\mathbf{B}, \mathbf{B}\right], \qquad \zeta = kT\left[F, F\right], \qquad p_{rel} = kT\left[F, G\right]. \tag{40}$$

In these formulae, $[A, B]$ (where A, B are arbitrary functions of molecular velocities) denotes a bilinear form depending on the linearized integral collision operator for rapid processes. In the kinetic theory, such bilinear forms are basically called bracket integrals. The bracket integrals in the expressions (40) are introduced in Nagnibeda & Kustova (2009) similarly to those defined in Ferziger & Kaper (1972) for a non-reacting gas mixture under the conditions of weak deviations from the equilibrium.

The diffusion velocity and the total energy flux in the considered approach are specified by the functions $\mathbf{D}^d_{cij}$, $\mathbf{A}^d_{cij}$ also depending on the cross sections of rapid processes and are studied in Kustova & Nagnibeda (2011).

Thus, the governing equations (10)–(12) with the first order transport terms describe a flow of reacting mixture of viscous gases with strong non-equilibrium chemical reactions in the Navier-Stokes approximation. Transport properties in the one-temperature approach in reacting gas mixtures are considered in Ern & Giovangigli (1994); Kustova (2009); Kustova et al. (2008); Nagnibeda & Kustova (2009).

The chemical reaction rate coefficients contributing to the production terms R_c^{react} in the equations (10) or to the reaction rates in the equations (15) in the first-order approximation are defined by the first order distribution functions (38) and depend on the cross sections of reactive collisions.

The chemical-reaction rate in Eqs. (15) in the first-order approximation has the form (23) where

$$k_{f,r} = k^{(0)}_{f,r}(T) - \bar{k}^{(1)}_{f,r}(\alpha_1, ..., \alpha_L, \rho, T) - \tilde{k}^{(1)}_{f,r}(\alpha_1, ..., \alpha_L, \rho, T), \tag{41}$$

$$k_{b,r} = k^{(0)}_{b,r}(T) - \bar{k}^{(1)}_{b,r}(\alpha_1, ..., \alpha_L, \rho, T) - \tilde{k}^{(1)}_{b,r}(\alpha_1, ..., \alpha_L, \rho, T). \tag{42}$$

Quantities $\bar{k}^{(1)}_{f,r}$, $\tilde{k}^{(1)}_{f,r}$, $\bar{k}^{(1)}_{b,r}$, $\tilde{k}^{(1)}_{b,r}$ express first-order corrections to the reaction-rate coefficients (17)–(20). The terms $\bar{k}^{(1)}_{f,r}$, $\bar{k}^{(1)}_{b,r}$ are due to deviations from Maxwell-Boltzmann distributions over velocities and internal energies whereas the terms $\tilde{k}^{(1)}_{f,r}$, $\tilde{k}^{(1)}_{b,r}$ are due to spatial non-homogeneity. If internal degrees of freedom are neglected, the coefficients $\tilde{k}^{(1)}_{f,r}$ and $\tilde{k}^{(1)}_{b,r}$ vanish.

The first-order corrections to the reaction-rate coefficients are defined by the expressions:

$$\nu_{ex,c}\,\bar{k}^{(1)}_{f,ex} = -\frac{N_A}{n}\sum_{iki'k'}\sum_{jlj'l'}\int \frac{f^{(0)}_{cij} f^{(0)}_{dkl}}{n_c n_d}\left(G_{cij} + G_{dkl}\right) g\,\sigma^{c'd',i'j'k'l'}_{cd,ijkl}\, d^2\Omega d\mathbf{u}_d d\mathbf{u}_c, \tag{43}$$

$$v_{ex,c}\,\tilde{k}^{(1)}_{f,ex} = -\nabla\cdot\mathbf{v}\,\frac{\mathcal{N}_A}{n}\sum_{iki'k'}\sum_{jlj'l'}\int\frac{f^{(0)}_{cij}f^{(0)}_{dkl}}{n_c n_d}\left(F_{cij}+F_{dkl}\right)g\,\sigma^{c'd',i'j'k'l'}_{cd,ijkl}\,d^2\Omega d\mathbf{u}_d d\mathbf{u}_c, \tag{44}$$

$$v_{ex,c}\,\bar{k}^{(1)}_{b,ex} = -\frac{\mathcal{N}_A}{n}\sum_{iki'k'}\sum_{jlj'l'}\int\frac{f^{(0)}_{c'i'j'}f^{(0)}_{d'k'l'}}{n_{c'}n_{d'}}\left(G_{c'i'j'}+G_{d'k'l'}\right)g'\,\sigma^{cd,ijkl}_{c'd',i'j'k'l'}d^2\Omega d\mathbf{u}_{d'}d\mathbf{u}_{c'}, \tag{45}$$

$$v_{ex,c}\,\tilde{k}^{(1)}_{b,ex} = -\nabla\cdot\mathbf{v}\,\frac{\mathcal{N}_A}{n}\sum_{iki'k'}\sum_{jlj'l'}\int\frac{f^{(0)}_{c'i'j'}f^{(0)}_{d'k'l'}}{n_{c'}n_{d'}}\left(F_{c'i'j'}+F_{d'k'l'}\right)g'\,\sigma^{cd,ijkl}_{c'd',i'j'k'l'}d^2\Omega d\mathbf{u}_{d'}d\mathbf{u}_{c'}, \tag{46}$$

$$v_{diss,c}\,\bar{k}^{(1)}_{f,diss} = -\frac{\mathcal{N}_A}{n}\sum_{iki'k'}\sum_{jlj'l'}\int\frac{f^{(0)}_{cij}f^{(0)}_{dkl}}{n_c n_d}\left(G_{cij}+G_{dkl}\right)g\,\sigma^{diss}_{cij,d}\,d\mathbf{u}_c\,d\mathbf{u}_d\,d\mathbf{u}_{c'}\,d\mathbf{u}_{f'}\,d\mathbf{u}'_{d}, \tag{47}$$

$$v_{diss,c}\,\tilde{k}^{(1)}_{f,diss} = -\nabla\cdot\mathbf{v}\,\frac{\mathcal{N}_A}{n}\sum_{iki'k'}\sum_{jlj'l'}\int\frac{f^{(0)}_{cij}f^{(0)}_{dkl}}{n_c n_d}\left(F_{cij}+F_{dkl}\right)g\,\sigma^{diss}_{cij,d}\,d\mathbf{u}_c\,d\mathbf{u}_d\,d\mathbf{u}_{c'}\,d\mathbf{u}_{f'}\,d\mathbf{u}'_{d}, \tag{48}$$

$$v_{diss,c}\,\bar{k}^{(1)}_{b,diss} = -\frac{\mathcal{N}_A^2}{n}\sum_{ik}\sum_{jl}\int\frac{f^{(0)}_{c'}f^{(0)}_{f'}f'^{(0)}_{dkl}}{n_{c'}n_{f'}n_d}\left(G_{c'}+G_{f'}+G_{dkl}\right)\sigma^{rec,cij}_{c'f'd}\,d\mathbf{u}_c\,d\mathbf{u}_d\,d\mathbf{u}_{c'}\,d\mathbf{u}_{f'}\,d\mathbf{u}'_{d}, \tag{49}$$

$$v_{diss,c}\,\tilde{k}^{(1)}_{b,diss} = -\nabla\cdot\mathbf{v}\,\frac{\mathcal{N}_A^2}{n}\sum_{ik}\sum_{jl}\int\frac{f^{(0)}_{c'}f^{(0)}_{f'}f'^{(0)}_{dkl}}{n_{c'}n_{f'}n_d}\left(F_{c'}+F_{f'}+F_{dkl}\right)\sigma^{rec,cij}_{c'f'd}\,d\mathbf{u}_c\,d\mathbf{u}_d\,d\mathbf{u}_{c'}\,d\mathbf{u}_{f'}\,d\mathbf{u}'_{d}. \tag{50}$$

It can be noted that the first-order corrections for the reaction rate coefficients depend on the same functions F_{cij} and G_{cij} which define the additional diagonal elements of the pressure tensor connected to the bulk viscosity and relaxation pressure.

Algorithms for the calculation of vector and tensor transport properties and first order corrections to reaction rate coefficients are described in details in Nagnibeda & Kustova (2009). In Ref. Alexeev & Grushin (1994), a procedure for the calculation of the first-order reaction rate coefficients has been developed for gases without internal degrees of freedom. In Ref. Kustova et al. (2008), the scalar functions F_{cij} and G_{cij} are considered, and transport linear systems for the calculation of bulk viscosity, chemical-reaction contribution to the normal mean stress and first-order reaction rate coefficients are derived taking into account internal energy of molecules. Numerical estimations of the first-order rate coefficients in reacting viscous gas flows remain an open question up to now. In the simulations of viscous flows, the first-order corrections to the rate coefficients are usually neglected as well as relaxation pressure and bulk viscosity. Some results in this field have been recently obtained in Ref. Kustova (2009) where numerical estimations of the normal mean stress and the first order corrections to the dissociation and recombination rates in the mixture N_2/N have been performed. It is shown that whereas the first-order contribution to the normal mean stress remains small, the first-order corrections to the reaction rates are not negligible in both shock heated and expanding flows.

3. State-to-state model for vibrational–chemical coupling

3.1 Distribution functions. Governing equations

In this section, chemical kinetics in multi-component reacting gas mixture flows are studied under the conditions of strong vibrational and chemical non-equilibrium. Experimental results on the relaxation times of various processes demonstrate that, in a wide temperature range, the equilibration of translational and rotational degrees of freedom proceeds much faster compared to the vibrational relaxation and chemical reactions. The characteristic relaxation times satisfy the relation

$$\tau_{el} < \tau_{rot} \ll \tau_{vibr} \sim \tau_{react} \sim \theta. \tag{51}$$

where τ_{rot}, τ_{vibr} are relaxation times for rotational and vibrational degrees of freedom. Under such conditions, the integral operators in the kinetic equations (2) take the form:

$$J^{rap}_{cij} = J^{el}_{cij} + J^{rot}_{cij}, \qquad J^{sl}_{cij} = J^{vibr}_{cij} + J^{react}_{cij}. \tag{52}$$

In this case, the vibrational-chemical coupling in reacting flows becomes important.

The kinetic equations for the distribution functions in the zero-order Chapman-Enskog approximation have the form:

$$J^{el(0)}_{cij} + J^{rot(0)}_{cij} = 0. \tag{53}$$

In this case, the system of collision invariants for the most frequent collisions includes along with the momentum and a particle total energy, any value independent of the velocity and rotational level j and depending arbitrarily on the vibrational level i and chemical species c. This values are conserved at the most frequent collisions because, according to the condition (51), vibrational energy transitions and chemical reactions are forbidden in the rapid processes. Based on the above set of the collision invariants, the solution of Eqs. (53) takes the form

$$f^{(0)}_{cij} = \left(\frac{m_c}{2\pi kT}\right)^{3/2} s^{ci}_j \frac{n_{ci}}{Z^{rot}_{ci}(T)} \exp\left(-\frac{m_c c_c^2}{2kT} - \frac{\varepsilon^{ci}_j}{kT}\right) \tag{54}$$

for molecular species, and

$$f^{(0)}_{c} = \left(\frac{m_c}{2\pi kT}\right)^{3/2} n_{c,a} \exp\left(-\frac{m_c c_c^2}{2kT}\right) \tag{55}$$

for atomic species. Here n_{ci} is the number density of molecules c at the i-th vibrational level, $n_{c,a}$ is the number density of atoms c, Z^{rot}_{ci} is the partition functions of rotational degrees of freedom:

$$Z^{rot}_{ci}(T) = \sum_j s^{ci}_j \exp\left(-\frac{\varepsilon^{ci}_j}{kT}\right), \tag{56}$$

ε^{ci}_j is the rotational energy of a molecule at the ith vibrational level, s^{ci}_j is the rotational statistical weight.

The solution (54) represents the local equilibrium Maxwell-Boltzmann distribution over the velocity and rotational energy levels with the temperature T and strongly non-equilibrium distribution over chemical species and vibrational energy levels. The distribution functions

(54), (55) are completely specified by the macroscopic gas parameters $n_{ci}(\mathbf{r}, t)$ ($c = 1, ..., L, i = 0, 1, ..., Lc$, L_c is the number of excited vibration levels of molecular species c), $T(\mathbf{r}, t)$, and $\mathbf{v}(\mathbf{r}, t)$ and correspond to the set of the collision invariants of rapid processes.

The set of equations for the macroscopic parameters $n_{ci}(\mathbf{r}, t)$, $\mathbf{v}(\mathbf{r}, t)$, and $T(\mathbf{r}, t)$ follows from Eq. (2) with collision operators (52). This system includes equations of state-to-state vibrational and chemical kinetics in a flow Kustova & Nagnibeda (1998); Nagnibeda & Kustova (2009):

$$\frac{dn_{ci}}{dt} + n_{ci} \nabla \cdot \mathbf{v} + \nabla \cdot (n_{ci} \mathbf{V}_{ci}) = R_{ci}, \qquad c = 1, ..., L, \ \ i = 0, ..., L_c, \tag{57}$$

coupled to the conservation equations for the momentum and total energy which formally coincide with Eqs. (11)–(12). Here, $\mathbf{V}_{ci}$ is the diffusion velocity of molecules c at the vibrational state i. The total energy per unit mass U is specified by level populations $n_{ci}(\mathbf{r}, t)$, atomic number densities $n_c(\mathbf{r}, t)$ and gas temperature.

The source terms in equations (57) characterize the variation of the vibrational level populations and atomic number densities caused by different vibrational energy exchanges and chemical reactions and are expressed via the integral operators of slow processes:

$$R_{ci} = \sum_j \int J^{sl}_{cij} d\,\mathbf{u}_c = R^{vibr}_{ci} + R^{react}_{ci}. \tag{58}$$

The equations (57), (11), (12) provide a detailed description of vibrational and chemical kinetics and flow dynamics for weak deviations from the equilibrium distributions over the velocity and rotational energy levels and arbitrary deviations from the equilibrium for the vibrational degrees of freedom and chemical species. Let us emphasize that for such an approach, the vibrational level populations are included to the set of main macroscopic parameters, and particles of various chemical species in different vibrational states represent the mixture components. The expressions (58) can be written in the form:

$$R^{vibr}_{ci} = \sum_{dki'k'} \left(n_{ci'} n_{dk'} k^{d,k'k}_{c,i'i} - n_{ci} n_{dk} k^{d,kk'}_{c,ii'} \right), \tag{59}$$

$$R^{react}_{ci} = R^{ex}_{ci} + R^{diss}_{ci},$$

$$R^{ex}_{ci} = \sum_{dc'd'} \sum_{ki'k'} \left(n_{c'i'} n_{d'k'} k^{d'k',dk}_{c'i',ci} - n_{ci} n_{dk} k^{dk,d'k'}_{ci,c'i'} \right), \tag{60}$$

$$R^{diss}_{ci} = \sum_{dk} n_{dk} \left(n_{c'} n_{f'} k^{dk}_{rec,ci} - n_{ci} k^{dk}_{ci,diss} \right). \tag{61}$$

Here the rate coefficients are introduced for the energy exchange:

$$A_{ci} + A_{dk} \rightleftharpoons A_{ci'} + A_{dk'}, \tag{62}$$

exchange chemical reactions:

$$A_{ci} + A_{dk} \rightleftharpoons A_{c'i'} + A_{d'k'} \tag{63}$$

and dissociation-recombination reactions:

$$A_{ci} + A_{dk} \rightleftharpoons A_{c'} + A_{f'} + A_{dk}. \tag{64}$$

The rate coefficients for the forward reactions (62)–(64) (for collisions of particles A_{ci} and A_{dk}) are introduced, respectively, as $k^{d,kk'}_{c,ii'}$, $k^{dk,d'k'}_{ci,c'i'}$, and $k^{dk}_{ci,diss}$, the recombination rate coefficient is denoted as $k^{dk}_{rec,ci}$. Note that if $k' = k$, then Eq. (62) describes VT(TV) transitions for a molecule A_{ci} during the collision with a molecule A_{dk} with the rate coefficient $k^{dk}_{c,ii'}$ of the forward transition. If d is an atom, then the corresponding rate coefficient of the forward transition (62) is $k^{d}_{c,ii'}$.

If $k \neq k'$ then the reaction (62) describes either VV_1 exchange of the vibrational energy between molecules of the same chemical species (for $c = d$) or VV_2 transitions between molecules of different chemical species (for $c \neq d$). Note that VV_1 and VV_2 transitions of the vibrational energy are almost always accompanied with the transfer of the part of vibrational energy into the translational or rotational modes. However, the probability of a simultaneous exchange between three and more energy modes during one collision is rather low, consequently, these exchanges are usually omitted in the production terms of the kinetic equations.

In the dissociation and recombination reactions (64), the particle A_{dk} can also be either a molecule or an atom. Therefore, different dissociation rate coefficients should be introduced: $k^{dk}_{rec,ci}$, $k^{d}_{rec,ci}$. The rate coefficients of the above processes depend on the order of the distribution function approximation.

The Chapman–Enskog method generalized for the conditions (51) gives the possibility to express, in any approximation, the transport and relaxation terms in Eqs. (57), (11), (12) as functions of the main macroscopic parameters $n_{ci}(\mathbf{r}, t)$, $\mathbf{v}(\mathbf{r}, t)$, and $T(\mathbf{r}, t)$ and thus to close completely the set of governing equations.

In the zero-order approximation (54), (55),

$$\mathbf{P}^{(0)} = nkT\mathbf{I}, \qquad \mathbf{q}^{(0)} = 0, \qquad \mathbf{V}^{(0)}_{ci} = 0 \quad \forall\, c, i, \tag{65}$$

and the governing equations contain the equations of state-to-state kinetics

$$\frac{dn_{ci}}{dt} + n_{ci} \nabla \cdot \mathbf{v} = R^{(0)}_{ci}, \qquad c = 1, ..., L, \quad i = 0, ..., L_c, \tag{66}$$

coupled to the conservation equations in the form (27), (28).

The right hand sides of Eqs. (66) $R^{(0)}_{ci}$ are specified by the zero-order distribution function. The expressions for R_{ci} contain the microscopic rate coefficients for vibrational energy exchanges and chemical reactions. The equations (66) describe detailed state-to-state vibrational and chemical kinetics in an inviscid non-conductive gas mixture flow in the Euler approximation. In the first-order approximation state-dependent transport properties and reaction rates in reacting non-equilibrium flows are studied in Kustova & Nagnibeda (1998); Kustova et al. (1999); Nagnibeda & Kustova (2009).

3.2 State dependent reaction rate coefficients

Let us consider state dependent rate coefficients for chemical reactions appearing in Eqs. (59)–(61). In the zero-order Chapman-Enskog approximation rate coefficients for exchange reactions have the form Nagnibeda & Kustova (2009):

$$k_{ci,c'i'}^{dk,d'k'} = \frac{4\pi}{Z_{ci}^{rot} Z_{dk}^{rot}} \left(\frac{m_{cd}}{2\pi kT}\right)^{3/2} \sum_{jlj'l'} \int \exp\left(-\frac{m_{cd} g^2}{2kT}\right) \times$$

$$\times s_j^{ci} s_l^{dk} \exp\left(-\frac{\varepsilon_j^{ci} + \varepsilon_l^{dk}}{kT}\right) g^3 \tilde{\sigma}_{cd,ijkl}^{c'd',i'j'k'l'} dg, \tag{67}$$

with $\tilde{\sigma}_{cd,ijkl}^{c'd',i'j'k'l'}$ designating the integral cross section of a collision resulting in a bimolecular reaction. The integral cross section is obtained integrating the corresponding differential cross sections over solid angles in which relative velocity appear before and after collision:

$$\tilde{\sigma}_{cd,ijkl}^{c'd',i'j'k'l'}(g) = \frac{1}{4\pi} \int \sigma_{cd,ijkl}^{c'd',i'j'k'l'}(\mathbf{g}, \Omega) d^2\Omega d^2\Omega'. \tag{68}$$

It is commonly supposed that the cross section depends on the absolute value g of the relative velocity rather than the vector $\mathbf{g}$. Then

$$\tilde{\sigma}_{cd,ijkl}^{c'd',i'j'k'l'}(g) = \int \sigma_{cd,ijkl}^{c'd',i'j'k'l'}(g, \Omega) d^2\Omega. \tag{69}$$

The recombination rate coefficients in the zero-order approximation can be represented in the form

$$k_{rec,ci}^{dk} = \frac{(m_{c'} m_{f'} m_d)^{3/2}}{(2\pi kT)^{9/2}} \sum_j \int \sigma_{c'f'd}^{rec,cij}(\mathbf{u}_{c'}, \mathbf{u}_{f'}, \mathbf{u}'_d, \mathbf{u}_c, \mathbf{u}_d) \times$$

$$\times \exp\left(-\frac{m_{c'} u_{c'}^2 + m_{f'} u_{f'}^2 + m_d u_d'^2}{2kT}\right) d\mathbf{u}_{c'} d\mathbf{u}_{f'} d\mathbf{u}'_d d\mathbf{u}_c d\mathbf{u}_d. \tag{70}$$

The zero-order dissociation rate coefficients take the form Kuščer (1991); Ludwig & Heil (1960)

$$k_{ci,diss}^{dk} = \frac{4\pi}{Z_{ci}^{rot}} \left(\frac{m_{cd}}{2\pi kT}\right)^{3/2} \sum_j \int \exp\left(-\frac{m_{cd} g^2}{2kT}\right) s_j^{ci} \exp\left(-\frac{\varepsilon_j^{ci}}{kT}\right) g^3 \tilde{\sigma}_{cij,d}^{diss} dg, \tag{71}$$

the integral dissociation reaction cross section is introduced by the formula

$$\tilde{\sigma}_{cij,d}^{diss} = \int \sigma_{cij,d}^{diss}(g, \mathbf{u}_{c'}, \mathbf{u}_{f'}, \mathbf{u}'_d) d\mathbf{u}_{c'} d\mathbf{u}_{f'} d\mathbf{u}'_d. \tag{72}$$

Since it is supposed that the cross sections of dissociation $\sigma_{cij,d}^{diss}$ and recombination $\sigma_{c'f'd}^{rec,cij}$ do not depend on the vibrational state k of the partner A_{dk} in the reaction (64), then:

$$k_{ci,diss}^{dk} = k_{ci,diss}^{d}, \qquad k_{rec,ci}^{dk} = k_{rec,ci}^{d} \tag{73}$$

The relations connecting the rate coefficients of forward and backward collisional processes follow from the microscopic detailed balance relations for reactive collisions (8)-(9) after averaging them with the Maxwell–Boltzmann distribution over the velocity and rotational energy. Thus for the rate coefficients of forward and backward reactions we obtain

$$K_{c'i',ci}^{d'k',dk} = \frac{k_{c'i',ci}^{d'k',dk}}{k_{ci,c'i'}^{dk,d'k'}} = \frac{s_i^c s_k^d}{s_{i'}^{c'} s_{k'}^{d'}} \left(\frac{m_c m_d}{m_{c'} m_{d'}}\right)^{3/2} \frac{Z_{ci}^{rot} Z_{dk}^{rot}}{Z_{c'i'}^{rot} Z_{d'k'}^{rot}} \times$$

$$\times \exp\left(\frac{\varepsilon_{i'}^{c'} + \varepsilon_{k'}^{d'} - \varepsilon_i^c - \varepsilon_k^d}{kT}\right) \exp\left(\frac{D_c + D_d - D_{c'} - D_{d'}}{kT}\right), \tag{74}$$

$$K_{rec-diss,ci}^{d} = \frac{k_{rec,ci}^{d}}{k_{ci,diss}^{d}} = s_i^c \left(\frac{m_c}{m_{c'} m_{f'}}\right)^{3/2} h^3 (2\pi kT)^{-3/2} Z_{ci}^{rot} \exp\left(-\frac{\varepsilon_i^c - D_c}{kT}\right). \tag{75}$$

In the last formula, $m_c = m_{c'} + m_{f'}$.

For diatomic gases, the vibrational statistical weight $s_i^c = 1$. Moreover, for the rigid rotator model, the rotational partition function is independent of the vibrational state $Z_{ci}^{rot} = Z_c^{rot}$. In this case, the ratio of the backward and forward reaction rate coefficients takes the reduced form. The expression (74) can be simplified if the collision partner is an atom.

For the application of Egs. (66), (27), (28) to particular problems of non-equilibrium fluid dynamics, the analytical expressions for the dependence of the reaction rate coefficients on the vibrational states of molecules participating in the reactions are needed.

As for vibrational energy transitions, a number of theoretical and experimental estimates for rate coefficients of these transitions are available in the literature in different temperature intervals. These data can be found, for example, in Nagnibeda & Kustova (2009); Phys-Chem (2002; 2004). The comparison of rate coefficients for vibational energy transitions of N_2 molecules obtained using different models is given in Nagnibeda & Kustova (2009).

The rate coefficients for dissociation from different vibrational levels have been studied much less widely than for vibrational energy transitions. Two models are commonly used for calculations: the ladder-climbing model assuming dissociation only from the last vibrational level (see, for instance, Armenise et al. (1996; 1995); Capitelli et al. (1997); Osipov (1966)), and that of Treanor and Marrone Marrone & Treanor (1963) allowing for dissociation from any vibrational state.

In the frame of ladder climbing model, the rate of dissociation is specified by the number of molecules occurring on the last vibrational level. Consequently, the dissociation rate is totally specified by the probabilities for the vibrational energy transitions to the last level. In the case when dissociation can occur from any vibrational level, the expression for the rate coefficient for dissociation of a molecule on the vibrational level i can be written in the form Nagnibeda & Kustova (2009):

$$k_{i,diss}^{d} = Z_i^d(T) k_{diss,eq}^{d}(T). \tag{76}$$

Here, $k_{diss,eq}^{d}(T)$ is the thermal equilibrium dissociation rate coefficient obtained by averaging the state-dependent rate coefficient with the one-temperature Boltzmann distribution; Z_i^d is the non-equilibrium factor. Using the Treanor–Marrone model Marrone & Treanor (1963), the expression for $Z_i^d(T)$ was obtained in Nagnibeda & Kustova (2009):

$$Z_i^d(T) = Z_i(T, U) = \frac{Z^{\text{vibr}}(T)}{Z^{\text{vibr}}(-U)} \exp\left[\frac{\varepsilon_i}{k}\left(\frac{1}{T} + \frac{1}{U}\right)\right], \tag{77}$$

Z_{vibr} is the equilibrium vibrational partition function

$$Z^{vibr}(T) = \sum_i s_i^c \exp\left(-\frac{\varepsilon_i}{kT}\right), \tag{78}$$

U is a parameter of the model.

Thus, the state-dependent dissociation rate coefficient $k^d_{i,diss}$ is expressed in terms of the averaged thermal equilibrium coefficient $k^d_{diss,eq}(T)$ and non-equilibrium factor (77). To calculate $k^d_{\rm diss,eq}(T)$, the empirical Arrhenius law can be applied:

$$k^d_{\rm diss,eq} = AT^n \exp\left(-\frac{D}{kT}\right), \tag{79}$$

the coefficients A and n are generally obtained as a best fit to experimental data. The tables of the coefficients in the Arrhenius formula for various chemical reactions can be found in Refs. Gardiner (1984); Kondratiev & Nikitin (1974); Park (1990); Phys-Chem (2002); Stupochenko et al. (1967).

In Ref. Esposito, Capitelli, Kustova & Nagnibeda (2000), the dissociation rate coefficients $k^d_{i,diss}$ calculated within the framework of the Treanor–Marrone model are compared with those obtained from trajectory calculations Esposito, Capitelli & Gorse (2000), some recommendations for the optimum choice for the parameter U for the specific reactions are given. Figure 1 presents the temperature dependence of the state-dependent dissociation rate coefficients $k^{N_2}_{i,diss}$ in an (N_2, N) mixture. The coefficients are calculated for different values of the parameter U for two vibrational quantum numbers: $i = 0$ and $i = 20$. The results of trajectory calculation for $k_{i,diss}$ taken from Ref. Esposito, Capitelli & Gorse (2000) are also plotted. We can see that for low vibrational levels, the choice for $U = \infty$ results in significant overestimation for $k_{i,diss}$, which confirms the common assumption of the preferential dissociation from high vibrational states.

With the increase in the vibrational quantum number, for $U = \infty$ we obtain more realistic values for $k_{i,diss}$, and for $i > 40$, we have the best agreement with the results of accurate trajectory calculations. $U = D/(6k)$ and $U = 3T$ provide good consistency for $k_{i,diss}$ at intermediate levels ($20 < i < 40$). Furthermore, $U = D/(6k)$ results in better consistency for low temperatures, whereas $U = 3T$ is good in the high temperature range ($T > 6000$ K).

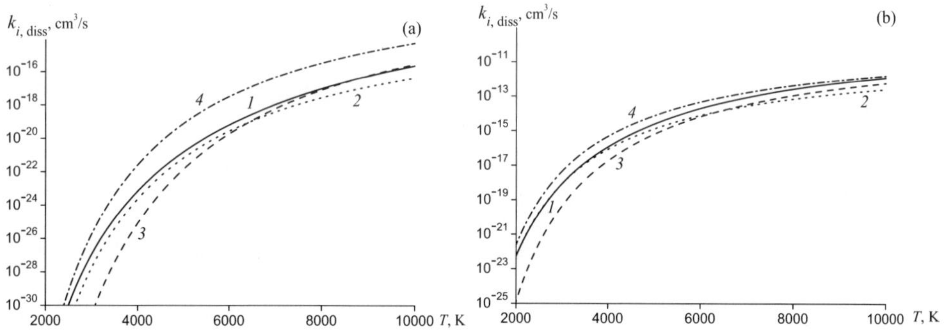

Fig. 1. The temperature dependence of the dissociation rate coefficient $k^{N_2}_{i,\rm diss}$ for $i = 0$ (*a*) and $i = 20$ (*b*). The curve *1* represents the results obtained in Ref. Esposito, Capitelli & Gorse (2000), curves *2*–*4* correspond to $U = D/(6k)$, $U = 3T$, and $U = \infty$.

It should be emphasized that using the same value for the parameter U for any i and T can result in considerable errors in the calculation for the state-to-state dissociation rate coefficients. The choice for the parameter should be specified by the conditions of a particular problem (the temperature range, basic channels of dissociation, etc.). In some studies Armenise et al. (1996); Candler et al. (1997); Capitelli et al. (1997), a possibility for dissociation from any vibrational state is suggested within the framework of the ladder-climbing model. To this end, it is supposed that a transition to the continuum occurs as a result of multi-quantum vibrational energy transfers.

The rate coefficients for bimolecular exchange reactions depending on the vibrational states of reagents and products have been less thoroughly studied than those for dissociation processes. Theoretical and experimental studies for the influence of the vibrational excitation of reagents on reaction rates were started by J. Polanyi Polanyi (1972); some experimental results were also obtained in Birely & Lyman (1975). The accurate theoretical approach to this problem primarily requires a calculation for the state-dependent differential cross sections for collisions resulting in chemical reactions, and their subsequent averaging over the velocity distributions. In the recent years, the dynamics of atmospheric reactions has been studied, and quasi-classical trajectory calculations for the cross sections and state-dependent rate coefficients for the reactions $N_2(i) + O \rightarrow NO + N$ and $O_2(i) + N \rightarrow NO + O$ have been carried out by several authors Gilibert et al. (1992; 1993).

At present time, two kinds of analytical expressions are available in the literature. The first kind includes analytical approximations for numerical results obtained for particular reactions (see Refs. Bose & Candler (1996); Capitelli et al. (1997; 2000); Phys-Chem (2002)). These expressions are sufficiently accurate and convenient for practical use; however, their application is restricted by the considered temperature range. Another approach is based on the generalizations of the Treanor–Marrone model to exchange reactions suggested in Refs. Aliat (2008); Knab (1996); Knab et al. (1995); Seror et al. (1997). These models can be used for more general cases, but the theoretical expressions for the rate coefficients contain additional parameters, which should be validated using experimental data. A lack of the data for these parameters restricts the implementation of the above semi-empirical models.

Therefore, the development of justified theoretical models for cross sections of reactive collisions and state-dependent rate coefficients for exchange reactions remains a very important problem of the non-equilibrium kinetics.

4. Multi-temperature models for vibrational-chemical kinetics

4.1 Governing equations

The approach proposed in the previous section makes it possible to develop the most rigorous model of reacting gas mixtures, since it takes into account the detailed state-to-state vibrational and chemical kinetics in a flow. However, practical implementation of this method leads to serious difficulties. The first important problem encountered in the realization of the state-to-state model is its computational cost. Indeed, the solution of the fluid dynamics equations coupled to the equations of the state-to-state vibrational and chemical kinetics requires numerical simulation of a great number of equations for the vibrational level populations of all molecular species. The second fundamental problem is that experimental and theoretical data on the state-specific rate coefficients and especially on the cross sections of inelastic processes are rather scanty. Due to the above problems, simpler models based on quasi-stationary vibrational distributions are rather attractive for practical applications. In quasi-stationary approaches, the vibrational level populations are expressed in terms of a few macroscopic parameters, consequently, non-equilibrium kinetics can be described by a considerably reduced set of governing equations.

It is known from experiments Gordiets et al. (1988) that in a vibrationally excited gas, near-resonant vibrational energy exchanges between molecules of the same chemical species proceed much faster than non-resonant transitions between different molecules, as well as transfers of vibrational energy to other modes and chemical reactions. Therefore the following relation between the characteristic relaxation times is fulfilled:

$$\tau_{el} \lesssim \tau_{rot} < \tau_{VV_1} \ll \tau_{VV_2} < \tau_{TRV} < \tau_{react} \sim \theta, \tag{80}$$

τ_{VV_1} is the mean time between the collisions of the same species; τ_{VV_2} is the characteristic time of the vibrational energy exchange between different molecules. In the multi-component reacting gas mixture under the condition (80) the integral operators in the kinetic equations (2) includes the operator of VV_1 vibrational energy transitions between molecules of the same species along with the operators of elastic collisions and collisions with rotational energy exchanges:

$$J_{cij}^{rap} = J_{cij}^{el} + J_{cij}^{rot} + J_{cij}^{VV_1}. \tag{81}$$

The operator of slow processes J_{cij}^{sl} consists of the operator of VV_2 vibrational transitions between molecules of different species, the operator describing the transfer of vibrational energy into rotational and translational modes J_{cij}^{TRV}, as well as the operator of chemical reactions J_{cij}^{react}:

$$J_{cij}^{sl} = J_{cij}^{VV_2} + J_{cij}^{TRV} + J_{cij}^{react}. \tag{82}$$

Governing equations of the reacting flows and distribution functions in the zero-order and first-order approximations, under condition (80) are studied in details in Nagnibeda & Kustova (2009). The distribution function is totally specified by the macroscopic parameters n_c, $\mathbf{v}$, T, and T_1^c, where the parameter T_1^c is the vibrational temperature of the first vibrational level of molecules c. The parameter T_1^c is associated to the additional collision invariant i_c which reflects the conservation of the number of vibrational quanta of each molecular species in rapid processes. The zero-order distribution functions in this case may be written in the form (54) where level populations n_{ci} are described by the relation:

$$n_{ci} = \frac{n_c}{Z_c^{vibr}(T, T_1^c)} s_i^c \exp\left(-\frac{\varepsilon_i^c - i\varepsilon_1^c}{kT} - \frac{i\varepsilon_1^c}{kT_1^c}\right). \tag{83}$$

with vibrational partition function

$$Z_c^{vibr}(T, T_1^c) = \sum_i s_i^c \exp\left(-\frac{\varepsilon_i^c - i\varepsilon_1^c}{kT} - \frac{i\varepsilon_1^c}{kT_1^c}\right). \tag{84}$$

ε_1^c is the vibrational energy of a molecule c at the first level. Here the vibrational energy is counted from the energy of the zeroth level.

The expression (83) yields the non-equilibrium quasi-stationary Treanor distribution Treanor et al. (1968) generalized for a multi-component reacting gas mixture taking into account anharmonic molecular vibrations and rapid exchange of vibrational quanta.

The closed set of governing equations for the macroscopic parameters $n_c(\mathbf{r},t)$, $\mathbf{v}(\mathbf{r},t)$, $T(\mathbf{r},t)$, and $T_1^c(\mathbf{r},t)$ derived in Chikhaoui et al. (2000; 1997) includes the equations of the multi-temperature chemical kinetics for the species number densities

$$\frac{dn_c}{dt} + n_c\nabla\cdot\mathbf{v} + \nabla\cdot(n_c\mathbf{V}_c) = R_c^{react}, \quad c = 1,...,L, \tag{85}$$

relaxation equations for the specific numbers of vibrational quanta W_c in each molecular species c:

$$\rho_c\frac{dW_c}{dt} + \nabla\cdot\mathbf{q}_{w,c} = R_c^w - W_c m_c R_c^{react} + W_c\nabla\cdot(\rho_c\mathbf{V}_c), \quad c = 1,...,L_{\mathrm{m}}. \tag{86}$$

along with the conservation equations for the momentum and the total energy, L_m is the number of molecular species in the mixture. The latter equations formally coincide with the corresponding equations (11) and (12) obtained in the two previous approaches. One should however bear in mind that in the multi-temperature approach, the total energy is a function of T, T_1^c, and n_c, and the transport terms are expressed as functions of the same set of macroscopic parameters T, T_1^c, and n_c.

The source terms in Eqs. (85) are determined by the collision operator of chemical reactions

$$R_c^{react} = \sum_{ij}\int J_{cij}^{react} d\mathbf{u}_c. \tag{87}$$

The production terms in the relaxation equations (86) are expressed as functions of collision operators of all slow processes: VV_2 and TRV vibrational energy transfers and chemical reactions,

$$R_c^w = \sum_{ij} i\int J_{cij}^{sl} d\,\mathbf{u}_c = R_c^{w,VV_2} + R_c^{w,TRV} + R_c^{w,react}. \tag{88}$$

The value $\mathbf{q}_{w,c}$ in Eq. (86) has the physical meaning of the vibrational quanta flux of c molecular species and is introduced on the basis of the additional collision invariant of the most frequent collisions i_c:

$$\mathbf{q}_{w,c} = \sum_{ij} i\int \mathbf{c}_c f_{cij} d\mathbf{u}_c.$$

It is obvious that the system of governing equations in the multi-temperature approach is considerably simpler than the corresponding system in the state-to-state approach, since it contains much fewer equations. In the zero-order approximation of the Chapman-Enskog method, the system of governing equations takes the form typical for inviscid non-conductive flows. In this case equations (85), (86) read:

$$\frac{dn_c}{dt} + n_c\,\nabla\cdot\mathbf{v} = R_c^{react(0)}, \qquad c = 1,...,L, \tag{89}$$

$$\rho_c\frac{dW_c}{dt} = R_c^{w(0)} - m_c W_c R_c^{react(0)}, \quad c = 1,...,L_{\mathrm{m}}. \tag{90}$$

4.2 Multi-temperature reaction rate coefficients

The production terms in Eqs. (89) may be written in the form (13), (14) similar to the equations obtained in the one-temperature approximation. However, the coefficients in these expressions differ from those in the one-temperature approach and contains the multi-temperature rate coefficients $k_{cc'}^{dd'}$ of the reaction (63) (during a collision of two molecules or a molecule and an atom A_d), the two-temperature coefficients of dissociation $k_{c,diss}^{d}$, and recombination rate coefficients $k_{rec,c}^{d}$.

In the zero-order approximation, the multi-temperature rate coefficients of exchange and dissociation reactions can be expressed in terms of the state-specific rate coefficients considered in section 3.2:

$$k_{cc'}^{dd'\,(0)} = \frac{1}{n_c n_d} \sum_{iki'k'} n_{ci} n_{dk}\, k_{ci,c'i'}^{dk,d'k'\,(0)}(T), \tag{91}$$

$$k_{c,diss}^{d\,(0)} = \frac{1}{n_c} \sum_{i} n_{ci}\, k_{ci,diss}^{d\,(0)}(T), \tag{92}$$

where n_{ci} denotes some non-equilibrium quasi-stationary distribution.

For the generalized Treanor distribution (83), the multi-temperature rate coefficients of exchange reactions occurring as a result of collisions of two molecules take the form

$$k_{cc'}^{dd'\,(0)}(T, T_1^c, T_1^d) = \frac{1}{Z_c^{vibr}(T, T_1^c) Z_d^{vibr}(T, T_1^d)} \sum_{iki'k'} s_i^c s_k^d \exp\left(-\frac{\varepsilon_i^c - i_c \varepsilon_1^c}{kT} - \right.$$
$$\left. -\frac{\varepsilon_k^d - k_d \varepsilon_1^d}{kT} - \frac{i_c \varepsilon_1^c}{kT_1^c} - \frac{k_d \varepsilon_1^d}{kT_1^d}\right) k_{ci,c'i'}^{dk,d'k'\,(0)}(T). \tag{93}$$

The rate coefficient for the exchange reaction in a collision of a diatomic molecule and an atom, as well as the dissociation rate coefficient, depends on two temperatures (T and T_1^c):

$$k_{cc'}^{dd'\,(0)}(T, T_1^c) = \frac{1}{Z_c^{vibr}(T, T_1^c)} \sum_{ii'} s_i^c \exp\left(-\frac{\varepsilon_i^c - i_c \varepsilon_1^c}{kT} - \frac{i_c \varepsilon_1^c}{kT_1^c}\right) k_{ci,c'i'}^{dd'\,(0)}(T), \tag{94}$$

$$k_{c,diss}^{d\,(0)}(T, T_1^c) = \frac{1}{Z_c^{vibr}(T, T_1^c)} \sum_{i} s_i^c \exp\left(-\frac{\varepsilon_i^c - i_c \varepsilon_1^c}{kT} - \frac{i_c \varepsilon_1^c}{kT_1^c}\right) k_{ci,diss}^{d\,(0)}(T). \tag{95}$$

The total recombination rate coefficient $k_{\text{rec},c}^{d\,(0)}$ is defined in terms of the state-specific rate coefficients as follows

$$k_{\text{rec},c}^{d\,(0)}(T) = \sum_{i} k_{\text{rec},ci}^{d\,(0)}(T) \tag{96}$$

and depends on the gas temperature T only. One should keep in mind that the superscript "0" in the notations for the state-to-state rate coefficients indicates that they are calculated by averaging the corresponding inelastic collision cross sections with the Maxwell–Boltzmann distribution over the velocity and rotational energy. The relations connecting the multi-temperature rate coefficients of forward and backward reactions can be obtained applying the microscopic detailed balance relations for the collision cross sections. For bimolecular reactions we find

$$k_{c'c}^{d'd\,(0)}(T,T_1^{c'},T_1^{d'}) = \frac{1}{Z_{c'}^{vibr}(T,T_1^{c'})Z_{d'}^{vibr}(T,T_1^{d'})} \sum_{iki'k'} s_{i'}^{c'} s_{k'}^{d'} \exp\left(-\frac{i'_{c'}\varepsilon_1^{c'}}{kT_1^{c'}} - \right.$$

$$\left. - \frac{k'_{d'}\varepsilon_1^{d'}}{kT_1^{d'}} - \frac{\varepsilon_{i'}^{c'} - i'_{c'}\varepsilon_1^{c'}}{kT} - \frac{\varepsilon_{k'}^{d'} - k'_{d'}\varepsilon_1^{d'}}{kT}\right) k_{ci,c'i'}^{dk,d'k'\,(0)} K_{c'i',ci}^{d'k',dk\,(0)}(T), \tag{97}$$

whereas for dissociation-recombination we can write

$$k_{rec,c}^{d\,(0)}(T) = \sum_i k_{rec,ci}^{d\,(0)}(T) = \sum_i k_{ci,diss}^{d\,(0)}(T) K_{rec-diss,ci}^{d\,(0)}(T). \tag{98}$$

In these formulae, the ratios for the state-to-state rate coefficients $K_{c'i',ci}^{d'k',dk\,(0)}(T)$, $K_{rec-diss,ci}^{d\,(0)}(T)$ are defined in (74), (75).

In the zero-order approximation, $R_c^{w(0)}$ includes the vibrational distributions (83) and the state-to-state rate coefficients of VV_2, VT vibrational energy transitions and chemical reactions.

If anharmonic effects are neglected then the Boltzmann vibrational distributions with the vibrational temperature T_v^c are valid, and the multi-temperature rate coefficients of the reactions (93)–(95) take the form

$$k_{cc'}^{dd'\,(0)}(T,T_v^c,T_v^d) = \frac{1}{Z_c^{vibr}(T_v^c)Z_d^{vibr}(T_v^d)} \times$$

$$\times \sum_{iki'k'} s_i^c s_k^d \exp\left(-\frac{\varepsilon_i^c}{kT_v^c} - \frac{\varepsilon_k^d}{kT_v^d}\right) k_{ci,c'i'}^{dk,d'k'\,(0)}(T), \tag{99}$$

if d is a molecule,

$$k_{cc'}^{dd'\,(0)}(T,T_v^c) = \frac{1}{Z_c^{vibr}(T_v^c)} \sum_{ii'} s_i^c \exp\left(-\frac{\varepsilon_i^c}{kT_v^c}\right) k_{ci,c'i'}^{dd'\,(0)}(T), \tag{100}$$

if d is an atom, and

$$k_{c,\text{diss}}^{d}(T,T_v^c) = \frac{1}{Z_c^{vibr}(T_v^c)} \sum_{i} s_i^c \exp\left(-\frac{\varepsilon_i^c}{kT_v^c}\right) k_{ci,\text{diss}}^{d\,(0)}(T). \tag{101}$$

For the calculation of two-temperature dissociation rate coefficients in the most studies (see Marrone & Treanor (1963); Phys-Chem (2002))), the two-temperature dissociation rate coefficient k_{diss}^d is associated with the equilibrium averaged coefficient $k_{diss,eq}^d$ by introducing the two-temperature non-equilibrium factor $Z(T,T_1,U)$ rather than the state-to-state factor $Z_i(T,U)$:

$$k_{diss}^d = Z(T,T_1,U) k_{diss,eq}^d(T). \tag{102}$$

where

$$Z(T,T_1,U) = \frac{1}{n_{\text{m}}} \sum_i n_i Z_i(T,U). \tag{103}$$

Using the Treanor distribution (83) for n_i, the factor Z is given by the relation

$$Z(T,T_1,U) = \frac{Z^{vibr}(T)}{Z^{vibr}(-U)Z^{vibr}(T,T_1)} \sum_i s_i \exp\left[\frac{i\varepsilon_1}{k}\left(\frac{1}{T}-\frac{1}{T_1}\right)+\frac{\varepsilon_i}{kU}\right]. \quad (104)$$

For the harmonic oscillator model, the non-equilibrium factor is specified by the vibrational temperature T_v and can be calculated using the expression:

$$Z(T,T_v,U) = \frac{Z^{vibr}(T)Z^{vibr}(T_f)}{Z^{vibr}(-U)Z^{vibr}(T_v)}, \quad (105)$$

where the effective temperature T_f is defined as

$$T_f = \left(\frac{1}{T_v} - \frac{1}{T} - \frac{1}{U}\right)^{-1},$$

Figure 2 presents the temperature dependence of the non-equilibrium factor $Z(T, T_1, U)$ in nitrogen for fixed vibrational temperature values. The non equilibrium factor is calculated for both anharmonic (104) and harmonic (105) oscillator models. We can see that for minor deviations from the equilibrium ($T_1/T \sim 1$), both models yield similar results, whereas for the ratio T_1/T essentially different from unity, the values of Z for harmonic and anharmonic oscillators differ considerably. In particular, for the selected dissociation model, the non-equilibrium factor and hence the dissociation rate coefficient of harmonic oscillators at $T_1/T > 1$ significantly exceed Z and k^d_{diss}, respectively, when calculated for anharmonic oscillators. For $T_1/T < 1$, the use of the harmonic oscillator model yields lower Z and k^d_{diss} than those obtained taking into account anharmonic effects.

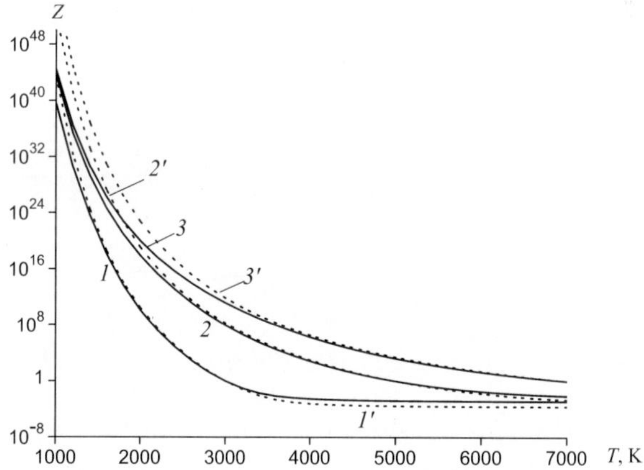

Fig. 2. The non-equilibrium factor Z in N_2 as a function of temperature T for fixed temperatures T_1 and $U = D/(6k)$. The solid lines represent anharmonic oscillators, dashed — harmonic oscillators. The curves *1, 1'* — $T_1 = 3000$; *2, 2'* — $T_1 = 5000$; *3, 3'* — $T_1 = 7000$ K.

Note in addition that the ratio of the dissociation and recombination rate coefficients $K_{\text{rec–diss}}$ under the non-equilibrium conditions can also be expressed in terms of the averaged non-equilibrium factor:

$$K_{rec-diss} = \frac{k^d_{rec}}{k^d_{diss}} = \frac{1}{Z} K^{eq}_{rec-diss}(T), \tag{106}$$

where $K^{eq}_{rec-diss}(T)$ is the ratio of the dissociation and recombination rate coefficients in a thermal equilibrium gas. Calculating Z from the state-to-state or quasi-stationary vibrational distributions n_i/n for various dissociation models, we can find $K_{rec-diss}$ under thermal non-equilibrium conditions and estimate its deviation from the equilibrium constant.

The equations of non-equilibrium reacting flows derived in the state-to-state, multi-temperature and one-temperature approaches were applied for calculations of distributions and macroscopic parameters in particular flows of air components behind shock waves, in nozzles, in non-equilibrium boundary layer (see Nagnibeda & Kustova (2009) and references in this book). On the basis of obtained distributions, global reaction rates (92) were calculated in relaxation zone behind the shock wave Kustova & Nagnibeda (2000) and in nozzle expansion Kustova et al. (2003) in different approaches. The results obtained for the relaxation zone behind the shock wave at the following free stream conditions: $T_0 = 293$ K, $p_0 = 100$ Pa, $M_0 = 15$ are presented in Fig. 3.

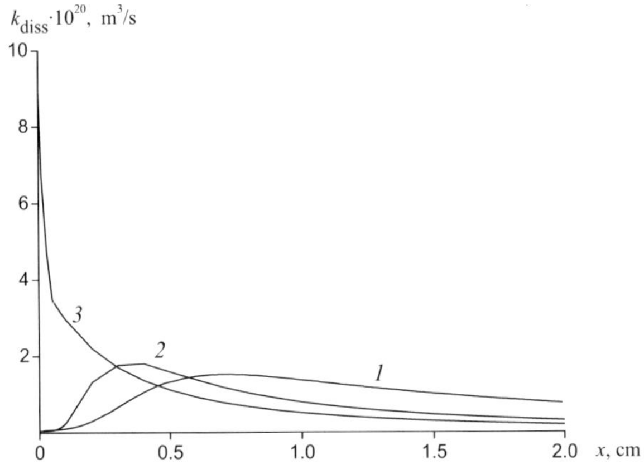

Fig. 3. The averaged dissociation rate coefficient $k^{N_2}_{diss}$ as a function of x. Curves *1, 2, 3* are, respectively, for the state-to-state, two-temperature, and one-temperature approaches.

It is seen that the one-temperature model describes the behavior of the dissociation rate coefficient inadequately, particularly close to the shock front. The two-temperature approach provides more realistic values for the dissociation rate coefficient, overestimating however $k^{N_2}_{diss}$ in comparison to the state-to-state approximation at $x < 0.5$ cm.

The averaged dissociation rate coefficient k^{mol}_{diss} calculated for O_2/O and N_2/N mixtures in a conic nozzle in four approaches using state-to-state, multi-temperature and one-temperature distributions, is presented in Fig. 4. The following conditions in the throat are considered: for O_2/O mixture, $T_* = 4000$ K, $p_* = 1$ atm; for N_2/N mixture, $T_* = 7000$ K, $p_* = 1$ atm. Two kinds of multi-temperature distributions are applied: the Boltzmann distribution for harmonic

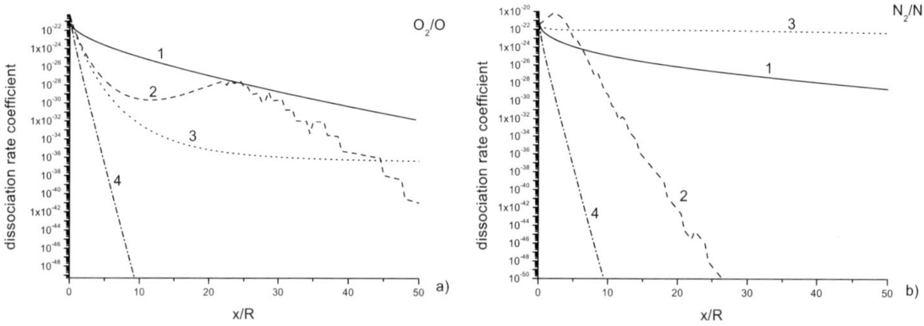

Fig. 4. Averaged dissociation rate coefficient $k_{diss}^{(mol)}$ (m^3/s) versus x/R in a conic nozzle. **(a)** O_2/O, $T_* = 4000$ K, $p_* = 1$ atm; **(b)** N_2/N, $T_* = 7000$ K, $p_* = 1$ atm. Curves 1: state-to-state model; 2: two-temperature anharmonic oscillator model; 3: two-temperature harmonic oscillator model; 4: one-temperature model.

oscillators and a complex distribution for anharmonic oscillators studied in Kustova et al. (2003). One can see a quite strong influence of the kinetic model on the averaged dissociation rate coefficients, all quasi-stationary models give the values of k_{diss}^{mol} rather far from those obtained in the rigorous state-to-state approximation, the same effect is obtained for k_{diss}^{at}. In all considered cases, k_{diss}^{at} is higher than k_{diss}^{mol}, i.e., atoms are more efficient as partners in the dissociation process.

5. Conclusions

In this Chapter, the theoretical models for non-equilibrium chemical kinetics in multi-component reacting gas flows are proposed on the basis of three approaches of the kinetic theory. In the frame of the one-temperature approximation the chemical kinetics in thermal equilibrium flows or deviating weakly from thermal equilibrium is studied. The coupling of chemical kinetics and fluid dynamics equations is considered in the Euler and Navier-Stokes approximations. Chemical kinetics in vibrationally non-equilibrium flows is considered on the basis of the state-to-state and multi-temperature approaches. Different models for vibrational-chemical coupling in the flows of multi-component mixtures are derived. The influence of non-equilibrium distributions on reaction rates in the flows behind shock waves and in nozzle expansion is demonstrated.

6. Acknowledgements

We are grateful to the Russian Foundation for Basic Research (Grant 11-01-00408) and Ministry of Education and Science of RF (Contract 13.G25.31.0076) for the support of this study.

7. References

Alexeev, B., Chikhaoui, A. & Grushin, I. (1994). Application of the generalized Chapman-Enskog method to the transport-coefficients calculation in a reacting gas mixture, *Phys. Review E* 49: 2809.

Alexeev, B. & Grushin, I. (1994). *Transport Processes in Reacting Gases and Plasma*, Energoatomizdat, Moscow.

Aliat, A. (2008). State-to-state dissociation–recombination and chemical exchange rate coefficients in excited diatomic gas flows, *Physica A* 387: 4163–4182.

Armenise, I., Capitelli, M., Colonna, G. & Gorse, C. (1996). Nonequilibrium vibrational kinetics in the boundary layer of re-entering bodies, *J. Thermophys. Heat Transfer* 10(3): 397–405.

Armenise, I., Capitelli, M. & Gorse, C. (1995). On the coupling of non-equilibrium vibrational kinetics and dissociation-recombination processes in the boundary layer surrounding an hypersonic reentry vehicle, *in* J. Hunt (ed.), *Aerothermodynamics for Space Vehicles*, ESA Publication Division, ESTEC, Noordwijk, The Netherlands.

Belouaggadia, N. & Brun, R. (1997). Chemical rate constants in nonequilibrium flows, *AIAA Paper* 97-2555.

Birely, J. & Lyman, J. (1975). Effect of reagent vibrational energy on measured reaction rate constants, *J. Photochem.* 4: 269.

Bose, D. & Candler, G. (1996). Thermal rate constants of the N_2+O→ NO+N reaction using *ab initio* $^3A''$ *and* $^3A'$ potential energy surfaces, *J. Chem. Phys.* 104(8): 2825.

Candler, G., Olejniczak, J. & Harrold, B. (1997). Detailed simulation of nitrogen dissociation in stagnation regions, *Phys. Fluids* 9(7): 2108–2117.

Capitelli, M., Armenise, I. & Gorse, C. (1997). State-to-state approach in the kinetics of air components under re-entry conditions, *J. Thermophys. Heat Transfer* 11(4): 570–578.

Capitelli, M., Ferreira, C., Gordiets, B. & Osipov, A. (2000). *Plasma Kinetics in Atmospheric Gases*, Vol. 31 of *Springer series on atomic, optical and plasma physics*, Springer-Verlag, Berlin.

Chikhaoui, A., Dudon, J., Genieys, S., Kustova, E. & Nagnibeda, E. (2000). Multi-temperature kinetic model for heat transfer in reacting gas mixture, *Phys. Fluids* 12(1): 220–232.

Chikhaoui, A., Dudon, J., Kustova, E. & Nagnibeda, E. (1997). Transport properties in reacting mixture of polyatomic gases, *Physica A* 247(1-4): 526–552.

Ern, A. & Giovangigli, V. (1994). *Multicomponent Transport Algorithms*, Lect. Notes Phys., Series monographs, M24, Springer-Verlag.

Ern, A. & Giovangigli, V. (1998). The kinetic chemical equilibrium regime, *Physica A* 260: 49–72.

Esposito, F., Capitelli, M. & Gorse, C. (2000). Quasi-classical dynamics and vibrational kinetics in $N_2(v) - N$ system, *Chem. Phys.* 257: 193–202.

Esposito, F., Capitelli, M., Kustova, E. & Nagnibeda, E. (2000). Rate coefficients for the reaction N_2(i)+N=3N: a comparison of trajectory calculations and the Treanor-Marrone model., *Chem. Phys. Lett.* 330: 207–211.

Ferziger, J. & Kaper, H. (1972). *Mathematical Theory of Transport Processes in Gases*, North-Holland, Amsterdam, London.

Gardiner, W. (ed.) (1984). *Combustion Chemistry*, Springer-Verlag.

Gilibert, M., Aguilar, A., Gonzales, M., Mota, F. & Sayos, R. (1992). Dynamics of the $N(^4S_u) + NO(X^2\Pi) \rightarrow N_2(X^1\Sigma_g^+) + O(^3P_g)$ atmospheric reaction on the $^3A''$ ground potential energy surface. I. Analytical potential energy surface and preliminary quasiclassical trajectory calculation, *J. Chem. Phys.* 97: 5542–5552.

Gilibert, M., Aguilar, A., Gonzales, M. & Sayos, R. (1993b). A quasiclassical trajectory study of the effect of the initial rovibrational level and relative translational energy on the dynamics of the $N(^4S_u) + O_2(^3\Sigma_g^-) \rightarrow NO(^2\Pi_u) + O(^3P_g)$ atmospheric reaction on the $^2A'$ ground potential energy surface, *Chem. Phys.* 178: 287–303.

Gordiets, B., Osipov, A. & Shelepin, L. (1988). *Kinetic Processes in Gases and Molecular Lasers*, Gordon and Breach Science Publishers, Amsterdam.

Knab, O. (1996). A physically consistent vibration-chemistry-vibration coupling model, *in* M. Capitelli (ed.), *Molecular Physics and Hypersonic Flows*, Kluwer Acad. Publishers, Netherlands, pp. 691–702.

Knab, O., Frühauf, H. & Messerschmid, E. (1995). Theory and validation of the physically consistent coupled vibration-chemistry-vibration model, *J. Thermophys. Heat Transfer* 9(2): 219–226.

Kondratiev, V. & Nikitin, E. (1974). *Kinetics and Mechanism of Gas Phase Reactions*, Nauka, Moscow.

Kuščer, I. (1991). Dissociation and recombination in an inhomogeneous gas, *Physica A* 176: 542–556.

Kustova, E. (2009). On the role of bulk viscosity and relaxation pressure in non-equilibrium flows, *in* T. Abe (ed.), *Rarefied Gas Dynamics: 26th International Symposium*, Vol. 1084 of *AIP Conference Proceedings*, pp. 807–812.

Kustova, E. & Nagnibeda, E. (1998). Transport properties of a reacting gas mixture with strong vibrational and chemical nonequilibrium, *Chem. Phys.* 233: 57–75.

Kustova, E. & Nagnibeda, E. (2000). The influence of the state-to-state distributions behind shock wave on the dissociation rates, *in* G. Ball, R. Hillier & G. Roberts (eds), *Proc. of the 22d International Symposium on Shock Waves*, Vol. 1, University of Southhampton, Southhampton, UK. 783–788.

Kustova, E. & Nagnibeda, E. (2011). Different approaches for modelling of heat transfer in non-equilibrium reacting gas flows, *in* A. Ahsan (ed.), *Evaporation, Condensation and Heat transfer*, InTech, ISBN: 978-953-307-583-9, Available from: http://www.intechopen.com/articles/show/title/different-approaches-for-modelling-of-heat-transfer-in-non-equilibrium-reacting-gas-flows, pp. 439–464.

Kustova, E., Nagnibeda, E., Alexandrova, T. & Chikhaoui, A. (2003). Non-equilibrium dissociation rates in expanding flows, *Chem. Phys. Lett.* 377(5-6): 663–671.

Kustova, E., Nagnibeda, E. & Chauvin, A. (1999). State-to-state nonequilibrium reaction rates, *Chem. Phys.* 248(2-3): 221–232.

Kustova, E., Nagnibeda, E. & Giordano, D. (January 2008). Mutual influence between flow compressibility and chemical-reaction rates in gas mixtures, *Esa str-255*, ESA Communication Production Office, ESTEC, Noordwijk, The Netherlands.

Ludwig, G. & Heil, M. (1960). Boundary layer theory with dissociation and ionization, *Advances in Applied Mechanics*, Vol. VI, Academic Press, New York.

Marrone, P. & Treanor, C. (1963). Chemical relaxation with preferential dissociation from excited vibrational levels, *Phys. Fluids* 6(9): 1215.

Nagnibeda, E. & Kustova, E. (2009). *Nonequilibrium Reacting Gas Flows. Kinetic Theory of Transport and Relaxation Processes*, Springer-Verlag, Berlin, Heidelberg.

Osipov, A. (1966). Thermal dissociation of diatomic molecules at high temperatures, *Teor. Exp. Khim.* 2(11): 649.

Park, C. (1990). *Nonequilibrium Hypersonic Aerothermodynamics*, J.Wiley and Sons, New York, Chichester, Brisbane, Toronto, Singapore.

Phys-Chem (2002). *Physical and Chemical Processes in Gas Dynamics: Cross Sections and Rate Constants for Physical and Chemical Processes. Volume I*, Vol. 196 of *Progress in Astronautics and Aeronautics.*

Phys-Chem (2004). *Physical and Chemical Processes in Gas Dynamics: Physical and Chemical Kinetics and Thermodynamics. Volume II*, Vol. 197 of *Progress in Astronautics and Aeronautics*.

Polanyi, J. (1972). Some concepts in reaction dynamics, *Acc. Chem. Res.* 5: 161–168.

Present, R. (1960). Chapman-Enskog method in chemical kinetics, *J. Chem. Phys.* 48: 4875–4877.

Prigogine, I. & Xhrouet, E. (1949). On the perturbation of Maxwell distribution function by chemical reaction in gases, *Physica* 15: 913–932.

Rydalevskaya, M. (1977). Formal kinetic description of gas mixtures with dissociation and recombination, *Aerodinamika Razrezhennykh Gazov*, Vol. IX, Leningrad University Press, Leningrad. (in Russian).

Seror, S., Druguet, M., Schall, E. & Zeitoun, D. (1997). A new vibration-exchange reaction coupling model for hypersonic air flows, *AIAA Paper* 97-2556.

Shizgal, B. & Karplus, M. (1970). Nonequilibrium contributions to the rate of reaction. I. Perturbation of the velocity distribution function, *J. Chem. Phys.* 52: 4262–4278.

Stupochenko, Y., Losev, S. & Osipov, A. (1967). *Relaxation in Shock Waves*, Springer-Verlag, Berlin, Heidelberg, New York.

Treanor, C., Rich, I. & Rehm, R. (1968). Vibrational relaxation of anharmonic oscillators with exchange dominated collisions, *J. Chem. Phys.* 48: 1798.

5

Model Reduction Techniques for Chemical Mechanisms

Terese Løvås
Department of Energy and Process Engineering
Norwegian University of Science and Technology
Norway

1. Introduction

To be able to meet the increasing demands for efficiency in energy producing systems (engines, turbines and furnaces), changes in the geometry of combustion devices or fuel composition are necessary. Such changes should be based on a thorough understanding of both the physical and chemical processes involved. Today, computer simulations are one of the most important tools for research to address these issues. This is increasingly employed for testing and characterizing the many features of the combustion process, along with or sometimes replacing the considerably more expensive experiments. Numerous types of reliable software are available for simulations of car engines, gas turbines, heaters and boilers. However, one limitation in using computer simulations is the degree to which one is forced to rely on the available computer capacity. Since most cases of combustion involve turbulent processes and numerous chemical reactions, this can be a serious drawback if one wishes to carry out a detailed simulation. Codes for turbulent flow situations are developed to account for turbulent motion between small regions, often called cells, where combustion within the cell is assumed to be homogenous. To deal with complex interaction between the physical and chemical processes in reactive systems, it is necessary to find methods that simplify modeling in such a way that it becomes both more comprehensible and practically useful.

The starting point for any reduction of chemical model is the detailed mechanism itself. Detailed chemical mechanisms have been investigated extensively during the history of combustion physics since the chemistry involved plays a key role in the outcome of any combustion process. By understanding the chemistry one can predict the rate of production and consumption of different species and thus also predict the total change in enthalpy during the combustion process. This in turn provides the values for the energy output, the end gas temperature and the emission characteristics allowing one to describe the overall combustion system.

The chemical system consists of a mechanism containing a set of differential equations representing the evolution of the concentrations of the individual species during the combustion process, thus representing the species conservation equation. The system itself is most often described in terms of molar fractions, X_i, or mass fractions, Y_i, of the following form:

$$\frac{\partial \mathbf{Y}}{\partial t} = \mathbf{P}(\mathbf{Y},\mathbf{u},\mathrm{T}) + \boldsymbol{\omega}(\mathbf{Y},\mathrm{T}) \tag{1}$$

where **P(Y,u,T)** represents the spatial differential operator (advection, convection and diffusion; it is thus depending on the velocity field, **u**, and the temperature, T) and ω**(Y,T)** represents the chemical source term, which includes chemical production and consumption of the species. **Y** is the N_S-dimensional vector of mass fractions of a mechanism containing N_S species.

A long list of different detailed mechanisms have been presented in literature, ranging from simple hydrogen-oxygen mechanisms (Lewis & von Elbe, 1987);(Li et al., 2004) to complex fuel mechanisms which involve hundreds of species that interact in thousands of reactions (Côme et al., 1996) or even thousand of species reacting in tens of thousands of reactions (Westbrook et al., 2009). Discussions related to the nature of these detailed mechanisms in the literature is dating back to the beginning of combustion science. Some of these mechanisms have been developed and extended by hand, the validation of the detailed mechanism coming through experimental measurements, a very time consuming procedure. One very well known mechanisms for methane kinetics is the GRI-Mech 3.0 mechanism (Bowman et al., 2004). This mechanism is the result of collaboration between several groups and is under constant revision. This mechanism contains 49 species and considers 277 reactions for the C_1 chain only.

Detailed mechanisms can also be obtained through an automatic generation process carried out by computer software. One way to automatically generate detailed mechanisms is described in works by Blurock (Blurock, 1995); (Blurock, 2000). Large and detailed chemical mechanisms including species larger than C12-hydrocarbons are generated by the use of *reaction classes* associated with the reacting substructure in the species and a set of reaction constants. As Blurock (Blurock, 2000) indicates this "allows for a wide variety of arbitrarily branched and substituted species far beyond straight-chained hydrocarbons". This is an advantage when performing numeric computations of the combustion process, since only the reacting part of a class of species is of importance for the computations. This allows a symbolically generated mechanism to be studied that is substantially larger and more detailed than mechanisms previously carried out by hand. Mechanism generation tools are also freely available, such as the "Reaction Mechanism Generator" (RGM) developed by W. Green and co-workers (Green et al., 2011). This is a very extensive tool which generates mechanisms based on knowledge on how molecules react through elementary reactions.

As much as such tools are needed to develop mechanisms for complex chemical processes such as for e.g. combustion of bio-fuels from various biomass sources, the models become increasingly unmanageable due to their size. The detailed mechanism is therefore the object of different reduction procedures aimed at obtaining smaller mechanisms to be used in more complex simulations of combustion systems. The reduced mechanisms can be and to a large extent have been, worked out by hand on the basis of the total sum of the experience and knowledge available. This can result in compact and accurate mechanisms subsequently validated by experimental data. However, these mechanisms are often restricted to a narrow range of conditions. It is advantageous therefore to find general procedures that can reduce mechanisms automatically by using physical quantities associated with different reactions and species. Through identifying a set of selection criteria it is possible to detect species and reactions that play a minor role in the overall reaction process and can thus be excluded from the mechanism. This can be done by use of *reaction flow* and *sensitivity analysis* or by using *directed relation graph* (DRG) methods, which result in what is hereafter referred to as a skeletal mechanism.

Furthermore, mathematical procedures can be applied to the detailed mechanism or the skeletal mechanism which reduces the mechanism even more. These mathematical procedures do not exclude species, but rather the species concentrations are calculated by the use of simpler and less time-consuming algebraic equations or they are tabulated as functions of a few preselected progress variables. The part of the mechanism that is left for detailed calculations is substantially smaller than the original mechanism. These methods often make use of the wide range of time scales and are thus called *time scale separation methods*. The most common methods are those of (i) *Intrinsic Low Dimensional Manifolds* (ILDM), (ii) *Computational Singular Perturbation*(CSP), and (iii) *level of importance* (LOI) analysis, in which one employs the Quasy Steady State Assumption (QSSA) or a partial equilibrium approximation (e.g. rate-controlled constraints equilibria, RCCE) to treat the steady state or equilibrated species.

In Figure (1) a schematic overview of the different reduction paths is laid out. As can be seen, different paths and possibilities for reducing the mechanisms are possible. Which method is adopted is determined mainly by the nature of the problem to be solved. The starting point is a detailed mechanism generated by hand or by the software available and validated for the current conditions. These mechanisms can contain up to hundreds of active species and thus need to be reduced for practical use. However, smaller detailed mechanisms can successfully be applied in stationary combustion situations, and in situations in which speed-up is of less concern. This could be the development of flamelet libraries or simple zone models, for example. Larger mechanisms are the object of reaction flow and sensitivity analysis in which minor and major pathways of the mechanism are identified. Species that are only involved in the minor paths and do not appear as species sensitive to the governing parameters, are selected for removal from the system. The result is a smaller mechanism containing the major pathways and the sensitive species, termed a skeletal mechanism. This mechanism is complete in the sense that it can be applied in combustion simulations. For reasons of speed-up it is favorable for use in stationary combustion situations. If the mechanism is small enough, it can also be applied in non-stationary situations such as in the calculation of interactive flamelets and transported probability density functions (PDF) for turbulent motion simulations. However, these calculations require very compact mechanisms and in most cases a further reduction through a lifetime analysis is necessary. This reduces the number of active species in the mechanism and accounts for the contributions of the remaining species selected as steady state species. The resulting reduced mechanism can be successfully applied in flow codes, and is applicable in simpler systems for speed-up reasons as well. The lifetime analysis and the resulting reduced mechanism is employed when on-line reduction is carried out, since the number of active species involved can change during the computational run.

In the following, reaction flow analysis, sensitivity analysis and the directed relation graph method will be presented as static and dynamic reduction procedures. Thereafter will the main features of ILDM (including extensions such as flamelet generated manifolds (FGM) and reaction-diffusion manifolds (REDIM)), CSP and the LOI be discussed, including the fundamentals of the quasi steady state elimination procedure and the rate-controlled constrained equilibria (RCCE) approach.

2. Static and dynamic analysis tools

The static and dynamic analysis tools available provide important information that is useful for reduction procedures and includes reaction flow and sensitivity analysis procedures. Reaction flow analysis detects minor and major flows in the reaction system, where the species involved in the minor flows can be neglected in further investigation. Under given physical

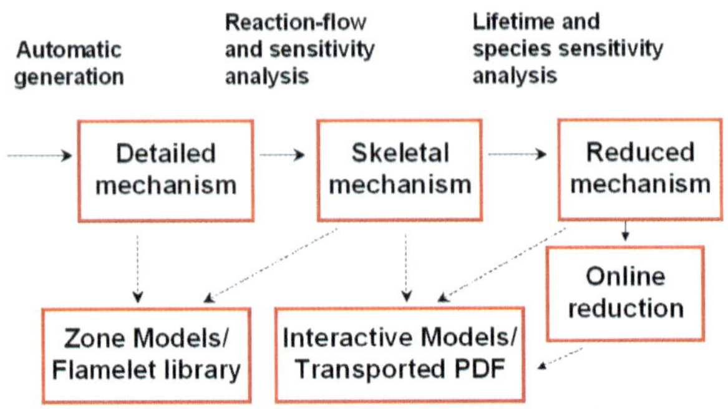

Fig. 1. A figure over the reduction methods and their relations. The dashed lines represent suggested uses of the different mechanisms. As shown in the figure, reduced mechanisms are applicable to both static and dynamic problems. Detailed mechanisms, in contrast, are not practical for dynamic systems.

conditions these will represent static properties of the mechanism. However, some species in the minor flows may exhibit a strong influence on the quantities under investigation and should thus not be neglected. These reactions and species are found through sensitivity analysis, in which the dynamic properties of the system are investigated. This can be formalized into one reduction tool called the directed relation graph (DRG) methodology. These three methods will now be discussed below.

2.1 Reaction flow analysis

Reaction flow analysis describes the importance of reaction paths in the mechanism under specified conditions. It is performed by calculating the transfer rate of certain atomic species such as C,O, N and H between molecular species. The flow of atoms between the reacting molecules is used as a measure of the relevance of the species in the reaction mechanism. The reaction flow of atomic species a between species i and species j can be described very simply by (Nilsson, 2011)

$$f_{ij}^{a} = \sum_{k=1}^{N_R} r_k (n_i^a \nu_{ik}'' - n_j^a \nu_{jk}'), \tag{2}$$

where the sum is taken over the number of reactions N_R. n_i^a and n_j^a are the numbers of the atom a in molecule i and j, and ν_{ik}'' and ν_{jk}' are the stoichiometric coefficients for the molecules i and j in reaction k. r_k is the reaction rate, ν_{jk}' and ν_{ik}'' are the stoichiometric coefficients of the reactants and the products in reaction k.

A more adequate method of determining the reaction flow, is described in more detail by Soyhan et al. (Soyhan et al., 2001); (Soyhan et al., 2001) and optimized further . In this work, forward and backward reactions are treated separately so as to capture reversible reaction pairs in which the flow of atoms is high in both directions but where the net flow is not necessarily high. This procedure results in the two new flow parameters shown below in which f_{ij}^a is the normalized flow of atom a by the formation of species i from species j relative to the total production of species i, and c_{ij}^a is the flow of atom a by the consumption of species i to species j relative to the total consumption of species i:

$$f_{ij}^a = \frac{\sum_{k=1}^{N_R} r_k \nu'_{jk} \nu''_{ik} \frac{n_i^a}{\triangle n_k^a}}{\sum_{k=1}^{N_R} r_k \nu'_{jk}}, \tag{3}$$

$$c_{ij}^a = \frac{\sum_{k=1}^{N_R} r_k \nu''_{jk} \nu'_{ik} \frac{n_i^a}{\triangle n_k^a}}{\sum_{k=1}^{N_R} r_k \nu''_{jk}}. \tag{4}$$

The number of atoms n_j^a is now normalized to the total number of atoms a transported in the reaction $\triangle n_k^a = \sum_{i=1}^{N_S} n_k^a(\nu''_{ik} - \nu'_{ik})$. The flow parameters are normalized to the total formation or consumption rate of species i in order to achieve a non-dimensional range between 0 and 1 for the flow parameters.

An example of the scheme of such an analysis is given in Figure (2) which shows the flow of C atoms in a reaction mechanism for a CH_4-fueled homogeneous reactor. This analysis was performed under specific conditions in which the engine speed was set to 1400 revolutions per minute (RPM), the fuel-air ratio was set to 0.412 and the compression ratio was set to 17.30. In the figure, the major reaction flows are marked by thick arrows and the minor flows by thinner arrows.

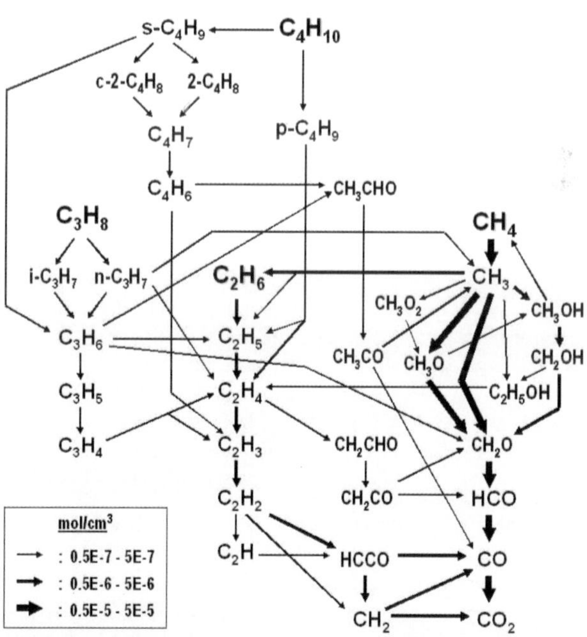

Fig. 2. Reaction flows of C atoms in a natural-gas mechanism for CH_4 as fuel in a homogeneous reactor (Nilsson, 2011).

Figure (2) shows that the major paths represents the high-temperature hydrocarbon oxidation of CH_4 through the relatively stable radicals C_2H_5 and CH_3 shown in the lower right corner of the figure. Flows with a lower transport rate than 5×10^{-7} mol/cm^3 can be considered minor flows. These are shown for the most part in the upper left corner of Figure (2). These flows can thus be neglected in further calculations. Note that the situation is different if natural gas is used as a fuel, in which some of the fuel components may be selected for removal. Thus some of the species involved in minor flows may be important for the desired results and should be retained in the reaction mechanism. These are selected by the sensitivity analysis, as described below.

2.2 Sensitivity analysis

Sensitivity analysis involves investigating the change in a quantity of interest due to small changes in the controlling parameters. Investigating this is of interest in itself for gaining insight into the reaction model. In addition, it is a very useful tool for reduction of reaction mechanisms. After the minor flows have been detected by reaction flow analysis, it is important to ensure that the species involved in the minor flows do not influence the result significantly, in which case they should not be excluded in the further calculations. In local sensitivity analysis, this is described by the partial derivative of the investigated quantity with respect to the controlling parameters. Emanating from Equation (1), investigation of how the concentration of a species i is influenced by a perturbation $\mathbf{\Delta}k$ of the rate coefficient k can be expressed by differentiating the original set of chemical differential equations with respect to k_j and expanding the right hand side giving

$$\frac{d}{dt}\frac{\partial \mathbf{Y}}{\partial k_j} = \frac{\partial \mathbf{P}}{\partial \mathbf{Y}}\frac{\partial \mathbf{Y}}{\partial k_j} + \frac{\partial \mathbf{P}}{\partial k_j} + \frac{\partial \omega(\mathrm{t})}{\partial \mathbf{Y}} + \frac{\partial \mathbf{Y}}{\partial k_j}\frac{\partial \omega(\mathrm{t})}{\partial k_j}, \quad j = 1, ..., N_S. \tag{5}$$

If considering a homogeneous reaction system, P$\equiv$ 0, the equation above results in the following expression:

$$\frac{d}{dt}\frac{\partial \mathbf{Y}}{\partial k_j} - \mathbf{J}(t)\frac{\partial \mathbf{Y}}{\partial k_j} + \frac{\partial \omega(\mathrm{t})}{\partial k_j}, \quad j = 1, ..., N_S, \tag{6}$$

where $\mathbf{J}(t) = \partial\omega(\mathrm{t})/\partial\mathbf{Y}$ is recognized as the Jacobian matrix and the initial condition for $\partial\mathbf{Y}/\partial k_j$ (recognized as the sensitivity matrix) is a vector containing only zeros (Tomlin et al., 1997). In order to solve Equation (6), the concentrations in the original set of equations must be known, which is not always the case. The most efficient way of overcoming this problem is to solve the two systems in succession. This method is called the decoupled direct method. It first takes one step in solving Equation (1) and then performs an equal step in solving Equation (6). This can be done since both sets of differential equations have the same Jacobian matrix $\mathbf{J}$ (Tomlin et al., 1997).

The same method can be applied to investigate the sensitivities of such parameters of the system as the flame temperature for premixed flames or the ignition timing in such ignition systems as in engine simulations as outlined below. The information obtained through this analysis is the basis for reduction of the mechanism. After the sensitivity analysis, the next step is to order the species and select those that are redundant. Tomlin et al. (Tomlin et al., 1997) classifies the species involved in a mechanism into three categories. The *important species* are those needed for the current investigation, such as the reaction products when investigating pollution or the initial reactants defining the fuels. The *necessary species* are those needed to provide for an accurate calculation of the concentration profiles of the important species, of temperature profiles and of other important features. The remaining species are the *redundant species* that are candidates for removal from the mechanisms without loss of important information. Tomlin et al. eliminated a reaction from the mechanisms if the redundant species played simply the role of being reactants in the reaction, since only the reactants are present in the equation for the rate of change of species concentrations. Even if a particular reaction needs to be retained in the mechanism the redundant species can be eliminated from the list of products if it does not violate the conservation of atoms and mass in the calculations.

The approach to finding redundant species described by Tomlin et al. (Tomlin et al., 1997) is to investigate the matrix $\mathbf{J}(t) = \partial\omega(\mathrm{t})/\partial\mathbf{Y}$ (for homogeneous systems; $\mathrm{P}\equiv 0$), where the element $\partial\omega_i/\partial Y_j$ describes the change of the rate of production of species i caused by a change of concentration of species j. A species is considered redundant if a change in its concentration does not affect the rate of production of important species significantly. A slightly different approach is taken by Soyhan et al. who let the sensitivities being transported through the mechanism in the sense that a species is rated according to its own importance and its involvement in producing or consuming important species (Soyhan et al., 1999);(Soyhan et al., 2001). Thus, the method can be considered as representing a simultaneous reaction flow and sensitivity analysis, called *necessity analysis*. First the reaction sensitivity represents a variable ψ's sensitivity towards a chosen reaction coefficient A_k in reaction k is changed by a factor x (e.g. 1 percent):

$$S^r_{\psi k} = \frac{\partial\psi}{\partial A_k} A_k x \tag{7}$$

The species sensitivity can be taken either as the sum of the reaction sensitivities in which the species are involved, or can be derived directly in the same manner as the reaction sensitivity; investigating how much a variable ψ is changed when the concentration of species i is changed by a small factor ϵ_i (again e.g. 1 percent):

$$S^s_{\psi i} = \frac{1}{c_i}\frac{\partial\psi}{\partial\alpha_i} \tag{8}$$

where $S^S_{\psi i}$ contains the information on how sensitive a chosen target variable, ψ, such as the mass fraction of a particular species or temperature, is to the species i. The factor in which the concentrations are allowed to change is small and $\alpha_i = 1 + \epsilon_i$ where ϵ_i is e.g. 1 percent. Therefore, α_i can be considered an error term for the concentrations which become $c_i^* = c_i\alpha_i$.

A species is assigned a relative necessity index which represents how important the species is for changes in variable ψ in relation to the other species. The redundancy index is based on the species sensitivity in the following way:

$$I_i = \max\left(\frac{S^S_{\psi i}}{\max_{k=1,N_s}\left(S^S_{\psi k}\right)}, Z_i\right) \tag{9}$$

where Z_i takes the value 1 or 0 depending on wheather the species has been preselected as an important species (fuel, oxidant etc.). Even if a species has a low necessity it can be assigned a high overall necessity index if there is a significant flow of atoms to or from an important species. The overall necessity is determined as follows:

$$\bar{I}_i = \max\left(I_j f_{ij}^a, \quad I_j c_{ij}^a, \quad I_i; j = 1, N_s, a = 1, N_a\right) \tag{10}$$

where f_{ij}^a and c_{ij}^a, as defined previously, are the flow of atom a by formation or consumption of species i from or to species j. This equation needs to be solved iteratively with a preset value of $\bar{I}_i$. Species with a low overall $\bar{I}_i$ are considered to be redundant. This procedure has been used extensively to perform reduction on large hydrocarbon mechanisms, e.g. up to C-8 reaction chains where together with a lumping procedure the mechanism was reduced from about 246 species to 47 (Zeuch et al., 2008). Also, this reduction procedure is been made available in reaction kinetics simulation tools such as DARS (DARS, 2011) where the reduction is performed entirely automatically. The computed necessity index ranks the species accordingly, and a user set cut-off limit will generate a skeletal mechanism according to desired accuracy of the resulting skeletal mechanism; i.e. the more species which are excluded from the mechanism the less accurate the mechanism will be to predict the combustion process.

2.3 Directed relation graph methodology

The step wise reduction procedure described above can been automated by the use of the Directed Relation Graph method (Lu and Law, 2005);(Lu and Law, 2006). This procedure quantifies the coupling between species, and assigns an "pair wise" error which contains the information of how much error is introduced to a species A by elimination of a species B:

$$r_{AB} \equiv \frac{\max \mid \nu_{Ai}\omega_i\delta_{Bi} \mid}{\max \mid \nu_{Ai}\omega_i \mid}, \delta_{Bi} = \begin{cases} 1 \text{ if the } i\text{th reaction involves B.} \\ 0 \text{ otherwise.} \end{cases} \tag{11}$$

Note that the denominator contains the maximum reaction rate contributing to the production of A, whereas the numerator contains the maximum reaction rate contributing to the production of A that also involves species B . The original formulation used a summation over *all* reactions which did not prove to be efficient when e.g. dealing with larger isomergroups (Luo et al., 2010). This formalism is not unsimilar to Equation (9). However, both the reaction flow and an error estimate are included when the species dependence is expressed in the following *graph* notation:

$$A \rightarrow B \text{ if } r_{AB} > \varepsilon. \tag{12}$$

Species A is thereby connected to species B only if the pair wise error is above a user set error threshold. The starting point if the directed relation graph would be one of the important species, such as the fuel species. When species with low connectivity (below the threshold) is eliminated the result will be a skeletal mechanism similar to what is obtained by a necessity analysis.

This procedure will not be discussed further here, but the DRG methodology has proven to be easy to implement and to fully automate. Hence, it has become very popular to use for reduction of larger mechanisms. In its simplest form DRG has however proved to have some limitations. These have been addressed in extended versions of the procedure. This includes DRG with error propagation (DRGEP) (Pepiot-Desjardins & Pitsch, 2008), DRG aided sensitivity analysis (DRGASA) (Zheng et al., 2007) and DRGEP and sensitivity analysis (Niemeyer et al., 2010). The reader is referred to these works for further discussion.

3. Time scale separation methods

In the following section the methods based on time scale separation analysis will be discussed. Employing these methods relies on the fact that the chemical system consists of a number of species that react with each other on time scales that range over several orders of magnitude. Thus, some of the reactions can be considered as being fast compared with the physical processes involved, such as diffusion, turbulence and other reactions that are considered slow. This is illustrated in Figure (3).

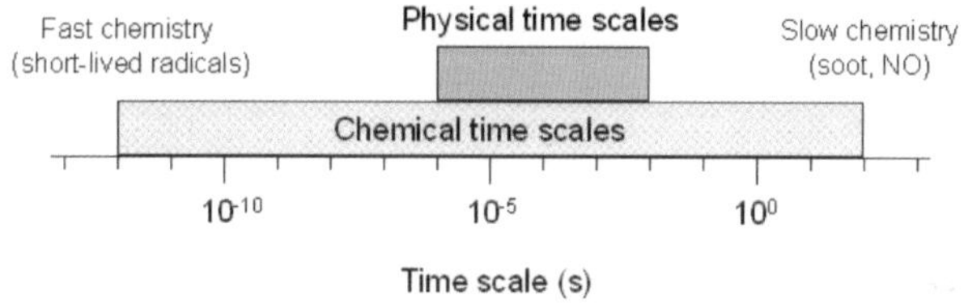

Fig. 3. Comparison of typical chemical and physical time scales. The chemical time scales span several orders of magnitude (Nilsson, 2011).

A time scale separation method makes use of the fact that the physical and chemical time scales have only a limited range of overlap. The time scales of some of the more rapid chemical processes can thus be decoupled and be described in approximate ways by the Quasi Steady State Assumption (QSSA) or partial equilibrium approximations for the selected species. This reduces the species list to only the species left in the set of differential equations. Also, eliminating the fastest time scales in the system solves the numerical stiffness problem that these time scales introduce. Numerical stiffness arises when the iteration over the differential equations need very small steps as some of the terms lead to rapid variations of the solution, typically terms involving the fastest time scales.

Three time-scale separation methods will be described below. These are the Intrinsic Low Dimensional Manifold method (ILDM), Computational Singular Perturbation (CSP), and the lifetime analysis based on the Level Of Importance (LOI).

Since the methods are all concerned with determining the processes involved on the shortest time scales, they have many similarities. Although it could be argued that they in reality are virtually the same, they have different coatings and different ways of presenting the solutions. In the overall picture here one can describe the differences as follows: the key difference between ILDM and CSP is the sub-space created to describe the new manifold. ILDM employs partial equilibrium approximations for the species selected and creates a species sub-space. CSP employs steady state approximations and creates a reaction sub-space. It does not indicate a preference for QSSA as to opposed to partial equilibrium approximation. Including the partial equilibrium approximation in selecting the "steady state" species represents a more general criterion than using only the QSSA (Goussis, 1996). However, this introduces all the species in the stoichiometry vector, often making the algorithm more complicated. The difference between CSP and lifetime analysis is that CSP includes coupled time scales, whereas lifetime analysis assumes that on a short time scale no coupling is significant, it is thus operating with a diagonal Jacobian. Details of this are described below.

Once the "fast" and the "slow" components are identified, several of these methods use the quasi-steady state assumption (QSSA) as the basis for reduction. Together with a chemical equilibrium assumption or as an alternative to it, this procedure makes it possible to mathematically eliminate species from the set of differential equations. They are treated separately through use of approximative algebraic relations. Their concentrations still contribute to the reaction rates of the non-reduced species. The basic idea of developing reduced chemical mechanisms by introducing the assumption of a steady state is not new and has, in fact, been used in chemistry since the 1950s (See (Peters, 1990)) and further references therein). However, not until the early 1990s was this strategy for solving complex chemical problems introduced in combustion physics.

Until rather recently, these reduced schemes were mainly developed by hand using QSSA and an à priori definition of which species were to be considered in steady state, a particularly time-consuming procedure. Before presenting the various time scale separation methods, the basic steps of the QSSA reduction procedure will be presented in the subsection below followed by the theory rate-controlled constraints equilibria (RCCE). Thereafter are the time scale separation methods outlined.

3.1 Manual reduction by means of QSSA

The underlying assumption for QSSA is that some species can be treated as being in steady state. This means that, if one ignores physical terms as convection and diffusion, their concentrations remain constant. It follows then from Equation (1) that the change in species concentration of species i is

$$\frac{dX_i}{dt} = \sum_{k=1}^{r} \nu_{i,k} r_k = \omega_i = 0, \tag{13}$$

where ω_i is the chemical source term and the summation is over all reactions of the product $\nu_{i,k} r_k$. This equation corresponds to Equation (1) for chemical treatment only, where the reaction rate r_k can be expressed by the following general definition:

$$r_k = k_k \prod_{j=1}^{n} X_j^{\nu'_{jk}}, \tag{14}$$

and the net stoichiometric coefficient being $\nu_i = \nu_i'' - \nu_i'$. The physical meaning of this assumption is that the reactions that consume the species are very much faster than the reactions producing the species. Thus, the concentration remain low just as their time derivative.

The H_2-O_2 system will be used as an example (Peters, 1990);(Peters et al., 1993). The reactions needed for the present analysis are (following the numbering in the original mechanism)

$$\begin{array}{llll} H + O_2 & \leftrightarrow OH + O, & (ii) \\ O + H_2 & \leftrightarrow OH + H, & (iii) \\ OH + H_2 & \leftrightarrow H_2O + H, & (iv) \\ H + O_2 + M & \rightarrow HO_2 + M, & (vii) \end{array}$$

where the backward reactions are treated as being separate reactions. Additional reactions in the H_2-O_2 reaction system are also included in the present example:

$$\begin{aligned} OH + OH &\leftrightarrow H_2O + O, && (x) \\ H + HO_2 &\rightarrow OH + OH, && (xi) \\ H + HO_2 &\rightarrow O_2 + H_2, && (xii) \\ OH + HO_2 &\rightarrow H_2O + O_2. && (xiii) \end{aligned}$$

Equation (13) indicated that the time derivatives of all the species concentrations can be expressed in terms of the concentrations of species that consume and that produce that particular species. As noted above, the derivatives not only contain a chemistry-term, but in the case of inhomogeneous systems, can also contain diffusive and convective terms, often being denoted in such cases by the L-operator. Here, only the chemical contribution is included, resulting in the following set of equations:

$$\begin{aligned} \omega_H &= -r_{\text{ii}} + r_{\text{iii}} + r_{\text{iv}} - r_{\text{vii}} - r_{\text{xi}} - r_{\text{xii}}, \\ 0 = \omega_{OH} &= r_{\text{ii}} + r_{\text{iii}} - r_{\text{iv}} - 2r_{\text{x}} + 2r_{\text{xi}} - r_{\text{xiii}}, \\ 0 = \omega_O &= r_{\text{ii}} - r_{\text{iii}} + r_{\text{x}}, \\ \omega_{H_2} &= -r_{\text{iii}} - r_{\text{iv}} + r_{\text{xii}}, \\ \omega_{O_2} &= -r_{\text{ii}} - r_{\text{vii}} + r_{\text{xii}} + r_{\text{xiii}}, \\ \omega_{H_2O} &= r_{\text{iv}} + r_{\text{x}} + r_{\text{xiii}}, \\ 0 = \omega_{HO_2} &= r_{\text{vii}} - r_{\text{xi}} - r_{\text{xii}} - \omega_{\text{xiii}}. \end{aligned} \tag{15}$$

where OH, O and HO_2 are all set to steady state and their derivatives are set equal to zero, transforming the corresponding differential equations conveniently into algebraic relations. Since the system is already reduced, the steady state concentrations can be found. However, in obtaining a set of global reactions and optimizing the reduction, the corresponding number of reaction rates can be eliminate from the system. A rule of thumb is for each species to eliminate the fastest reaction rates at which this species is consumed. This is r_{iv} for OH, r_{iii} for O and r_{xii} for HO_2, them being placed on the right-hand side of the equations and expressed in terms of the remaining reaction rates on the left-hand side (Peters, 1990). However, the reaction rates that are eliminated from the system are arbitrary and result in the same global reactions. After some algebra, the system is as follows:

$$\begin{aligned} \omega_H &= 2r_{\text{ii}} - 2r_{\text{vii}} + 2r_{\text{xi}}, \\ \omega_{H_2} &= -3r_{\text{ii}} + r_{\text{vii}} - 3r_{\text{xi}}, \\ \omega_{O_2} &= -r_{\text{ii}} - r_{\text{xi}}, \\ \omega_{H_2O} &= 2r_{\text{ii}} - 2r_{\text{xi}}. \end{aligned} \tag{16}$$

By arranging the right-hand side so that rates with the same stoichiometric coefficients are added together one obtains

$$\begin{aligned} \omega_H &= 2(r_{\text{ii}} + r_{\text{xi}}) - 2r_{\text{vii}}, \\ \omega_{H_2} &= -3(r_{\text{ii}} + r_{\text{xi}}) + r_{\text{vii}}, \\ \omega_{O_2} &= -(r_{\text{ii}} + r_{\text{xi}}), \\ \omega_{H_2O} &= 2(r_{\text{ii}} + r_{\text{xi}}), \end{aligned} \tag{17}$$

resulting in the following global reactions:

$$\begin{aligned} 3H_2 + O_2 &= 2H + 2H_2O, && \text{I} \\ 2H + M &= H_2 + M, && \text{II} \end{aligned}$$

with the reaction rates being $r_I = (r_{ii} + r_{xi})$ and $r_{II} = r_{vii}$. This procedure shows how a set of eight elementary reactions can be reduced to just two global reactions and two corresponding reaction rates, which are sufficient to describe the system. The resulting system is also called a two-step mechanism.

The computations above are quite straightforward once a choice is made of which species are to be considered to be in steady state. In the H_2-O_2 system, the three species OH, O and HO_2 are conveniently set to steady state. Although, in the manual reduction procedure the choice of steady state species often stems simply from the experience of which species can be approximately calculated. However, the choice is often based on an analysis of the intermediate species' mole fraction. The argument is that no species at high concentration, and no reactant or product species either, can be a steady state candidate. The algorithm is such that the conservation equations are dealt with only for the species included in detail in the mechanism. The steady state species only appear through their contribution to the reaction rates determining the non-steady state species. Thus, species of high concentrations or high enthalpy content need to be kept in the mechanism so as to not violate the conservation of mass fraction and enthalpy. In the case of the methane-air mechanism that was reduced by Peters (Peters, 1990), the computation of mole fractions in a premixed stoichiometric methane-air flame was the basis for defining the steady state species.

In the flame calculations accounting for the physical processes diffusive and convective terms must also be small in order for the differentials to be set equal to zero. Nevertheless, in the reactive inner layer of the flames, the diffusive terms turn out to be dominant as compared with the convective terms. Consequently, since the species concentrations are strongly influenced by the diffusion, obtaining an order-of-magnitude estimate for selection of the steady state species requires that the mole fractions be weighted to the molecular weight of the inert species N_2, W_{N_2}, the resulting weighting factor being

$$\sqrt{W_{N_2}/W_{i,N_2}} \tag{18}$$

where W_{i,N_2} is given by

$$W_{i,N_2} = \frac{2W_i W_{N_2}}{W_i + W_{N_2}}. \tag{19}$$

The H radical, for example, diffuses through the flame quickly and displays a low concentration profile. However, it is not a species in steady state and it is highly sensitive to the desired result. The species for the methane-air flame fall into two distinct groups: those in which the corresponding weighted mole fraction has a value well below 1% and those in which the corresponding weighted mole fraction has a value well above 1%. Thus, the choice is clear, the first group being selected as steady state species candidates.

The final step is to calculate the values of the reaction rates for the species and to then determine their concentrations. The reaction rates are expressed in the form of rate constants, stoichiometric coefficients and concentrations, as defined in Equation (13) and (14). However, the reaction rates also contain concentrations of the steady state species. As shown in Equation (13), these can be calculated from their balance equation with $\omega_i = 0$. The concentration of OH, for example, can be calculated as follows:

$$0 = r_{ii} + r_{iii} - r_{iv} - 2r_x + 2r_{xi} - r_{xiii}, \tag{20}$$

where r_{iv}, r_{ii} and r_{iii} all include both forward and backward reactions. The equation can be solved by setting r_{iv}, for example, on the left-hand side and inserting all the rate constants and concentrations.

A very powerful and important step in the reduction process is the *truncation of the steady state relations,* such as that shown in Equation (20). By investigating the reaction rates, both the forward and the backward rates, for a stoichiometric flame over the typical physical range of calculations one can track down the one or two reaction rates that are dominant. Peters (Peters, 1990) could show that in the case of OH only r_{iv} is dominant, allowing the other reaction rates to be neglected in the further calculations. The advantage of performing truncation is that the most rapid reaction rates are excluded from the system, reducing the stiffness of the problem considerably and enhancing the accuracy. Thus, Equation (20) can easily be solved, the resulting [OH] being found to be

$$[\mathrm{OH}] = \frac{k_{\mathrm{iv}b}[\mathrm{H_2O}][\mathrm{H}]}{k_{\mathrm{iv}f}[\mathrm{H_2}]} \tag{21}$$

Similar calculations for the other steady state species need to be performed. In the next step then these relations are used to calculate the remaining set of differential equations which govern the non-steady state species. The overall reaction rate for each remaining species is thus determined by means of an *inner iteration loop*, a simple fixed-point iteration procedure is often employed. The remaining set of differential equations can be solved in different ways, and several numerical solvers for stiff differential equations are freely available.

This procedure has proven successful, many authors having presented work in which reduced mechanisms resemble detailed mechanisms very closely (See e.g. work presented in (Peters & Rogg, 1993);(Smooke, 1991)). Similarly reduced mechanisms have been produced for a variety of fuels, for example the three-step mechanism for CO-H_2-N_2/air diffusion flames by Chen et. al. (Chen et al., 1993) and four-step mechanisms for both ethylene/air and ethane/air flames by Wang and Rogg (Wang & Rogg, 1993).

Methane is the simplest of the carbon-containing fuels and extensive investigations of the reduced mechanisms for methane-air flames have been carried out, even before hydrogen flames as the C_1 chain provides a lower radical level, steady state relations thus being easier justified. The first reduced mechanisms for methane-air flame combustion originated from a skeletal mechanism consisting of 25 reactions for the C_1 chain, and 61 reactions including the C_2 chain evolved during the 1970-1980s (Kaufman, 1982);(Mauss & Peters, 1993);(Smooke, 1991);(Turns, 2000). A fully detailed mechanism can contain over 40 species and involve some 300 reactions. An example of such a mechanism is the GRI-Mech 3.0 mechanism obtained from Berkeley University (Bowman et al., 2004). Peters (Peters, 1990) and Mauss et al.(Mauss & Peters, 1993) demonstrated the reduction of the skeletal mechanism for methane-air flame combustion by use of the quasi steady state assumption, validating it for the range of lean to stoichiometric mixtures. The mechanism was reduced to a four-step mechanism containing 7 species, the reduction procedure following exactly the same underlying principles as for the H_2-O_2 system described above.

The investigation of higher carbon containing fuels such as acetylene for the purpose of reduction is of considerable importance for soot studies. Ring compounds and their growth through acetylene (C_2H_2) are important features for formation of soot under fuel-rich conditions (Turns, 2000). Mauss et al. (Mauss & Lindstedt, 1993) presented a 7 step reduced mechanism validated for acetylene-air premixed flames which originates from the skeletal mechanism described in Peters and Rogg (Peters & Rogg, 1993), including all 87 reactions for up to C_3−species. With use of the 7 step mechanism, both flame velocities and species concentrations were well predicted as compared to the results for the full mechanism. Some deviations were found in the reaction zone, where a steeper consumption of reactants was obtained for the reduced mechanism. However, this can also result from a steeper temperature profile in the same region, which would enhance the reaction rates. In Lindstedt et al. (Lindstedt & Mauss, 1993) the same mechanism for acetylene formation is applied to a diffusion flame system having 8 additional reaction steps. In the work, a five step reduced mechanism is generated and is validated for the entire range of strain rates up to the extinction point. As in the case of the premixed flame, the temperature profiles and species concentration profiles agree very well with the results of the full mechanism for a selected range of pressures.

Nevertheless, as noted, the calculations above and their validations are time-consuming, and since the demand for larger and more complex mechanisms is very strong from areas related to combustion modeling, automating the procedure is important. This will be discussed in the following section.

3.2 Rate-controlled constrained equilibria

The Rate-Controlled constrained equilibria (RCCE) approach incorporates the assumption of time scale separation in reactive systems in much the same way as the QSSA described above. However, in the case of RCCE the analytical expressions are derived from equilibrium assumptions rather than steady state. These equilibrium states are constrained by the leading or main species, hence the terminology of constrained equilibria. It means that if e.g. considering a simple chemical system such as CH_4-O_2, and O_2 is constrained, then O_2 will occupy all O-atoms in the present form as the amount of O_2 can not change, whereas both H and C atoms may be occupied by whatever CH-molecule are thermodynamically stable in the current state. The constraints are thus linear combinations of the species' concentrations. The RCCE method is in large developed by Jones and Rigopoulos for combustion systems (Jones and Rigopoulos, 2005);(Jones and Rigopoulos, 2007), and only briefly outlined here.

In order to derive the equilibrium states, the RCCE makes use of minimizing the Gibbs free energy subject to conservation of enthalpy, elements and mass for each constraint i:

$$h = \sum_{j=1}^{N_S} n_j H j^0(T) \tag{22}$$

$$E_i = \sum_{j=1}^{N_S} a^e_{ij} n_j, \ (i = 1, ...M_e) \tag{23}$$

$$C_i = \sum_{j=1}^{N_S} a^c_{ij} n_j, \ (i = 1, ...M_c) \tag{24}$$

where a^e_{ij} is the matrix of number of element i in the jth species, a^c_{ij} is the matrix of linear combination of concentration of the j species making up the ith constraint, and n_j is the concentration of the jth species.

It can be shown that two sets of equations arises when employing minimization of Gibbs free energy (Jones and Rigopoulos, 2005). One set becomes algebraic equations defining the constraints:

$$\mu_j^0(T) + RT\ln\frac{n_j}{n} + RT\ln\frac{P}{P_0} + \sum_{i=1}^{M_e}\lambda_i^e a_{ij}^e + \sum_{i=1}^{M_c}\lambda_i^c a_{ij}^c = 0,\ (j = 1, ...N_S) \tag{25}$$

where N_s is the number of species, and P_0 and μ_j^0 are the pressure and chemical potential in the standard state, where the chemical potential is a given function of temperature. These algebraic equations need to be solved simultaneously to compute the concentrations at the constrained equilibrium state. The second set becomes differential equations for the concentrations of the remaining constrained species where the matrix a_{ij}^c is now incorporated:

$$\frac{dC_i}{dt} = \sum_{j=1}^{N_S} a_{ij}^c \sum_{k=1}^{N_r} \nu_{jk} r_k(n_1, ..., n_{N_S}, T, \rho),\ (i = 1, ...M_c) \tag{26}$$

The algebraic-differential equation system is then solved in much the same manner as for the QSSA approach. Because the formulation of Equation (25) yields for all species, the RCCE is particularly attractive in adaptive chemistry systems.

3.3 Intrinsic Low Dimensional Manifolds

3.3.1 The standard approach to ILDM

Intrinsic Low Dimensional Manifolds is a method for reducing a chemical system by using *attractors* for the chemical kinetics involved. It is thought that fast reactions quickly bring the composition down to the attracting manifolds, an equilibrium solution space that fast chemical reactions relax towards, slow reactions moving within these manifolds (Maas, 1998);(Schmidt et al., 1998); (Yang & Pope, 1998). This represents a time separation of the fast chemical processes. In the work of Maas et al. (Maas & Pope, 1994) and developed further in Maas (Maas, 1998), the fundamental formalism behind the decoupling of the short time scales by use of ILDM is taken up, and this is to be referred here further.

Reacting flow and its scalar field evolve in time according to an N_u-dimensional partial differential equation system, where N_u is the number of unknown chemical and physical variables (See Equation (1) for comparison):

$$\frac{\partial \boldsymbol{\psi}(t)}{\partial t} = \mathbf{P}(\boldsymbol{\psi}, \nabla\boldsymbol{\psi}, \nabla^2\boldsymbol{\psi}) + \omega(\boldsymbol{\psi}), \tag{27}$$

$\boldsymbol{\psi}$ being the N_u-dimensional vector of the unknown scalars, $\omega(\boldsymbol{\psi})$ the vector of the source terms, including the chemical reaction rates, and $\mathbf{P}(\boldsymbol{\psi}, \nabla\boldsymbol{\psi}, \nabla^2\boldsymbol{\psi})$ being the spatial vector operator that governs the contributions of all other physical processes such as diffusion, convection, advection, etc. The time scales governed by $\omega(\boldsymbol{\psi})$ span over a large range. Some of the fastest can be decoupled from the system as desired.

The N_u variables form an N_u-dimensional space. A chemical reaction represents a movement along a trajectory from the initial state to the final state for $t \to \infty$. An example is given in Figure (4), which shows the trajectories in a CO-H_2 system as plotted in the CO_2-H_2O plane. In Figure (4) several cases involving differing initial conditions are plotted. However, one can clearly see in the figure that the trajectories all move towards an equilibrium condition, in this case at the far right end point of the main manifold. The equilibrium state can represent the chemical system as one single point if the computations do not include the chemical dynamics.

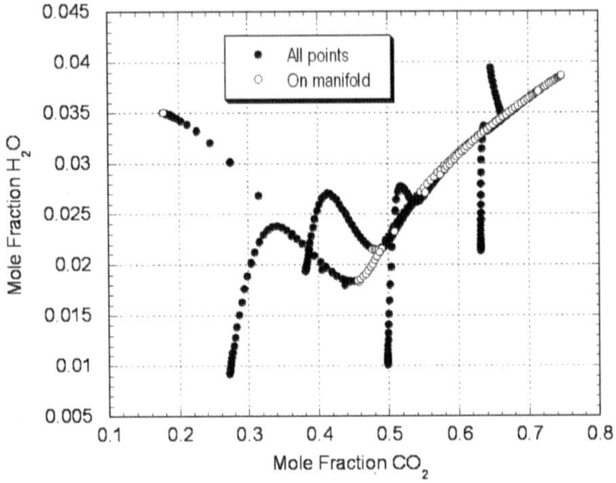

Fig. 4. Trajectories of the chemical reactions progress for a CO-H_2 system and its projection into the CO_2-H_2O plane (Nilsson, 2011).

The equilibrium process in this case takes about 5 ms If the physical processes are slower or have the same order of magnitude, the equilibrium point offers an approximate solution. This corresponds to neglecting chemical dynamics on time scales shorter than 5 ms. By neglecting chemical dynamics that take place on time scales shorter than say 100μs, the solution can be described by a single variable since the main equilibrium curve remains in the state space, which is a one-dimensional manifold. This is shown by the open circles in Figure (4). It is a consequence of the fast relaxation process leading to the reactions being in partial equilibrium and the species involved being in steady state. One can thus conclude that after the relaxation period of 5 ms the system can be described in an approximate way by the equilibrium value, which is a single point. If time scales shorter than 100μs can be neglected, the system can be described by using a single reaction progress variable, a one-dimensional manifold. If even shorter time scales are needed, several additional reaction progresses need to be included, which results in a higher-dimensional manifold.

After identifying the low-dimensional manifolds in the N_u-dimensional state space that the thermodynamic state of the system has been relaxed to, the reduced system consisting of $S = N_u - R$ variables (R is the degree of reduction), can be represented as $\mathbf{\Phi}=(\mathbf{\Phi}_1, ..., \mathbf{\Phi}_S)^T$. Thus the original system $\psi=\psi(\mathbf{\Phi})$ can be projected onto the S-dimensional sub-space

$$\frac{\partial \mathbf{\Phi}}{\partial t} = \mathbf{\Pi}(\mathbf{\Phi}, \nabla\mathbf{\Phi}, \nabla^2\mathbf{\Phi}) + \mathbf{\Omega}(\mathbf{\Phi}), \tag{28}$$

where $\mathbf{\Omega}$ and $\mathbf{\Pi}$ are the corresponding S-dimensional vectors for the source terms and from the other physical processes, respectively. The low-dimensional manifold described by equation (28) represents the chemical system in a further calculation.

The advantage of the ILDM method is that it requires no information concerning which reactions are to be set in equilibrium or which species are in steady state: "The manifold method is based on a more intrinsic study of the chemical reaction process happening in combustion" (Yang & Pope, 1998). The use of attractors is sufficient to find a solution. Since computer simulations of combustion processes involving ILDM reduction speed up calculations by a factor of ten, the method is applicable to numerical problems in particular. The results of the calculations of the manifolds are stored and *tabulated* in a preprocessing step. Since the tabulated data consist of the relevant data (such as the reduced reaction rates) the information is assessed through a table look-up during the computational run. This method however requires significant amounts of storage memory, which becomes problematic in higher dimensional manifold calculations. An alternative storage method is proposed by Niemann et al. (Niemann et al., 1996). Whereas the classic approach employs an interpolation procedure within small tabulation cells and a local mesh refinement, Niemann et al. employs a higher order polynomial approximation within large coarse cells. This decreases the storage requirement considerably; for an H_2-O_2 laminar flat flame calculation the storage requirements were reduced by a factor 200 (Niemann et al., 1996). However, since the method does not provide a set of rate equations, it cannot be related to a set of global reactions that provide information on the underlying kinetics involved (Tomlin et al., 1997). Furthermore, classic ILDM does not account for transport processes which may be important for diffusion flames. The two next sub-sections will be devoted to methods to account for transport in the ILDM framework.

3.3.2 Flamelet Generated Manifolds (FGM)

The Flamelet Generated Manifolds (FGM) approach aims to provide a tool for simplified treatment of the chemical system for flames where also transport in terms of diffusion is important. This is particularly the case for premixed flames where there are also less reactive parts on one side of the flame zone from which radicals diffuse towards the flame zone. The concept is based on two simplification procedures: one is the flamelet approach where a multi-dimensional flame is considered as an ensemble of one-dimensional flames, and another which is the consideration of a low-dimensional manifold in composition space.

van Oijen and co-workers have developed this technique for a set of different flames (van Oijen & de Goey, 2000);(van Oijen & de Goey, 2002). The first approach considers a premixed flame. The technique of FGM make use of premixed flames with detailed chemistry which are pre-calculated and tabulated. Then tables are generated, reflecting the solution of these flamelets as a function of one or more control variables. When solving equations for these control variables by the use of the ILDM, one can use the table of flamelets to retrieve quantities related to the composition that are not known. Since the major part of convection and diffusion processes are included in FGM through the flamelet calculations, the method is more accurate in the low-temperature region of a premixed flame than methods based on local chemical equilibria as the classic ILDM.

3.3.3 Reaction-Diffusion Manifolds (REDIM)

The Reaction-Diffusion Manifolds (REDIM) approach represent an extension to the formulation of the standard ILDM. Where the ILDM is in fact a relaxation of a set of ordinary differential equations (ODE's) describing a homogenous system, the REDIM formulation generalizes for a set of partially differential equation (PDE's) where also the coupling between the reaction and diffusion processes are accounted for. Bykov and Maas (Bykov & Maas, 2007) have performed the full derivation of this generalized system in the framework of ILDM and an optimized tabulation procedure of generalized coordinates. They present the method in three limiting cases: (1) where there is pure mixing and thus no chemical source term, (2) where there is a homogeneous system and thus no transport, and (3) where there is a case of known gradients of the local coordinates. This last limiting case will if the known gradients are found from detailed flame calculations become equivalent to the FGM approach as described in the previous sub section.

It is clear that REDIM represents a generalized form of applying known ideas from invariant manifold theory and have been shown to apply to a wide range of applications from homogeneous systems, premixed flames and diffusion flames (Bykov & Maas, 2009). It is less straight forward to implement, tabulation of the multi-dimensional manifolds need special attention and the interpretation of the results are non-trivial. However, once implemented REDIM represents a very general and powerful reduction tool.

3.4 Computational Singular Perturbation method

Computational Singular Perturbation (CSP) is an alternative method employing a time scale separation analysis, thereafter use being made of exhausting modes for the approximate treatment. The core of the technique is to rewrite the set of differential equations that govern the system, using a new set of basis vectors so defined that they represent the fast and the slow sub domains. These vectors thus contain a linear combination of the reaction rates involved in the original mechanism. By employing this method, the problem becomes one of an eigenvalue problem that can help in discarding fast "modes" which involve species that are candidates for steady state. Work on development of the CSP method can be examined in detail in a substantial selection of papers (Lam, 1993);(Lam et al., 1994); (Massias et al., 1999a); (Massias et al., 1999b);(Tomlin et al., 1997).

The method as a whole is described in terms of three major steps (Massias et al., 1999a); (Massias et al., 1999b). The first step concerns as usual identification of the detailed chemical and physical system and setting the limits for reduction. The next step involves finding the steady state species, and constructing the reduced mechanism that involve the simpler algebraic operations. The final step is to optimize the reduced mechanism through truncation of the algebraic relations or of the remaining differential equations and of the resulting global rates. This is done to enhance the computations and also provide a more accurate solution.

The *second* step which is of interest here consists of choosing the number of global steps that are desired for the reduced mechanism, noted here by G, and determining the *local CSP pointers* for each species. The definition of the size of the reduced mechanism is being based on experience and empirical considerations. A method is yet not presented that can determine the size of the reduced mechanism *a priori* based on the relevant physical situation. The number of steady state species, R, is given by $R = N_S - E - G$, where N_S is the total number of species in the detailed mechanism and E is the number of elements in the mechanism, such as C, O, H and N.

The local CSP pointers are generated through representation of the chemical system, Equation (1), by a set of basis vectors, **a**, defined such that (Massias et al., 1999b):

$$\frac{\partial \mathrm{Y}}{\partial t} = \mathbf{a}_r \mathbf{h}^r + \mathbf{a}_S \mathbf{h}^s, \tag{29}$$

where $\mathbf{a}_r$ is an R-dimensional vector for the R reduced species, $\mathbf{a}_S$ is an S-dimensional vector for the remaining species, and $\mathbf{h}^r$ and $\mathbf{h}^s$ are the corresponding vectors of the form

$$\mathbf{h}^r = \mathbf{b}^r(\mathbf{P} + \omega) \qquad \text{and} \quad \mathbf{h}^s = \mathbf{b}^s(\mathbf{P} + \omega), \tag{30}$$

where **P** contains the spatial differential operator, ω is the species source term from Equation (1). $\mathbf{a}_r$ and $\mathbf{a}_s$ are the stoichiometric vectors for the modified non-physical mechanism, and $\mathbf{b}^r$ and $\mathbf{b}^s$ form the corresponding inverse set of basis vectors . According to the definition of the basis vectors, the first term on the right hand side in Equation (29) should be assumed to be insignificant because of the steady state assumption that $h^i \approx 0$ for $i = 1, R$, resulting in the following expression:

$$\frac{\partial \mathbf{Y}}{\partial t} \approx \mathbf{a}_s \mathbf{h}^s. \tag{31}$$

The goal of CSP analysis is thus to find the set of basis vectors that can fulfill this requirement. A CSP analysis is performed on each species at each spatial point, the R elements to be considered as being in steady state are identified by the N_S diagonal elements of the *CSP pointer*, $D_i, i = 1, N_S$:

$$\mathbf{D} = diag[\mathbf{a}_1\mathbf{b}^1 + \mathbf{a}_2\mathbf{b}^2 + ... + \mathbf{a}_R\mathbf{b}^R]. \tag{32}$$

The pointer takes a value between zero and one. It is a function of the space, thus describing the influence of the R shortest chemical time scales on each of the species i at this particular point in space. When D_i takes on a value close to unity, species i is completely influenced by the shortest time scales and is a candidate for being set to steady state. The opposite occurs when D_i becomes close to zero, the species in question is not being influenced at all by the shortest chemical time scales and thus not being in steady state.

Some species have local pointers for which the value can go from zero to unity within the range of the calculation. These species are treated wrongly if the local pointer of a certain point in space is the basis of the reduction. Thus, the local pointers are integrated over the computational domain L. The *third step* involves an integration over the space to find the overall value on the influence on the time scale for each species. These integrated pointers are weighted with the species' mole fraction. This is done so that species at high concentrations are not set to steady state, since the resulting errors in calculating their concentrations as steady state species could affect the results too much.

Massias et. al. (Massias et al., 1999b) propose three different integration procedures for capturing the steady state candidates in the most appropriate way. However, they take the form similar to

$$I^I = \frac{1}{L}\int_0^L D_i \frac{1}{X_i}\frac{q_i}{q_{i,\max}} dx, \tag{33}$$

where q_i is the production rate of species i, $q_{i,\max}$ is the maximum production rate over the computational range, and X_i is the mole fraction of the species. Caution is in order as both X_i and q_i can take on the value zero (inert species), so that small terms ϵ_1 and ϵ_2 are added to the respective denominators so as to avoid numerical problems. The R species with the highest values for I^I are selected as steady state species. Note that since for most species $q_{i,\max}$ is situated in the reaction zone, the largest contribution to the integrated pointer comes from the value in the reaction zone since $q_i/q_{i,\max}$ there is unity.

The elementary reaction rates are integrated over the space in order to determine the R fastest elementary reaction rates, which can then be eliminated from the system. The fastest reactions that consumes a steady state species, as identified in the previous step, are selected as to be the "fast reaction". For each steady state species, the fastest reaction consuming the species is found through use of the integral (Massias et al., 1999b):

$$H_k^i = \frac{1}{L} \int_0^L r_k, \quad (34)$$

where r_k is the reaction rate of the $k'th$ reaction. The remaining reactions are considered to be the "slow reactions", their reaction rates being retained in the mechanism. This procedure is carried out in order to optimize the computations when a reduced mechanism is applied. This step is not needed for accuracy.

Finally, the rates of the global reactions and their stoichiometric values are determined. The resulting global reactions consist of the major species found in the previous steps, their rates being determined by a linear combination of the rates of the "slow reactions", which depend both on the steady state species and in the non-steady state species.

Obtaining the solutions to the algebraic equations can still require a significant amount of computational time, and the system can still suffer from stiffness problems. If the result obtained in using the reduced mechanisms is found to be discrepant with the results of the detailed mechanism, a truncation is performed. An importance analysis of the reaction rates then can lead to some reaction rates being omitted. This can be understood as being similar to a reaction flow and reaction sensitivity analysis, where for each species the participation rate, ϵ_P, of each elementary reaction and its importance rate, ϵ_I, are ordered, the corresponding reaction rates for the elementary steps that produce negligible values of both ϵ_P and ϵ_I being truncated from the steady state relations. In the work of Massias et al. (Massias et al., 1999a) the number of species that needs to be calculated in greater detail after the CSP analysis is said to be small, often only two or three truncations needing to be carried out.

The advantage of CSP calculations in a simple eigenvalue analysis is that it provides information about which species and reactions are associated with the fastest modes. However, the method does not always represent a computationally efficient technique for repeated reduction, since the time saved by eliminating the slowest modes may be outweighed by the time required for recomputing the basis for each time step (Tomlin et al., 1997). The terminology employed in the CSP method to some extent hides the chemical information if this is not analyzed in detail. Skevis et al. (Skevis et al., 2002) provides an excellent presentation of the physical and chemical meaning of the CSP data. In this paper there are tables that show the contribution of the major elementary reactions to the CSP reactions, the slowest reactions moving the trajectories of the physical processes along the manifold created by the fast reactions. In the work, diffusion and convection processes were also included, demonstrating the CSP methodology being as much a tool for characterization of the combustion process as a tool for reduction of chemical mechanisms.

3.5 Level of importance

The success of the reduced mechanism depends on the reliability of the selection procedure in selecting steady state species. Whereas the CSP method selects species that take part in the fastest reactions, which is done by solving an eigenvalue problem, the level of importance (LOI) method concerns the individual chemical lifetime of a species - or a *function* of its lifetime - as the selection parameter. The line of argument used is that some species are in steady state as a result of that the reactions consuming the species are very much faster than those producing them. The species, when formed, are thus very short lived and are low in concentration. This approach has been developed by Løvås et al. (Løvås et al., 2000)-(Løvås et al., 2009). However, the method has been adopted into automatic reduction and optimization tools by e.g. Pepiot-Desjardins and Pitsch (Pepiot-Desjardins & Pitsch, 2008) and Shekar et al. (Shekar et al, 2011).

Since a chemical system is strongly non-linear, carrying out a lifetime analysis requires that the system is linearized around a starting point $\mathbf{Y_0}$, which results in the following equation, corresponding to Equation (1) where the spatial operator is neglected:

$$\frac{d\mathbf{Y}}{dt} = \omega(Y) \Longrightarrow \frac{d}{dt}(\mathbf{Y} - \mathbf{Y}_0) = \omega_0 + \mathbf{J}(\mathbf{Y} - \mathbf{Y}_0) \quad (35)$$

where the limit at which $\mathbf{Y} - \mathbf{Y_0} \to \mathbf{0}$ and $\mathbf{J}$ is the Jacobian matrix with respect to the source terms in ω. The Jacobian matrix holds information regarding the rate of change in the source terms of the species when a change in species concentrations occur. The error introduced by the steady state approximation to a species ΔY_i is calculated as (Tomlin et al., 1997)

$$\Delta Y_i = \frac{1}{J_{ii}} \frac{\mathbf{d}Y_i}{\mathbf{dt.}} \quad (36)$$

The fact that the dimensions of J_{ii} is 1/t[sec] means that the inverse of the Jacobian elements, $1/J_{ii}$, can be interpreted as the characteristic timescale of the species in question. From Equation (36) it can be seen that a short lifetime, i.e. a small $1/J_{ii}$, or a slow rate of change for a species, results in a small error in the calculated concentration.

In line with the argumentation above, and expanding the Jacobi elements accordingly, the chemical lifetime can be expressed as

$$\tau_i = 1/\frac{\partial \omega_i}{\partial c_i} = \frac{c_i}{\sum_{k=1}^{N_R}(\nu'_{ik} - \nu''_{ik})\nu'_{ik} r'_k}, \quad (37)$$

where ω_i represents the species source term in terms of concentrations, c_i is the species concentration, ν_{ik} is the stoichiometric coefficient, the prime denotes the reactant values, the double prime denotes the product values, and r_k is the reaction rate at which k is the Arrhenius reaction coefficient. The chemical lifetime can be understood in these terms as being a measure of how fast a particular species is consumed after being produced. Hence the species with the shortest lifetimes can be selected as steady state species alone. However, species with long lifetimes can still be insensitive to the desired result and can thus be approximated by steady state. On the other hand, species with short lifetimes can still be sensitive and should not be set to steady state. In order to capture these species a combined lifetime and species sensitivity measure termed the *level of importance*, LOI, is defined:

$$(\mathbf{LOI})_i = S^S_{A,i}\vartheta_i, \quad (38)$$

where $S^S_{A,i}$ is the relative species sensitivity, as defined in the previous section, of species i towards some parameter of interest, such as for example the burning velocity v or the temperature T. ϑ_i can be chemical lifetime itself, τ, or a wegithed function of the chemical lifetime:

$$\vartheta_i = \frac{\tau_i^{DW}}{\sqrt{(\tau_i^{DW})^2 + (\tau_F)^2}} \qquad \text{where} \qquad \tau_i^{DW} = \tau_i \frac{D_i}{D_{N_2}}. \quad (39)$$

The lifetime is here weighted to both the diffusion time in a manner similar to which is described for the manual reduction procedure by Equation (19), and the flame time, τ_F suitable for premixed flames. It can also be weighted to the scalar dissipation rate, $\boldsymbol{a}$, in diffusion flames.

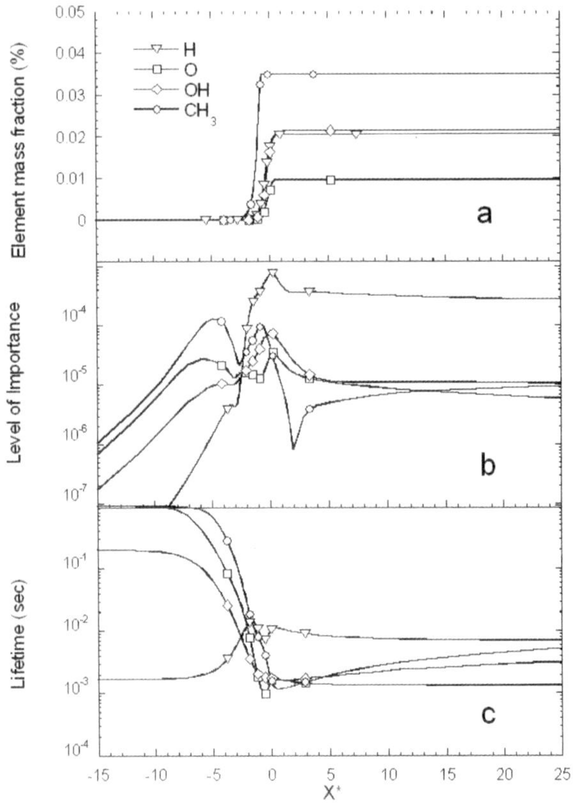

Fig. 5. Selection parameter profiles over the flame zone for a set of species (H, O, OH and CH_3): (a) element mass fraction as a function of the dimensionless flame coordinate x*, (b) LOI as a function of the dimensionless flame coordinate x*, and (c) weighted lifetime as a function of the dimensionless flame coordinate x*. (Løvås et al., 2000)

In Figure (5) the profiles of the selection parameters for various important radicals (H, O, OH and CH_3) in a stoichiometric methane flame have been plotted as functions of the dimensionless flame coordinate x* (Løvås et al., 2000). The upper plot shows the element mass fractions as a function of x*. After the reaction zone, the species all have high element mass fractions. The threshold limit is most commonly set to 1, leaving only O slightly under the threshold. In the two lower plots, b and c, in Figure (5), the effect of including the sensitivity in the selection procedure is evident. Since during and after the flame zone, the weighted lifetimes are generally short as compared with the cold unburned mixture in which the reactions have not yet started (plot c). An accumulated weighted lifetime over the entire flame zone favors the high values found in the pre-heat zone. However, the sensitivity contained in the LOI has clearly shown to counteract the high weighted lifetimes found at low temperatures (plot b). The weighted lifetime measure retains the species O, OH and CH_3 as active species, H being set to steady state with a maximum lifetime in the order of 10^{-2}. In employing the LOI measure, all the species except H are set to steady state. The high LOI for hydrogen is to a large extent caused by weighting the lifetime to the diffusion. Although H has a relatively high diffusion coefficient as compared with the other species, is nevertheless an important species to retain in the mechanism.

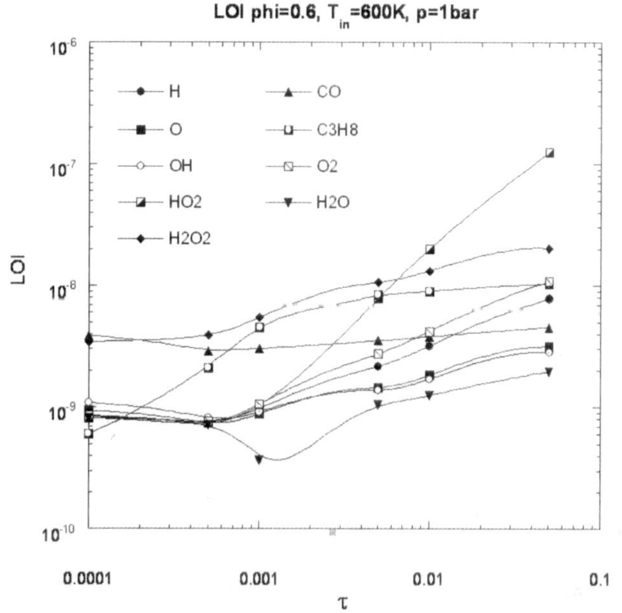

Fig. 6. The evolution of species' LOI as a function of the residence time, shown for certain selected species at a given equivalence ratio in PSR, $\phi = 0.6$. (Løvås et al., 2001)

For comparison, Figure 6 shows the evolution of the LOI for an ignition process in a reactor sequence as function of the residence time for a given equivalence ratio in the PSR (Løvås et al., 2001). As the residence time increases, species such as HO_2, H_2O_2 and H show a significantly high LOI and are thus retained the mechanism. The effect of the low equivalence ratio is also evident in the dominant role of O. Investigation of the evolution of the LOI as a function of the residence time becomes important when reduced mechanisms are applied in CFD calculations. Many of the CFD simulations model each computational cells as a small perfectly stirred reactor. Thus, the validity of the reduced mechanism needs to be considered over the range set for the CFD calculations. The time scale for the turbulent mixing needs to be included since it affects the chosen residence time for the specific computational cells. Although in the unburned regions, the residence time is much longer than the turbulent mixing times, in the reaction zone the turbulent mixing time is dominant. Thus, varying residence times need to be accounted for when reduced mechanisms are developed for this purpose.

By thorough investigation the optimum conditions for determining the level of importance can be found. For a simple methane flame, the LOI has been calculated from (1) the maximum accumulated values for the lifetime and the sensitivity, (2) the LOI in the reaction zone and (3) the LOI at the point where the species have a maximum mass fraction. The overall conclusion to be drawn is that the maximum values obtained for the lifetime or for LOI accumulated over the entire range investigated are reliable to some extent, the range involved being over the equivalence ratios, the mixture fractions for the flame calculations, or the time range for the ignition process. However, for the flame calculations a more accurate selection of steady state species is obtained if the values in the reaction zone or the values at maximum species mass fraction are used (Løvås et al., 2009). In ignition situations, the integrated LOI up to the point of ignition, defined as the point of maximum temperature gradient, is found to represent the most appropriate selection parameter (Løvås et al., 2002c). This result is of interest in comparing the LOI with Equation (33), which defines the selection criteria used in the CSP method. The integrated pointers consist of the CSP pointer, a factor weighting it by the species mass fraction and a factor including the production rate of the species. The production rate factor, $q_i/q_{i,\max}$, where q_i is the production rate and $q_{i,\max}$ is the maximum production rate over the integration range, is unity for most of the species in the reaction zone. Thus, the largest contribution to the integrated CSP pointer comes from that zone, corresponding to the finding that the LOI in the reaction zone is the most appropriate selection parameter.

4. Results

In the present section, the results from applications of reduced mechanisms mainly based on skeletal mechanisms and LOI analysis will be presented. For whatever system is chosen the degree of reduction is variable and user defined. It has been found that the strongly reduced mechanisms can be developed for simple premixed flames. Simulating an ignition process however requires a larger set of species in order to predict ignition timing and heat release in an adequate way. If emission rates are of primary concern, however, ignition timing is not necessarily an important feature to investigate. In this section results of developing reduced mechanisms for (i) a diffusion flame configuration, (ii) a reactor sequence for modeling NO emissions and (iii) an ignition process in a SI engine will be presented.

4.1 Diffusion flame configuration

In the case of a counterflow diffusion flame, the detailed mechanism in the present example containing 46 species was successfully reduced to 12 species, completely automatically through the LOI and placing restrictions on the element mass fraction, as described above. The chemical kinetic model involves a detailed C_1-C_2- mechanism (Bowman et al., 2004). The chemistry of H_2-O_2-CO-CO_2 combustion stems from Yetter et al.(Yetter et al., 1991). In the present case, the LOI was based on the values in the reaction zone. The results of applying reduced mechanisms with varying degrees of reduction to the simulation of a counterflow flame in a mixture fraction space of constant scalar dissipation rate and unity Lewis number is shown in Figure (7). According to the upper plot in the figure, the temperature profile over the mixture fraction range is very accurately reproduced. Most species profiles were in close agreement with the detailed mechanism, but some of the C_2-species showed a discrepancy as a result of all but a few of the C_2-species being set to steady state. The errors introduced into the computations of these species' concentrations have a knock-on effect on the species that are retained in the mechanism. This is shown in the lower plot in Figure (7). As can be seen for both the temperature profile and the species concentration profiles, the reduced mechanism perform very well as compared with the results from the detailed mechanism.

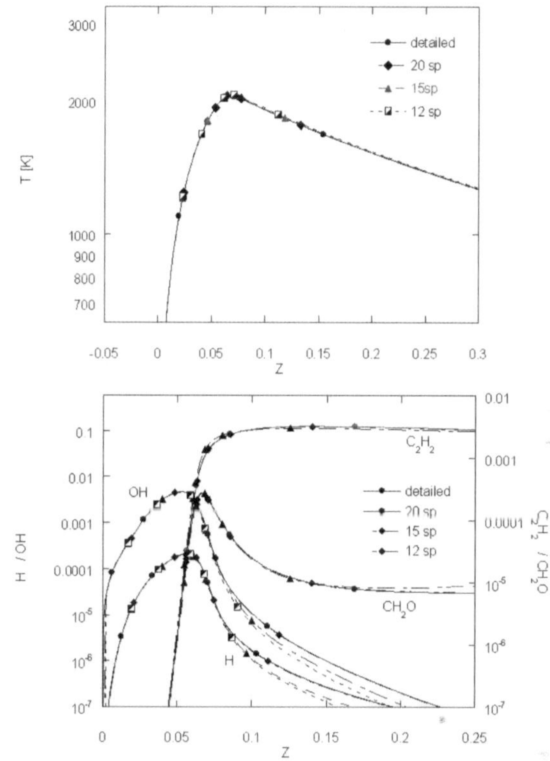

Fig. 7. Results of employing reduced mechanisms for simulating a methane/air counterflow diffusion flame with $\chi = \mathbf{0.54}$ at 1Bar. The detailed mechanism containing 46 species is reduced to one involving 12 species yet still able to reproduce the features of the flame.

4.2 Reactor sequence

For the simulation of emissions from a staged combustor, the reaction mechanism is extended to include 69 species that interact in 770 different reactions. In order to model NO emissions from such a device, the reactor is fueled with a mixture of ethylene (C_2H_4) doped with monomethylamine (CH_3NH_2) (Kantak et al., 1997); (Klaus et al., 1997). As stated in the previous section, the steady state species selected varies depending upon whether the lifetime alone or an extended lifetime which includes the species sensitivity is used. A reduction of the mechanism through fully automatic selection in terms of the species' LOI towards NO in the PSR has been carried out and presented by Løvås et al. (Løvås et al., 2001). Figure (8) shows the calculated NO concentrations after the PSR as function of the equivalence ratio. The results were obtained using a reduced mechanism containing as little as 31 of the detailed mechanism, the achieved accuracy of the reduced scheme being within an acceptable level of accuracy as compared with the detailed reaction mechanism. Three of the mechanisms are based on a selection according to chemical lifetime only, whereas the mechanism reduced the most is obtained with the LOI towards NO concentration.

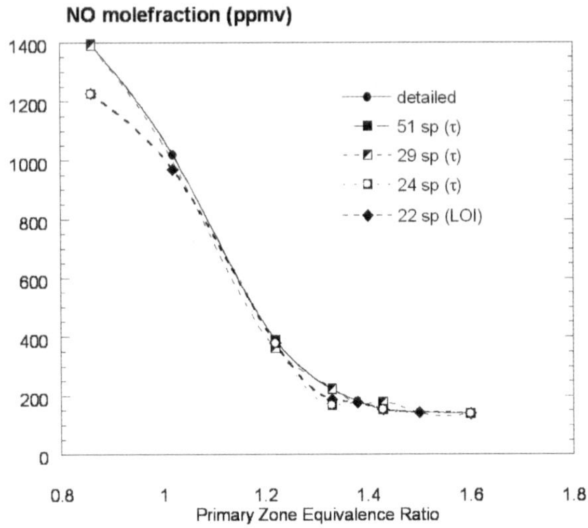

Fig. 8. The NO molefraction as a function of the equivalence ratio in the PSR. Results were obtained for reduced mechanism with increasing degrees of reduction. (Løvås et al., 2001)

4.3 SI engine

The degree of reduction depends strongly on the combustion system and on the degree of complexity involved. Ignition processes often require a more detailed mechanism than simple flame configurations. The on-set timing of the ignition is sensitive to the accuracy of species concentrations because of their dependency on the reaction rates.

In Figure (9), temperature and species profile plots obtained in an investigation of autoignition in the end-gas of an SI-engine, known as knock, as presented by Soyhan et al. (Soyhan et al., 2000), are shown. The calculations are obtained in employing a two-zone model (burnt and unburnt zones), the detailed mechanism for iso-octane and n-heptane mixtures being compiled from Chevalier (C_1-C_4) (Chavelier, 1993) and Muller (C_5-C_8) (Muller et al., 1992), consisting of 75 species and 510 reactions. In the work displayed in the figure, this mechanism was reduced with reaction flow and sensitivity analysis together with LOI. The results obtained with different reduced mechanisms are displayed in the figure, in which they are compared with the results of the detailed mechanism. The skeletal mechanism, obtained on the basis of the reaction flow and sensitivity analysis (denoted "skel" in the figure), was developed prior to the mechanisms from a reduction based on lifetime analysis (denoted "red" in the figure).

In the temperature profile for the end-gas as shown in Figure (9) one can note that at an inlet temperature of 1200K the end gas ignites at around -24 CAD. This is far ahead of the onset of the ignition by the spark plug, and even further ahead of the propagating flame front reaching the wall. Under such conditions, knocking occurs. The presented work concerns the performance of various reduced mechanisms and their performance as compared with the detailed mechanism. The comparison shows that over a large range of physical conditions the profiles of the chemical species and the temperature are the same for the various mechanism, except for changes in the ignition delay times. Thus, the basic characteristics of the detailed mechanism are preserved. The accuracy of the calculation of radicals such as the OH, HO_2

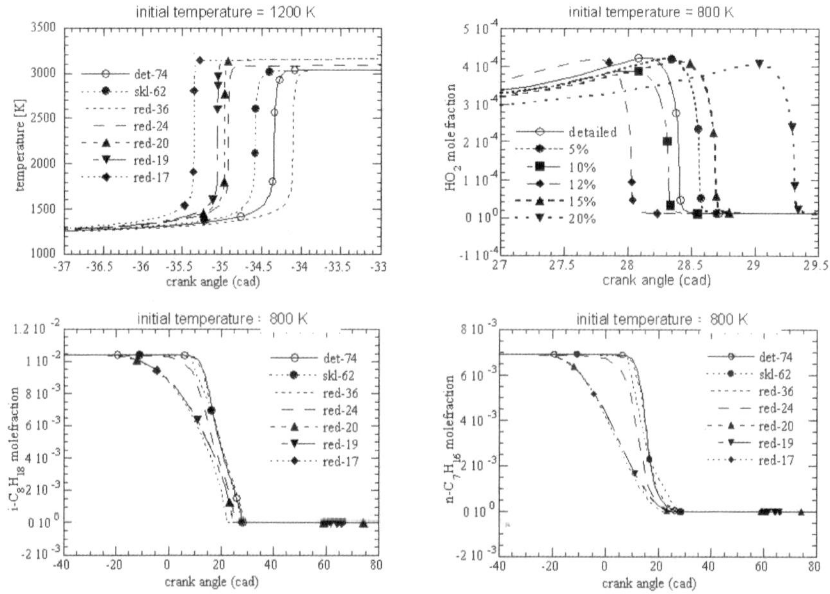

Fig. 9. Calculated temperatures and mole faction profiles for the end-gas of an SI-engine. Top left: temperature profile, top right: HO_2 molefraction representing a radical profile, bottom: fuel profiles, the iso-octane and the n-heptane. Different reduced mechanisms are compared with the detailed and skeletal mechanisms (Soyhan et al., 2000)

and CH_3 that participate in chain reactions, is important since the formation of HO_2, for example, is crucial for the formation of an initial radical pool (Westbrook et al., 1991). The plot at the top left in Figure (9) shows the profiles of HO_2 that result from employing the skeletal mechanisms as compared with the results from the detailed mechanism for inlet temperatures of 800K. The two lower plots show fuel decomposition as a function of CAD at the same inlet temperature. The plots reveal a close agreement between the reduced and the detailed mechanisms, showing clearly the positive effects on the ignition timing in the end-gas achieved by decreasing the inlet temperature.

The most obvious differences between the various reduced mechanisms in prediction of ignition delay times. Too early an onset of ignition results in both the decomposition of the fuel and the production of the radicals occurring earlier. However, since the errors in the ignition timing are within 1-2 CAD, the mechanisms are seen as performing well within the specified range.

5. Application of adaptive kinetics

In contrast to the previously discussed reduction schemes, in which chemical species only are selected if they are in steady state throughout the process, the *adaptive* method allows species to be selected at each operating point or domain separately, generating adaptive chemical kinetics. This is a dynamic reduction procedure that can be employed to ignition systems that are changing over time and to flame systems that change over the flame coordinate. As discussed for the LOI, in some cases the maximum accumulated value over the computational range was employed, but the values in the reaction zones were found to be a better choice of steady state candidates. However, this means that species that are of importance in the reaction zone are kept throughout the computation, also in regions in which the species may be in steady state. In order to improve the efficiency of the reduction procedure, it is desirable to only consider true steady state species at each point in the calculations. For this reason, methods of reducing the mechanism on-line or adaptively have been developed.

There are two main issues in developing an adaptive reduction procedure. One is the choice of a useful selection criterion for species or reactions to be removed, one that is accurate in selecting the correct species but does not require any considerable amount of CPU time as the analysis is repeated in the course of the computations. For true on-line reduction the selection of steady state species needs to be performed for each operating point or domain, allowing for the fact that species may move in and out of steady state in accordance with their lifetime under the conditions in hand. The second issue is that of implementation into flow codes, the question of how to implement the possibility of a mechanism changing in both size and matter during the simulation.

5.1 Selection criteria for adaptive kinetics

The first issue concerning adaptive kinetics is that of the selection criteria. This is rather straight forward for homogeneous ignition scenarios employing adaptive chemistry as only the time evolution of the chemistry needs to be considered. An on-the-fly reduction scheme was proposed by Liang et al. (Liang et al., 2009) for a homogeneous ignition scenario (HCCI), where the basis of the reduction was a modified version of the DRG procedure described earlier. Their procedure removes the locally redundant species from the detailed treatment, and "freezes" their mass fractions in the continuation of the computation. This is performed for each time step through the computation. The DRG analysis is sufficiently efficient that performing this on-line does not outperform the reduction compared to employing the detailed mechanism throughout.

A different approach to a similar problem can be to introduce a separation between vectors for *all* the species, containing specific species data that is kept available in module routines, and dynamic vectors for the *active* species, those being treated in detail. This is the approach proposed by Løvås et al. (Løvås et al., 2002a). The vector of the active species changes during the run according to an array of logicals that hold the information concerning the species' status as steady state. Initially the logicals are assigned their value based on an a priori LOI analysis. The species set to steady state are assigned the logical true such that the species concentrations are to be calculated using algebraic equations instead of the original differential equations. This implies that algebraic equations for *all* the species need to be available in the code for when/if the species is selected to be in steady state. From the list of active species, the source terms are calculated and used to complete the calculations at this point. The combustion process proceeds at each point and the physical conditions change accordingly. This suggests that a new analysis of the species' lifetimes should be performed to allow for modifications in the mechanism so as to account for these changes. The code assesses the new lifetimes based on the inverse of the Jacobian matrix already available; species that has a considerable change in chemical lifetime on the basis of the new conditions being added or removed accordingly. A buffer for numerical inaccuracy needs to be included so as to prevent species with lifetimes very close to the specified threshold limit from systematically going in and out of steady state without adding any accuracy of the computations. Redefining the mechanism at almost every operating point becomes tedious and can mean that the CPU time saved by applying the reduced mechanism is lost. Figure (10) shows temperature profiles resulting from employing this method of adaptive kinetics with varying threshold limits in selecting steady state species, which result in a greater degree of reduction. The profiles are compared with the corresponding profiles for the detailed mechanism (Løvås et al., 2002a). It is clear that as the level of reduction is increased, the reduced models reproduce the temperature profiles with increasing error. However, it seems to be a very clear cut-off when the reduced adaptive schemes can not reproduce ignition at all.

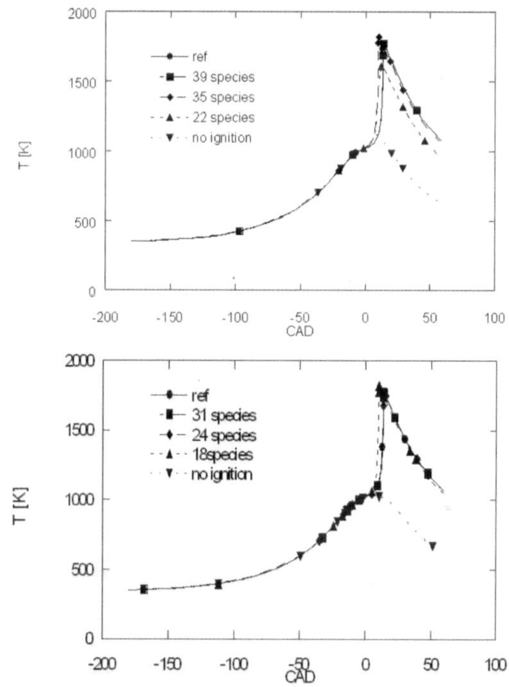

Fig. 10. Temperature profiles of a HCCI engine cycle, employing adaptive kinetics. The upper plot is a result of applying the pure chemical lifetime. The middle plot is a result from applying mass fraction weighted lifetime. The lower plot results from an initial temperature 356K +/- 2K applying mass fraction weighted lifetime. (Løvås et al., 2002a)

For 2D and 3D dynamic simulations such on-line reduction are very computationally costly. A less CPU time intensive approach is to pre-define the combustion domains or zones in which a certain sub-set of the detailed mechanism is used. This is often used for diffusion flame calculations where the domains can be defined by the fuel rich and the fuel lean zones. Hence, schemes that find the smallest chemical sub-set locally in time or space have been proposed e.g. by Schwer et al. (Schwer et al., 2003)). Here each computational cell was assigned a certain sub-mechanism based on a set of physical criteria such as temperature, pressure, species concentrations etc. For highly turbulent flames where these criteria can change rapidly and steeply from cell to cell, this method can be demanding. A single criterion was therefore proposed by Løvås et al. (Løvås et al., 2010), where the sub-mechanism was chosen based on *mixture fraction* alone. This approach will act as example of implementation of adaptive chemistry into turbulent combustion modeling and will be described in more detailed in the following sub section.

5.2 Implementation of adaptive kinetics

When simulation a highly turbulent diffusion flame details regarding both the flow field and the chemical interactions are important. In the present discussion a turbulent ethylene flame is simulated suing large eddy simulations (LES). It is not the scope here to discuss the implementation of turbulence models in CFD. However, it can be noted that LES describe the turbulent flow field by resolving the large scales, but employing a sub-grid model for the small unresolved scales. This is a rather CPU intensive approach, and with detailed chemistry the computations becomes cumbersome.

Løvås et al. (Løvås et al., 2010) therefore proposed to combine a hierarchy of methods to simplify the treatment of the chemistry in such large simulations of turbulent combustion. At first it was recognized that the turbulent flow needed a much finer grid than the chemical system. Therefore a coarser "super grid" for the chemistry was imposed onto the spatial CFD grid for which mixing and transport is treated. However, due to the turbulent nature of the flame it was not practical to let the super grid follow the physical 2D or 3D co-ordinates. Instead, the chemistry was solved in the 1D mixture fraction space with the mixture fraction ranging from 0 (pure oxidant) to 1 (pure fuel). The interaction between the turbulent mixing and chemical kinetics are often modeled employing either the flamelet approach (Peters, 1984) or the conditional moment closure (CMC) (Klimenko & Bilger, 1999) method, where the latter was the choice of Løvås et al.

The LES/CMC approach for turbulent reactive flow modeling has already been developed without reduction (Navarro-Martinez et al., 2005). Løvås et al. extended this approach to also include an adaptive chemistry treatment. At first, distinct domains had to be defined using a domain splitting method. In this case the domains were identified in mixture fraction space and the analysis was therefore conveniently limited to one dimension. However, more rigorous automatic domain splitting methods using clustering techniques can be employed (Blurock et al., 2003). Since the choice of selection parameter was the LOI, the mixture fraction space was divided into 4 domains in which the species' LOI was relatively unchanged towards each other. This is illustrated in Figure (11). In this case the cut off limit was chosen such that the number of species was constant throughout the domains. However, the species changed between domains according to the highest ranked species.

Once the domains and the active species within each domain was identified, the RCCE approach described in the previous sub chapter was employed to treat the chemical system. In the LES-CMC code the reduction procedure is implemented on the CMC grid. The adaptive procedure is as follows: the local mixture fraction from the LES-CMC selects the relevant LOI-domain and therefore determines which species are locally leading. The RCCE uses the LOI information to select which species to constrain for a user-given number of constraints and provides a reduced mechanism. Equation (25) is then solved using an iterative Newton solver while non-constrained species are obtained directly from Equation (26). Since concentrations of the non-constrained species are known, the transitions between domains are smooth.

Figure (12) shows the resulting flame simulation based on the LES-CMC LOI-RCCE approach as described above. Employing 4 spatial sub-domains, each with their optimally reduced model for the given conditions (fuel rich, reaction zone, post-reaction zone, and fuel lean)

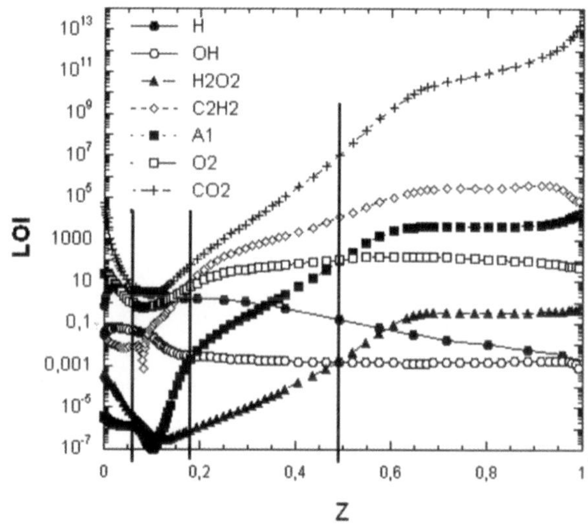

Fig. 11. The LOI profiles for selected species through the flame in mixture fraction space Z. The vertical lines indicate domain limits. (Løvås et al., 2010)

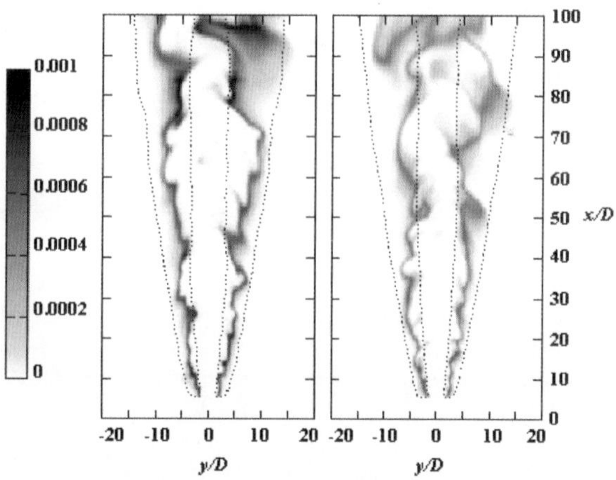

Fig. 12. Instantaneous contour plots of H2 in a turbulent ethylene diffusion flame resulting from adaptively reduced scheme with 15 species (left) in 4 sub-domains and direct integration of the full mechanism with 75 species (right). Average iso-lines are included to indicate the statistical similarities. (Løvås et al., 2010)

gives excellent correlation to the full treatment. Since these are instantaneous plots, the flame is not identical. However, the averaged values indicated by the stapled lines show clearly the close correlation. It was demonstrated that when adaptive chemistry is employed the number of species that need to be treated in detail is substantially reduced, only true steady state species being selected at each operating point.

6. Conclusion

The present chapter intended to outline the main model reduction techniques for chemical systems used in combustion modeling, with the end goal of presenting the recent developments of reducing chemical mechanisms through application of automatic and adaptive procedures. In the past, reduced mechanisms have been used extensively in simulations of combustion processes but they were carried out by hand, which is a tedious process. They were therefore often limited to very specific physical conditions and often represented very simple fuels. However, as chemical models of complex fuels have become very large and detailed, the need for automatic procedures and smart implementation into CFD is evident. These automatic procedures are however based on the ideas of the manual and analytical procedures developed in the past. Although the chapter emphasizes the classic fundamental reduction procedures, it was the goal here to demonstrate the usage of automatic reduction procedures suitable to a wide range of conditions and applicable to realistic multi-component fuels.

It is important to state that this field of research is under constant development, and there are still very promising and interesting techniques being proposed in literature which has not been discussed here. This is not a result of lack of importance, but rather the limitation of space. The reader is therefore encouraged to follow up from here, and based on the current review make a decision in his or her own mind for which approach is the most applicable to the problem in hand.

7. References

Blurock, E.S. (1995). Reaction: System for Modelling Chemical Reactions, *J. Chem. Info. Comp. Sci.*, Vol. 35, pp. 607-616.

Blurock, E.S. (2000). Generation and Subsequent Reduction of Large Detailed Combustion Mechanisms, *Proceedings of the Combustion Institute*, WIP 4-D19, p 331.

Blurock, E., Løvås, T. & Mauss, F. (2003). Steady State Reduced Mechanisms Based on Domain Splitting, In Proceeding: 19th International Colloquium on the Dynamics of Explosions and Reactive Systems (ICDERS), Hakone, Japan.

Bowman, C.T., Hanson, R.K., Davidson, D.F., Gardiner, W.C.,Jr., Lissianski, V., Smith, G.P., Golden, D.M., Frenklach, M. & Goldenberg, M., GRI-Mech Home Page, http://www.me.berkeley.edu/gri_mech/

Bykov, V. & Maas, U. (2007). The extension of the ILDM concept to reaction-diffusion manifolds, *Combustion Theory and Modelling* Vol. 11, No. 6, pp 839-862

Bykov, V. & Maas, U. (2009). Problem adapted reduced models based on Reaction-Diffusion Manifolds (REDIMs), *Proceedings of the Combustion Institute* Vol. 32, Issue 1, pp 561-568

Callahan, C., Held, T., Dryer, F., Minetti, R., Ribaucour, M., Sochet, L., Faravelli, T., Gaffuri, & P., Ranzi, E., (1996). Experimental Data and Kinetic Modeling of Primary Reference Fuel Mixtures, *Proceedings of the Combustion Institute* Vol. 26, Issue 1, pp 739-746

Chevalier, C. (1993). Entwicklung eines detaillierten Reak-tionsmechanismus zur Modellierung der Verbren-nungsprozesse von Kohlenwasserstof-fen bei Hoch- und Niedertemperatur-bedingungen, Ph.D.-Thesis, Universität Stuttgart, Germany.

Chen, J.-Y., Liu, Y. and Rogg, B. (1993). in: Peters, N. and Rogg, B. (Eds.), Reduced Kinetic Mechanisms for Application in Combustion Systems, *Lecture Notes in Physics*, New Series, m 15, Springer Verlag, pp. 196-223.

Côme, G.M., Warth, V., Glaude, P.A., Fournet, R., Battin-Leclerc, & F. Scacchi, G. (1996). Computer Aided Design of Gas Phase Oxidation Mechanisms - Application to the Modelling of n-Heptane and Iso-octane Oxidation, *Proceedings of the Combustion Institute*, Vol. 26, pp. 755-762.

DARS. Available from: http://www.diganars.com/; DigAnaRS: Delaware, USA, 2011.

Doute, C., Delfau, J., Akrich, R., & Vovelle, C., (1997). Experimental Study of the Chemical Structure of Low-Pressure Premixed n-Heptane-O2-Ar and iso-Octane-O2-Ar Flames, *Combustion Science and Technology*, Vol. 124, pp.249-276.

Fieweger, K., Blumenthal, R., & Adomeit, G.,(1997). Self-Ignition of SI Engine Model Fuels: A Shock Tube Investigation at High Pressure, *Combustion and Flame*, 109:599-619

Green, W.H., Allen, J.W., Ashcraft, R.W., Beran, G.J., Class, C.A., Gao, C., Goldsmith, C.F., Harper, M.R., Jalan, A., Magoon, G.R., Matheu, D.M., Merchant, S.S., Mo, J.D., Petway, S., Raman, S., Sharma, S., Song, J., Van Geem, K.M., Wen, J., West, R.H., Wong, A., Wong, H., Yelvington, P.E. & Yu, J., RMG - Reaction Mechanism Generator v3.3 Home Page, http://rmg.sourceforge.net/

Goussis, D.A., (1996). On the Construction and Use of Reduced Chemical Kinetic Mechanisms Produced on the Basis of Given Algebraic Relations, *Journal of Comp. Physics*, 128, pp. 261-273.

Jones, W.P. & Rigopoulos, S. (2005). Rate-controlled constrained equilibrium: Formulation and application to nonpremixed laminar flames, *Combustion and Flame* Vol. 142, pp 223-234.

Jones, W.P. & Rigopoulos, S. (2007). Reduced chemistry for hydrogen and methanol premixed flames via RCCE, *Combustion Theory and Modelling* Vol. 11 (5) pp 755-780.

Kantak, M.V., De Manrique, K.S., Aglave, R.H. & Hesketh, R.P. (1997). Methylamine Oxidation in a Flow Reactor: Mechanism and Modeling, *Combustion and Flame* Vol.108, pp. 235-265.

Kaufman, F., (1982). Chemical Kinetics and Combustion: Intricate Paths and Simple Steps, *Proceedings of the Combustion Institute*, Vol. 19, pp. 1-10.

Klaus, P., & Warnatz, J. (1997). A Further Contribution Towards a Complete Mechanism for the Formation of NO in Flames, VDI-Berichte 1313, VDI Verlag.

Klimenko, A. & Bilger R. (1999). Conditional Moment Closure for Turbulent Combustion, *Prog. Ener. Combustion*, Vol. 25, pp 595-687

Lam, S.H. (1993). Using CSP to understand complex chemical kinetics, *Combustion Science and Technology* Vol. 89, pp. 375-404.

Lam, S. H. & Gaussis, D.A., (1994). The CSP Method for Simplifying Kinetics, *International Journal of Chemical Kinetics*, 26, pp. 461-486.

Lewis, B. & von Elbe, G. (1987). Combustion, Flames and Explosions of Gases, Academic Press Inc., pp.25-78.

Li, J., Zhao, Z., Kazakov, A., & Dreyer, F.L.(2004). An updated comprehensive kinetic model of hydrogen combustion, *International Journal of Chemical Kinetics*, Vol. 36, pp566-75.

Liang, L., Stevens, J.G., & Farrell, J.T. (2009). A dynamic adaptive chemistry scheme for reactive flow computations, *Proceedings of the Combustion Institute* Vol. 32, pp 527-534.

Lindstedt, R. P. & Mauß, F. (1993). Reduced Kinetic Mechanisms for Acetylene Diffusion Flames, in: Peters, N. and Rogg, B. (Eds.), Reduced Kinetic Mechanisms for Application in Combustion Systems, Lecture Notes in Physics, New Series, m 15, Springer Verlag, pp. 259-283.

Løvås, T., Nilsson, D. & Mauss, F. (1999). Development of Reduced Chemical Mechanisms for Nitrogen Containing Fuels, Proceedings of the Fifth International Conference on Technologies and Combustion for a Clean Environment (Clean Air V), The Portuguese Section of the Combustion Institute, pp. 139-143.

Løvås, T., Nilsson D. & Mauss, F. (2000). Automatic Reduction Procedure for Chemical Mechanisms Applied to Premixed Methane-Air Flame, *Proceedings of the Combustion Institute* Vol. 28, pp. 1809-1815.

Løvås, T., Soyhan. H. & Mauss, F. (2001). Reduction of Complex Fuel Chemistry for Simulation of Combustion in an PSR-PFR reactor sequence, VDI-Berichte 1629, pp539-544.

Løvås, T., Mauss, F., Hasse, C. & Peters, N. (2002). Development of Adaptive Kinetics for Application in Combustion Systems, *Proceedings of the Combustion Institute* Vol. 29, pp. 1387-1393.

Løvås, T., Mauss, F., Hasse, C. & Peters, N. (2002). Modeling of HCCI Combustion using Adaptive Chemical Kinetics , SAE 2002-01-0426.

Løvås, T., Amneus, P., Mauss, F. & Mastorakos, E. (2002). Comparison of Automatic Reduction Procedures for Ignition Chemistry, *Proceedings of the Combustion Institute* Vol. 29, pp. 1403-1410.

Løvås, T. (2009). Automatic generation of skeletal mechanisms based on level of importance analysis, *Combustion and Flame* Vol. 156, pp. 1348-1358 .

Løvås, T., Navarro-Martinez, S., & Rigopoulos S. (2010). On adaptively reduced chemistry in large eddy simulations, *Proceedings of the Combustion Institute* Vol. 33, pp. 1339-1346

Lu, T.F. & Law, C.K. (2005). A Directed Relation Graph Method for Mechanism Reduction, *Proceedings of the Combustion Institute* Vol. 30, pp 1333-1341.

Lu, T.F. & Law, C.K. (2006). *Combustion and Flame* âĂIJLinear-Time Reduction of Large Kinetic Mechanisms with Directed Relation Graph: n-Heptane and iso-Octane, Vol. 144, pp 24-36.

Luo, Z.Y., Lu, T.F., Maciaszek, M.J., Som, S., & Longman, D.E. (2010). A Reduced Mechanism for High-Temperature Oxidation of Biodiesel Surrogates, *Energy and Fuels*, Vol. 24, pp 6283-6293

Maas, U. & Pope, S.B., (1994). Laminar Flame Calculations using Simplified Chemical Kinetics Bases on Intrinsic Low-Dimensional Manifolds, *Proceedings of the Combustion Institute* Vol. 25, pp. 1349-1356.

Maas, U. (1998). Efficient Calculation of Intrinsic Low Dimensional Manifolds for Simplification of Chemical Kinetics, *Comput. Visual Sci.* Vol. 1, pp. 69-81.

Massias, A., Diamantis, D., Mastorakos, E. & Goussis, D.A. (1999). Global Reduced Mechanisms for Methane and Hydrogen Combustion with Nitric Oxide Formation Constructed with CSP Data, *Combust Theory Modelling*, Vol. 3, pp. 233-257.

Massias, A., Diamantis, D., Mastorakos, E. & Goussis, D.A. (1999). An Algorithm for the Construction of Global Reduced Mechanisms With CSP Data, *Combustion and Flame* Vol. 117, p. 685-708.

Mauss, F. & Lindstedt, R. P. (1993). Reduced Kinetic Mechanisms for Premixed Acetylene-Air Flames, in: Peters, N. and Rogg, B. (Eds.), Reduced Kinetic Mechanisms for Application in Combustion Systems, Lecture Notes in Physics, New Series, m 15, Springer Verlag, pp. 102-122.

Mauss, F. and Peters, N. (1993). Reduced Kinetic Mechanisms for Premixed Methane-Air Flames, in: Peters, N. and Rogg, B. (Eds.), Reduced Kinetic Mechanisms for Application in Combustion Systems, Lecture Notes in Physics, New Series, m 15, Springer Verlag, pp. 58-75.

Mauß, F. Peters, N., Rogg, B. & Williams, F.A. (1993). Reduced Kinetic Mechanisms for Premixed Hydrogen Flames, in: Peters, N. and Rogg, B. (Eds.), Reduced Kinetic

Mechanisms for Application in Combustion Systems, Lecture Notes in Physics, New Series, m 15, Springer Verlag, pp. 29-43.

Müller, U.C., Peters, N. & Linan, A. (1992). Global Kinetics for n-Heptane Ignition at High Pressures, *Proceedings of the Combustion Institute* Vol. 24, pp. 777-784.

Navarro-Martinez, S., Kronenburg A. and di Mare, F. (2005). Conditional moment closure for large eddy simulations, *Flow, Turbulence and Combustion* Vol. 75, pp 245-274

Niemann, H., Schmidt, D. & Maas, U. (1996). An Efficient Storage Scheme for Reduced Chemical Kinetics Based on Orthogonal Polynomials, Konrad Zuse-Zentrum für Informationstechnik Berlin, Preprint SC 96-18.

Niemeyer, K., Sung, C. & Raju, M. (2010). Skeletal mechanism generation for surrogate fuels using directed relation graph with error propagation and sensitivity analysis, *Combustion and Flame* Vol. 157, pp 1760-1770.

Nilsson, D. (2001). Automatic Analysis and Reduction of Reaction Mechanisms for Complex Fuel Composition, Doctoral Thesis, Lund University, LRCP-68.

van Oijen, J. A. & de Goey, L. P. H. (2000). Modelling of premixed laminar flames using the flamelet-generated manifold, *Combustion Science and Technology*, Vol. 161, pp 113-137.

van Oijen, J. A. & de Goey, L. P. H. (2002). Modelling of premixed counterflow flames using the flamelet-generated manifold method, *Combustion Theory and Modelling*, Vol. 6, pp 463-478

Peters, N. (1990). Reducing Mechanisms, in: Smooke, M. D. (Eds.), Reduced Kinetic Mechanisms and Asymptotic Approximations for Methane-Air Flames,Lecture Notes in Physics, 384, pp48-68, Springer Verlag.

Peters, N. & Rogg, B. (Eds.) (1993). Reduced Kinetic Mechanisms for Application in Combustion Systems, Lecture Notes in Physics, New Series, m 15, Springer Verlag.

Peters N. (1984). Laminar diffusion flamelet models in non-premixed turbulent combustion, *Prog. Energy Combus. Sci.* 10, pp 319-339.

Pepiot-Desjardins, P. & Pitsch, H. (2008). An efficient error-propagation-based reduction method for large chemical kinetic mechanisms, *Combustion and Flame* Vol (154) pp 67-81

Shekar, S., Sander, M., Riehl, R., Smith, A.J., Braumann, A., Kraft, M. (2011) Modelling theflamesynthesisofsilicananoparticlesfromtetraethoxysilane, *Chemical Engineering Science*, In Press.

Schmidt, D., Blasenbrey, T. & Maas, U. (1998). Intrinsic Low-Dimensional Manifolds of Strained and Unstrained Flames, *Combustion Theory and Modelling* Vol 2, pp. 135-152.

Skevis, G., Mastorakos, E. & Gaossis, (2002). Analysis of Laminar Premixed CH4/O2/N2 Flames with CSP Data, *Proceedings of the Combustion Institute* Vol. 29, pp. 777-784.

Smooke M. D. (Ed.) (1991). Reduced Kinetic Mechanisms and Asymptotic Approximations for Methane-Air Flames, Lecture Notes in Physics 384, Springer Verlag.

Soyhan, H., Amnéus, P., Mauß, F. & Sorusbay, C. (1999). A Skeletal Mechanism for the Oxidation of iso-Octane and n-Heptane Validated under Engine Knock Conditions, SAE Technical Paper 1999-01-3484.

Soyhan, H. (2000). Chemical Kinetic Modelling of Autoignition Under Conditions Relevant to Knock in Spark Ignition Engines, Ph.D. Thesis, İstanbul Technical University.

Soyhan, H., Amnéus, P., Løvås, T., Nilsson, D., Maigaard, P., Mauß, F. & Sorusbay, C. (2000). Automatic Reduction of Detailed Chemical Reaction Mechanisms for Autoignition Under SI Engine Conditions, SAE Technical Paper 2000-01-1895.

Soyhan, H., Løvås, T., & Mauß, F. (2001). A stochastic simulation of an HCCI engine using an automatically reduced mechanism, ASME Fall Technical Conference, Technical Paper 2001-ICE-416.

Soyhan, H., Mauß, F. & Sorusbay, C. (2002). Chemical kinetic modeling of combustion in internal combustion engines using reduced chemistry, *Combustion Science and Technology* Vol. 174 (11-12) (2002) 73-91.

Schwer,D.A., Lu, P. & Green, W.H. (2003). An adaptive chemistry approach to modeling complex kinetics in reacting flows, *Combustion and Flame* Vol. 133, pp 451-465.

Tomlin, A.S. and Turányi, T. & Pilling, M.J. (1997). Mathematical tools for construction, investigation and reduction of combustion mechanisms, in : M.J.Pilling (Ed.), Low-Temperature Combustion and Autoignition, Comprehensive Chemical Kinetics, Vol. 35, Elsevier.

Turns, S. R. (2000). An Introduction to Combustion, 2nd Ed., Mc-GRAW-HILL INTERNATIONAL EDITIONS, Mechanical Engineering Series

Wang, W. & Rogg, B. (1993). Premixed Ethylene/Air and Ethane/Air Flames: Reduced Mechanisms Based on Inner Iteration, in: Peters, N. and Rogg, B. (Eds.), Reduced Kinetic Mechanisms for Application in Combustion Systems, Lecture Notes in Physics, New Series, m 15, Springer Verlag, pp. 76-101.

Warnatz, J., (1981). The Structure of Laminar Alkane-, Alkene-, and Acetylene- Flames, *Proceedings of the Combustion Institute* Vol. 18, pp. 369-384.

Warnatz, J. & Chevalier, C. (1995). in: Combustion Chemistry, Eds. Gardiner, WC jr., Springer Verlag.

Westbrook, C. K., Pitz, W. J., & Leppard, W. R, (1991). The Autoignition Chemistry of Paraffinic Fuels and Pro-Knock Additives: A Detailed Chemical Kinetic Study, SAE912314

Westbrook, C. K., Pitz, W. J., Herbinet, O., Curran, H. J. & Silke, E.J. (2009). A Detailed Chemical Kinetic Reaction Mechanism for n-Alkane Hydrocarbons from n-Octane to n-Hexadecane, *Combustion and Flame* Vol. 156 (1) pp 181-199

Yang, B. & Pope, B., (1998). An Investigation of the Accuracy of Manifold Methods and Splitting Schemes in the Computational Implementation of Combustion Chemistry, *Combustion and Flame* 112:16-32.

Yetter, R.A., Dryer, F. L. & Rabitz, H., (1991). Flow Reactor Studies of Carbon Monoxide/Hydrogen/Oxygen Kinetics, *Combust. Sci. and Tech.* pp 79:129.

Zeuch, T., Moerac, G., Ahmed, S.S. & Mauss, F. (2008). A comprehensive skeletal mechanism for the oxidation of n-heptane generated by chemistry-guided reduction , *Comb. and Flame* Vol 155, pp 651-674

Zheng, X.L., Lu, T.F., & Law, C.K. (2007). Experimental Counterflow Ignition Temperatures and Reaction Mechanisms of 1,3-Butadiene, *Proceedings of the Combustion Institute*, Vol. 31, pp 367-375.

6

Ignition Process in a Non-Homogeneous Mixture

Hiroshi Kawanabe
Graduate School of Energy Science,
Kyoto University,
Japan

1. Introduction

An auto-ignition process of a non-homogeneous mixture is investigated using a numerical calculation based on chemical kinetics and the stochastic approach. This type of auto-ignition phenomenon is considered as a fundamental process of the initial stage of diesel combustion (Ishiyama, et al., 2003) or homogeneous charged compression ignition (Shimasaki, et al., 2003). In order to investigate these combustion processes, many numerical calculations have been performed and for many of those it has been assumed that the ignition process is dominated by the turbulent mixing (Kong and Reitz, 2000).

However, the fuel-air mixing and chemical reaction progress happen simultaneously for these types of combustion processes. Due to the long ignition delay time and high homogeneity of the mixture, combustion characteristics, such as ignition delay and combustion duration, could be affected equally by non-homogeneity of the mixture, turbulent mixing rate and chemical reaction rate. Therefore, the understanding of those combustion mechanisms is incomplete due to the complexity of the phenomena in which the mixing and chemical processes interact with each other. The main purpose of this chapter is to estimate these effects quantitatively using a numerical method.

Here, n-heptane is assumed as a fuel and its reaction process is calculated by means of a reduced mechanism (Seiser et al., 2000). The non-uniform states of turbulent mixing are statistically described using probability density functions and the stochastic method, which was newly developed from Curl's model (Curl, 1963). Focusing on the effects of mixture heterogeneity on combustion characteristics, such as ignition delay and combustion intensity (rate of temperature rise), the evolution of chemical reactions was calculated for the mixture in which variance in fuel-mass fraction decreases at given rates from the initial value under a fixed mean fuel-mass fraction and a constant pressure. The results show that the start timing of the low-temperature oxidation and ignition delay period are hardly affected by the equivalence-ratio variation, however, combustion duration increases with increasing variance. Furthermore, the combustion duration is mainly affected by the non-homogeneity at the ignition and is not much affected by the mixing rate.

2. Numerical models

2.1 Mixing model

In order to describe the homogenization process of a fuel-air mixture by turbulent mixing, the statistical state of the mixture is expressed by means of probability density function (PDF) and the dissipation process is described by a particle-interaction model. In the particle-interaction model, the statistical state f of scalar ϕ at time t is represented by the N delta functions δ;

$$f(\phi;t)=\frac{1}{N}\sum_{n=1}^{N}\delta\left(\phi-\phi(n)\right) \tag{1}$$

Here, $\phi^*(n)$ indicates ϕ value on the nth particle. In the coalescence/dispersion model proposed by Curl (1963), the state of f at $t + \Delta t$ is calculated from the collision frequency ω. The compositions of a pair of particles, which are selected at random (denoted by n_1 and n_2), change as;

$$\phi^*(n_1)\big|_{t=t+\Delta t}=\phi^*(n_2)\big|_{t=t+\Delta t}=\frac{1}{2}\left(\phi^*(n_1)\big|_{t=t}+\phi^*(n_2)\big|_{t=t}\right) \tag{2}$$

Then, within the time interval Δt, this operation is repeated $\Delta tN\omega$ times.

The change in the value of ϕ^* is sometimes large, especially in the early stages of mixing, because it is calculated as the average of significantly different quantities of two particles. This tends to cause unrealistic change in the progress of chemical reactions. The modified Curl's model (Janicka, Kolbe and Kollmann, 1979) is one possible method to mitigate this tendency. In this method, the scalar exchange of a pair of particles (n_1 and n_2) is calculated from a uniform random number C between 0 and 1;

$$\begin{aligned}\phi^*(n_1)\big|_{t=t+\Delta t}&=\phi^*(n_1)\big|_t+\frac{1}{2}C\left(\phi^*(n_2)\big|_{t=t}-\phi^*(n_1)\big|_{t=t}\right)\\ \phi^*(n_2)\big|_{t=t+\Delta t}&=\phi^*(n_2)\big|_t-\frac{1}{2}C\left(\phi^*(n_2)\big|_{t=t}-\phi^*(n_1)\big|_{t=t}\right)\end{aligned} \tag{3}$$

This operation is repeated $3/2\Delta tN\omega$ times and can describe statistically the same process as Curl's model. However, the value of $\phi^*_{t+\Delta t}$ still changes significantly if C is near 1. Here, in order to avoid a significant difference between ϕ^*_t and $\phi^*_{t+\Delta t}$, C is fixed to a value sufficiently smaller than unity and the replacement procedures are repeated $\Delta tN\omega/(2C)$ times. In order to confirm the consistency between the present model and Curl's model, a mixing process was calculated starting from the initial state in which fuel and air are perfectly separated.

Time change of variance v_m for fuel-mass fraction mf distribution is shown in Fig. 1. Here, v_m is normalized with respect to initial variance v_{mi} and dimensionless time $t^* = \omega t$ is used. C = 0.05 and N = 1000 are adopted. As shown, the time changes of v_m/v_{mi} calculated by these three methods are completely equivalent. Meanwhile, Figure 2 shows the time change in m_f-PDF. The distributions at smaller t calculated by the present model are similar to Gaussian rather than to the PDFs by the Curl's and modified Curl's models.

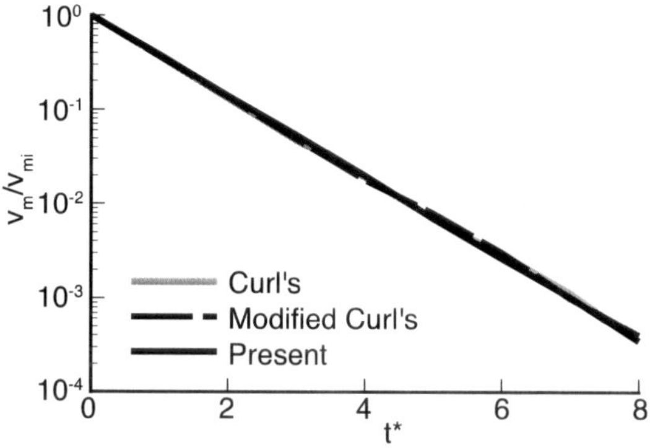

Fig. 1. Course of normalized variance v_m/v_{mi} against non-dimensional time t^*

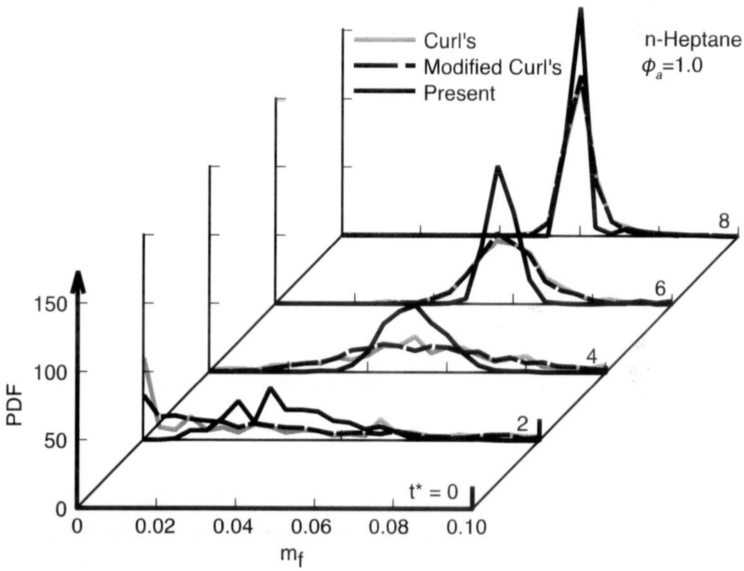

Fig. 2. Temporal change in PDF of fuel-mass fraction m_f

2.2 Chemical reaction model

Here, n-heptane is assumed as a fuel and a chemical reaction system is described by a semi-detailed kinetic mechanism (Seiser et al., 2008[Web]). This system consists of 160 chemical species and 1540 elemental reactions, and is selected for reducing computation time.

3. Results and discussion

By means of the above-mentioned procedure, an ignition process of non-homogeneous mixture with a constant mixing rate is calculated. For simplicity, the calculation is performed under a constant pressure. The initial temperature T_i and pressure p are set to

T_i = 900K and p = 4MPa. The initial distribution of fuel-mass fraction is Gaussian with a mean value m_{fa} and a variance v_{mi}. Figure 3 shows time histories of mean temperature T_a and variance v_m for the initial condition of $m_f = 6.22\times10^{-2}$ and $v_{mi} = 4.34\times10^{-5}$, corresponding to a mean equivalence ratio ϕ_a of unity and the standard deviation of ϕ of approximately 0.1. The collision frequency ω is varied within the range of 0 s^{-1} to 10000 s^{-1}. For comparison, the result for the case of the homogeneous mixture is also shown. Collision frequency ω is usually given by $\omega = C_m\ \varepsilon/k$ for the PDF model combined with CFD using the k-ε turbulence model.

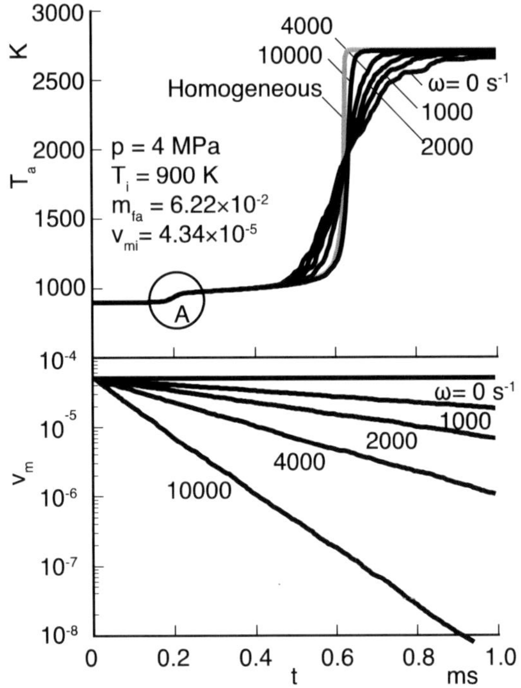

Fig. 3. Courses of mean-temperature T_a and v_m for the non-homogeneous mixture (ϕ_a = 1.0)

Here, k and ε represent turbulence energy and its dissipation rate, respectively. C_m is fixed at 2, therefore, ω = 2000 s^{-1} corresponds approximately to turbulence intensity of 5 m/s and scale of 3 mm. For these calculations, the number of fluid particles is fixed to N = 100. Generally, as collision frequency increases, the start of heat release by hot flame delays and maximum heat release rate increases simultaneously to approach the result of a homogeneous mixture. Meanwhile, the time when the temperature reaches 50% of adiabatic flame temperature is approximately constant regardless of the collision frequency ω. The reason will be discussed later in Fig. 8. Furthermore, Fig. 4 shows a magnified view of Fig. 3 around the starting points of heat release by cool flame (marked as 'A'). The change in mean temperature T_a is exactly the same, in spite of the change of ω.

Next, in order to clarify the effect of mean equivalence ratio, calculations are performed for lean and rich cases. Fig. 5 shows T_a and v_m under the conditions of (a) $m_{fa} = 3.87\times10^{-2}$ (ϕ_a = 0.6) and (b) $m_{fa} = 1.17\times10^{-1}$ (ϕ_a = 2.0) for the same ω as in Fig. 3. Here, initial value of variance

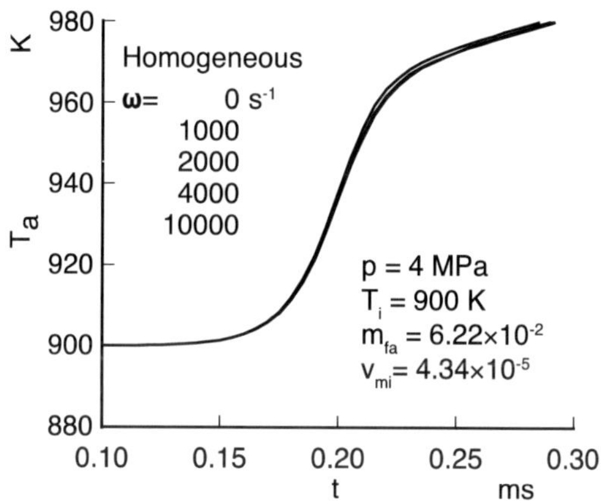

Fig. 4. Temporal changes of Ta due to low temperature oxidation

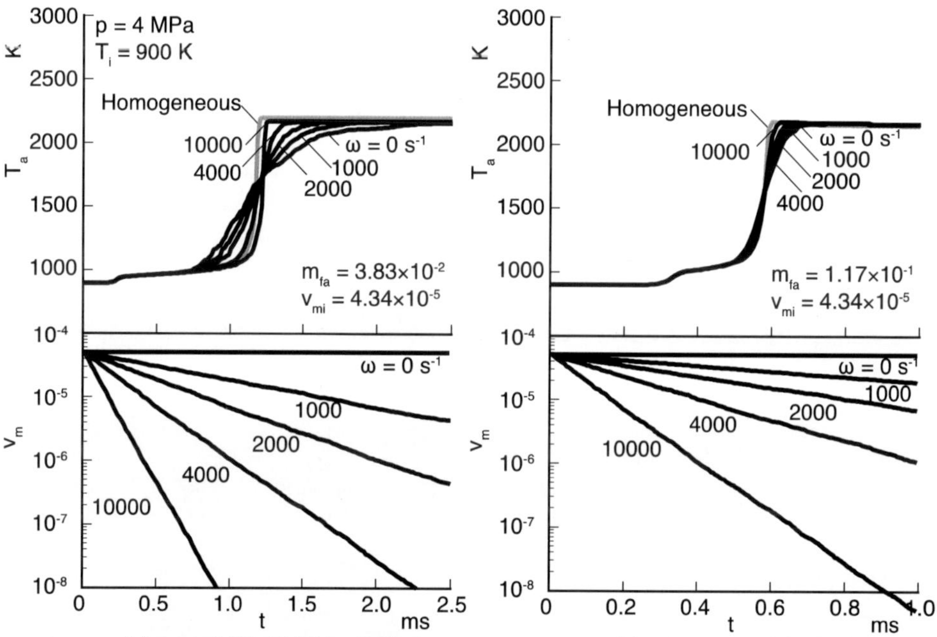

(a) m_{fa} = 3.83×10-2 (ϕ_a = 0.6) (b) m_{fa} = 1.17×10-1 (ϕ_a = 2.0)

Fig. 5. Effect of mean mass-fraction m_{fa}

is fixed to v_{mi} = 4.34×10-5. For the two conditions, histories of the mean temperature T_a are similar to the result of ϕ_a = 1.0 in Fig. 3. For the lean case (a), due to the longer delay of hot flame heat release, the mixture is thought to be more homogeneous and to provide rapid temperature rise. However, the temperature-rising rate at ignition is lower compared to the result of ϕ_a = 1. Meanwhile, for the rich case (b), the variance v_m at the ignition is comparably large, whereas the temperature rise at the ignition is steep, similar to the homogeneous case.

In order to clarify the reason why the temperature-rising rate of the non-homogeneous mixture becomes smaller than in the homogenous case, the temporal change of temperature T and mass fraction of fuel mf in each fluid particle are examined. Fig. 6 shows the data of

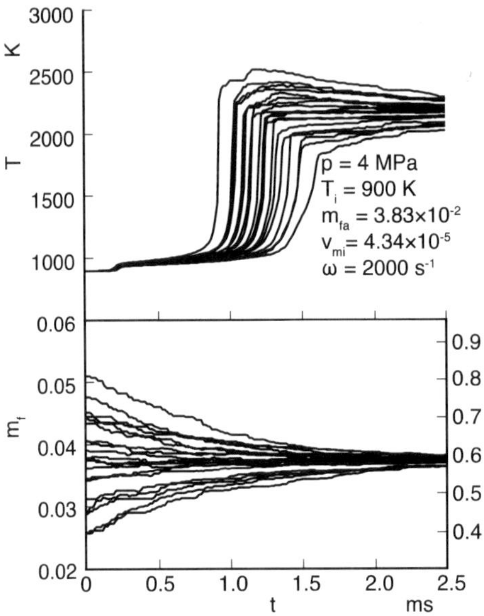

(a) m_{fa} = 3.83×10-2 (ϕ_a = 0.6)

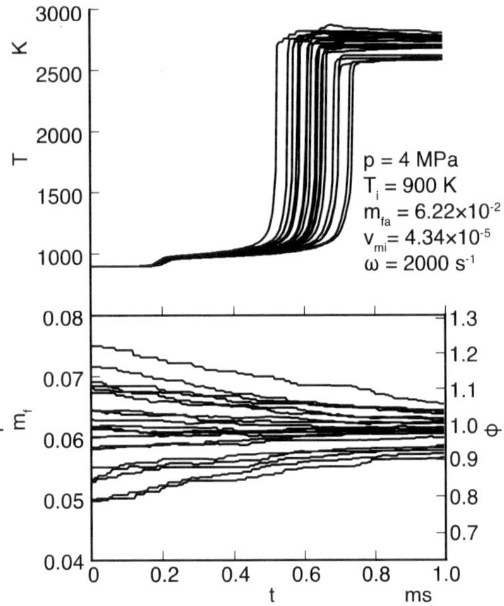

(b) m_{fa} = 6.22×10-1 (ϕ_a = 1.0)

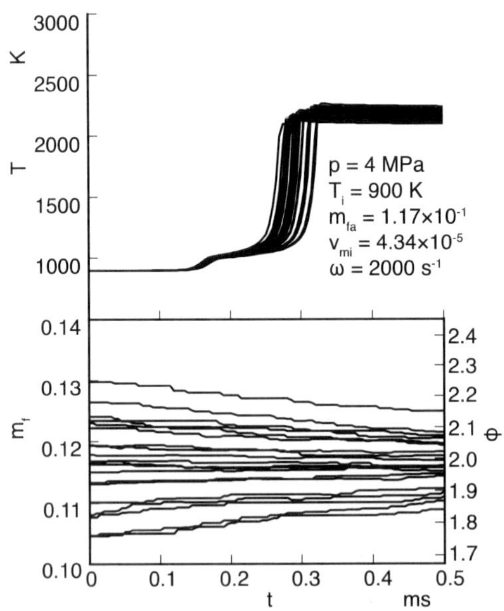

(c) m_{fa} = 1.17×10-1 (ϕ_a = 2.0)

Fig. 6. Time history of T and m_f for each stochastic particle

20 fluid particles, which are selected randomly, for (a) m_{fa} = 3.83×10^{-2} (ϕ_a = 0.6), (b) m_{fa} = 6.22×10^{-2} (ϕ_a = 1.0) and (c) m_{fa} = 1.17×10^{-1} (ϕ_a = 2.0) at p = 4 MPa, T = 900 K and ω = 2000 s^{-1}. In each fluid particle, hot flame occurs with rapid temperature rise when mf approaches m_{fa}. For every case of mean fuel-mass fraction, the hot flame ignition delay varies over a wide range, because the mixture contains a variety of fuel-mass fractions. However, the particle-to-particle variation of the hot flame start time is not determined by the variation in fuel-mass fraction.

In order to examine the relation between non-homogeneity and temperature rise rate quantitatively, some characteristic times of temperature rise process are defined as shown in Fig. 7. Firstly, the time at 50% temperature rising between the initial and adiabatic temperatures is expressed as τ_{50} and that at 95% as τ_{95}. Next, using these values, temperature rise period τ_i and ignition delay time τ_s are defined as below;

$$\tau_i = 2 \times (\tau_{50} - \tau_{95}) \tag{4}$$

$$\tau_s = \tau_{95} - \tau_i \tag{5}$$

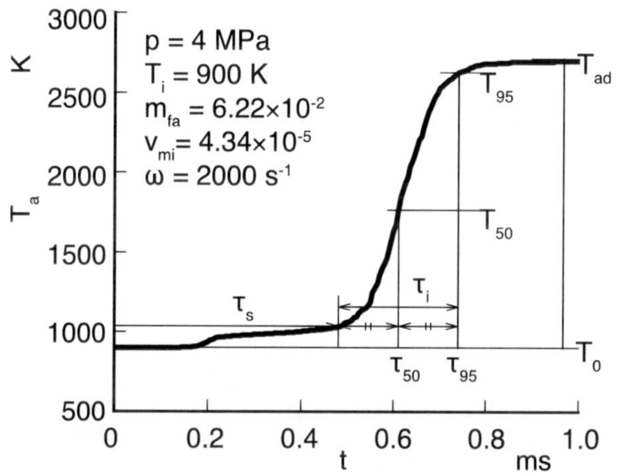

Fig. 7. Definition of ignition delay time τ_s and combustion duration τ_i

Based on these values, the ignition processes of non-homogeneous and homogeneous mixture are discussed. τ_s, τ_{95} and τ_i (marked by an arrow) are displayed for non-homogeneous mixtures with average equivalence ratios ϕ_a of 0.6, 1.0, and 2.0. In Fig. 8, PDF for mf at t = τ_{50} is also displayed for each mixture. In addition, the curves of τ_s and τ_{95} calculated for homogeneous mixtures are drawn. Within this m_f-condition, ignition delay τ_s of the homogeneous mixture becomes shorter with increasing m_f. At the same time, τ_i becomes larger for the leaner and richer sides. Here, ignition delay time of each fluid particle varies due to the variation of equivalence ratio at ignition, therefore, the temperature rise period increases. In addition, m_f dispersion becomes larger for the richer condition, due to shorter ignition delay time. The change in ignition delay against mf around ϕ_a = 2.0 is small so that τ_i also becomes smaller in spite of the wide distribution of m_f. On the other hand, for the leaner side around ϕ_a = 0.6, the distribution width is narrow, whereas τ_s-change against mf becomes larger than in the stoichiometric case. Then τ_i becomes longer.

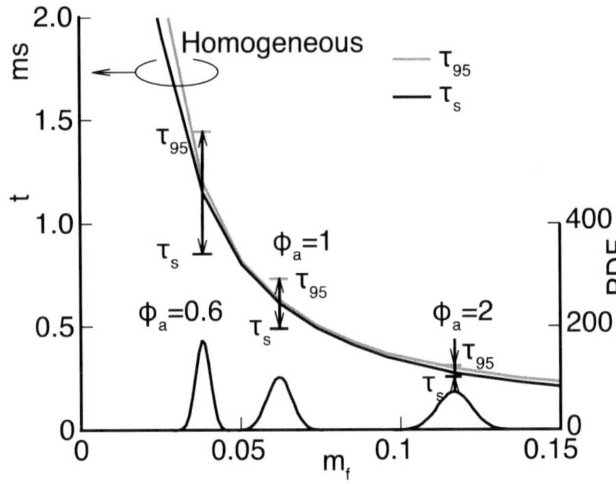

Fig. 8. Changes of ignition delay time τ_s and combustion duration τ_i

In order to confirm the effect of mixing rate on the combustion process, temperature histories are compared for different mixing rates at the same m_f-variance in the middle of hot flame temperature rise, as shown in Fig. 9. The calculation starts with ω = 2000 s^{-1}, then ω is suddenly increased to 10000 s^{-1} just before the ignition. The obtained temperature history differs from that of ω = 10000 s^{-1} and is similar to that of ω = 4000 s^{-1}, whose variance of m_f-PDF at τ_{50} is nearly equal to this ω jumping-up case. This result shows that the rate of temperature rise is strongly affected by the m_f-distribution at ignition rather than the mixing rate. Fig. 10 shows the correlation plots of (a) $\tau_i - \omega$ and (b) $\tau_i - v_{m50}$. Here, v_{m50} represents the variance of m_f-PDF at τ_{50}. In this case these plots are calculated for wide ranges of v_{mi}, T_i and ω with fixed p = 4.0 MPa and $m_{fa} = 6.22\times10^{-2}$ (ϕ_a = 1.0). For the plots on (a), τ_i scatters widely even at the same ω, however, for (b), the plots distribute on a certain curve. This indicates the great influence of m_f variance on combustion duration.

A similar calculation is performed for the case of longer ignition delay and lower temperature rise rate, which is set by $m_{fa} = 1.95\times10^{-2}$ (ϕ_a = 0.3), p = 2.0MPa and T_i = 900K.

In this case, the mixture is comparably lean and ambient pressure is low so that τ_s and τ_i become much longer than in the case shown in Fig. 3. Fig. 11 shows the results for ω = 0 s^{-1}, 200 s^{-1}, 400 s^{-1}, 1000 s^{-1} and 2000 s^{-1}. Here, the ignition delay time is longer, therefore, mixture at ignition becomes more homogeneous for the case of ω > 2000 s^{-1}. The ignition delay time τ_s and temperature rise rate become larger with increasing mixing rate, which is similar to the results shown in Fig. 3. Also, τ_{50} is almost constant against ω.

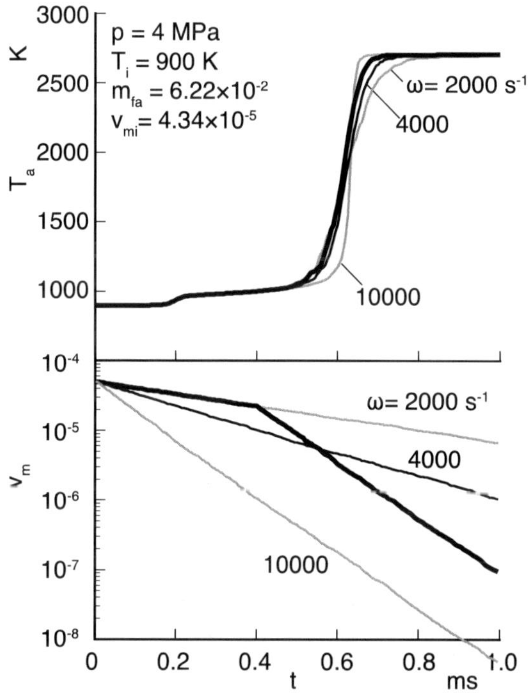

Fig. 9. Effect of collision frequency ω on combustion duration

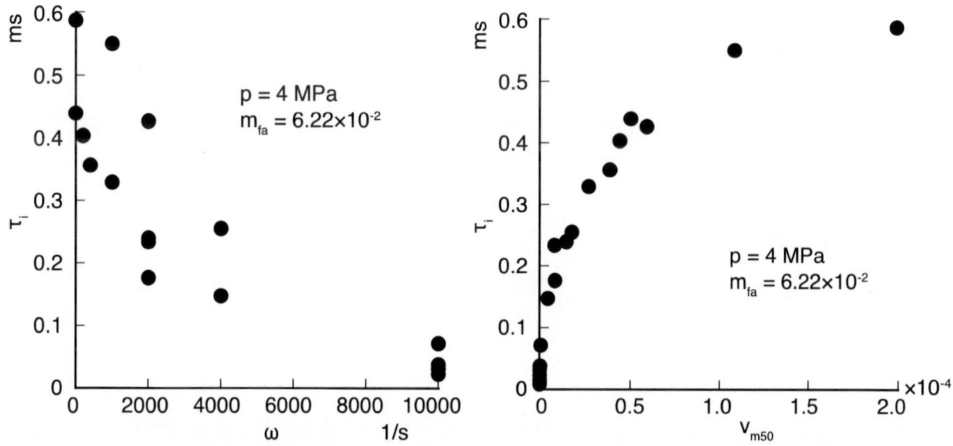

(a) τ_i-ω Correlation

(b) τ_i -v_{m50} Correlation

Fig. 10. Correlations between combustion duration τ_i - collision rate ω and τ_i - mass variation at t = τ_{50}

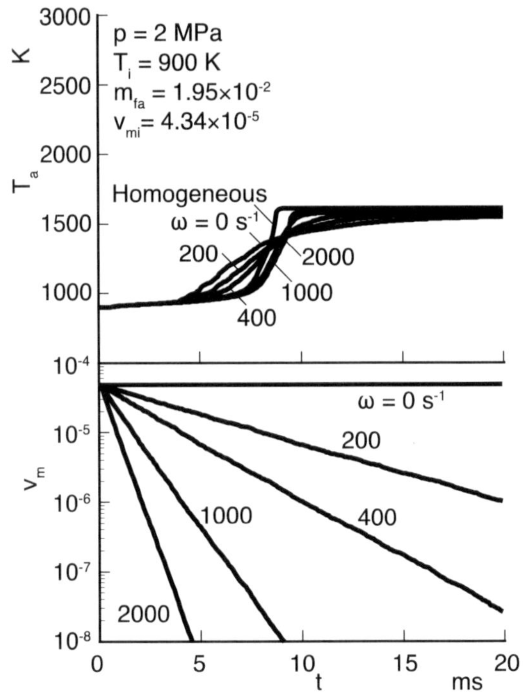

Fig. 11. Courses of mean-temperature T_a and v_m for PCCI-like condition

4. Conclusion

An auto-ignition process of a non-homogeneous mixture in fuel concentration was fundamentally investigated by means of a numerical calculation based on chemical kinetics and the stochastic approach. The auto-ignition process of n-heptane is calculated by means of a semi-detailed mechanism and the non-uniform state of turbulent mixing is statistically described by means of probability density functions and the stochastic method. The following conclusions are derived from the results:

1. For the auto-ignition process of a non-homogeneous mixture during the mixing process, ignition delay time of the cool flame is almost constant against the mixing rate. On the other hand, ignition delay time of hot flame becomes longer with increasing mixing rate. This is because the hot flame ignition delay is more sensible to equivalence ratio than the cool flame delay.
2. For the temperature rising process of hot flame, start points of heat release vary depending on equivalence ratio in a non-homogeneous mixture. Therefore, the rise period increases with increasing non-homogeneity. Also, the temperature rise rate due to heat release of hot flame increases with increasing mixing rate.
3. The tendencies described above are the same for the case of changing equivalence ratio, initial temperature and pressure.

4. Ignition delay time of each fluid particle varies due to the variation of equivalence ratio at ignition, therefore, the temperature rise period increases. In addition, the temperature rise rate becomes larger with decreasing variance of fuel-mass fraction distribution.

5. Nomenclature

C:	Coefficient of modified Curl's model
C_m:	Coefficient of turbulent mixing
f:	Statistical state function
m_f:	Fuel-mass fraction
m_{fa}:	Mean value of m_f
N:	Total number of fluid particles
t:	Time
t^*:	Dimensionless time
p:	Pressure
T:	Temperature
T_a:	Mean temperature
T_i:	Initial temperature
v_m:	Variance of m_f
v_{m50}:	vm at τ_{50}
v_{mi}:	Initial value of v_m
δ:	Delta function
ϕ:	Scalar
ϕ_a:	Mean equivalence ratio
τ_{50}:	Time at 50% temperature rise
τ_{95}:	Time at 95% temperature rise
τ_i:	Combustion duration
τ_s:	Ignition delay of hot flame
ω:	Collision frequency

6. References

Shimazaki, N., Tsurushima, T. and Nishimura, T., Dual-Mode Combustion Concept with Premixed Diesel combustion by Direct Injection near Top Dead Center, SAE Paper, 2003-01-0742.

Ishiyama, T., Shioji, M. and Ihara, T., Analysis of Ignition Processes in a Fuel Spray Using an Ignition Model Including Turbulent Mixing and Reduced Chemical Kinetics, *Int. J. of Engine Research*, Vol. 4, No. 3 (2003), 155-162.

Kong, S-C., Reitz, R. D., Modeling HCCI Engine Combustion Using Detailed Chemical Kinetics with Combustion of Turbulent Mixing Effects, ASME Paper 2000-ICE-306, 2000.

Curl, R. L., Dispersed Phase Mixing: I. Theory and Effects in Simple Reactors, *A. I. Ch. En. J.*, Vol. 9, No. 2 (1963), 175-181.

Janicka, J., Kolbe W, and Kollmann, W., Closure of the Transport Equation for the Probability Density Function of Turbulent Scalar Fields, *J. of Non-equilibrium Thermodynamics*, Vol. 4 (1979), 47.

Seiser, H., et al., Extinction and Autoignition of n-Heptane in Counterflow Configuration, *Proc. of the Combustion Institute* 28 (2000), pp. 2029-2037.

7

Numerical Analysis of the Effect of Inhomogeneous Pre-Mixture on Pressure Rise Rate in HCCI Engine by Using Multi-Zone Chemical Kinetics

Ock Taeck Lim[1] and Norimasa Iida[2]
[1]*University of Ulsan,*
[2]*Keio University,*
[1]*Republic of Korea*
[2]*Japan*

1. Introduction

In HCCI, a premixed air/fuel mixture is inhaled to the combustion chamber and ignited by adiabatic compression. The HCCI engine, which is using the bulk combustion, is promising concept of the high efficient and low emission engine. However, power produced in HCCI engine is limited by knocking cause of excessive heat release and pressure rise at local area in condition of high load. Therefore, the main investigation of the HCCI is avoiding knocking problem to be able to operate at a high load. Delaying the combustion angle and stratifying temperature or concentration of fuel resulting in dispersion of combustion timing is the well-known effective method. In this study, effect of the pressure increase rate in combustion chamber by stratified temperature and fuel concentration of pre mixture according to fuel characteristic was investigated. Numerical analysis in chemical reaction was conducted for investigating an emission property.

2. Experimental method

In this paper, DME(Di-Methyle Ether) and Methane were used as a fuel. The Numerical analysis was conducted for the purpose of investigating that fuel or temperature stratification effect on pressure rise rate and emission using the multi-zone code with detailed chemical kinetics. DME has two stages of heat reaction which is called HTR(High Temperature Reaction) and LTR(Low Temperature Reaction). In case of DME, proportion of LTR is more than those of HTR. It is known that the more DME concentration make heat release increase during the LTR. Due to those facts, existing of DME fuel stratification in combustion chamber is expected to contribute reduction of gas pressure rise rate because heat release difference in local area during LTR causes stratification of temperature before the HTR which makes combustion duration extend. On the other hand, Methane has only 1 stage heat release and self-ignition temperature is high. The detailed specifications of the test engine are presented in Table 1. The hermetic gas is used for calculation duration from

Process	Only 1 Compression & Expansion
Bore X Stroke	112mm X 115mm
Displacement	1132cc
Length of Conrod	205mm
Crank Radius	57.5mm
Intake Valve Close Timing	ATDC-132
Exhaust Valve Open Timing	ATDC-132
Compresstion Ratio	8.0(DME)/21.6(Methane)

Table 1. Engine specifications

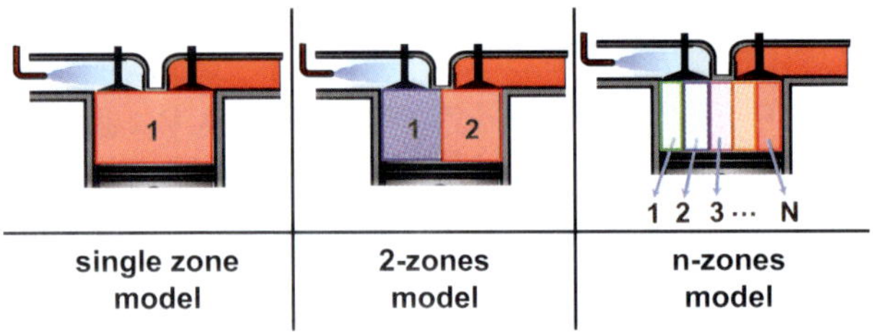

Fig. 1. Concept of multi-zone model

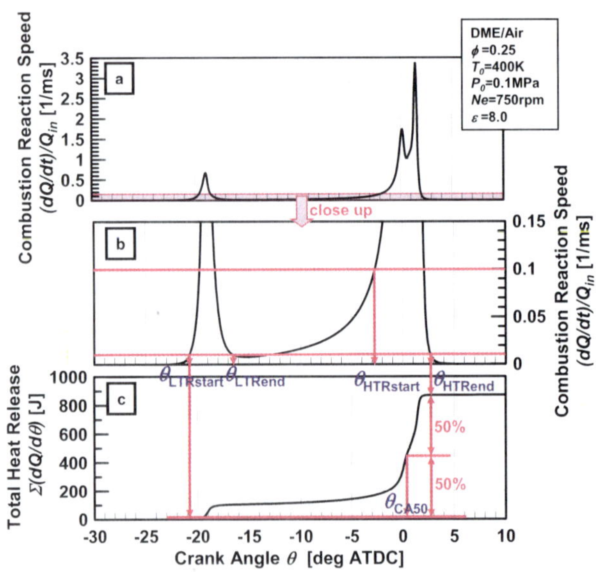

Fig. 2. Definitions of LTR start, LTR end, HTR start, HTR end and 50% heat release timing

the time that intake valve closed to the time that exhaust valve opened. As a calculation code, both CHEMKIN-II(5) and SENKIN(6) which is developed by Sandia National Laboratory is adjusted and then used. Curran for reaction of DME model, GRI-Mech3.0 for reaction of Methane model and Zeldvich for NOx model are used. The calculation is conducted following consumption. Heat loss and residual gas was neglected. All the chemical gases were considered to be ideal gas and mass of pre mixture is assumed to be conservative. Multi-zone model is able to make stratification of temperature and fuel concentration in combustion chamber by changing the gas temperature and equivalent ratio before each of zones are compressed. Shown in Fig. 1, each zone model that is equally gas temperature and homogenous chemical species is 0-demension. Between the each zone, there is not chemical species and heat transfer but pressure is constant. The definition of CA50, start and end timing of both LTR and HTR are shown in Fig. 2 Shown in Fig. 2(a)(b), the combustion reaction velocity((dQ/dt)/Qin) was defined as rate of heat production divided by quantity of heat into the 1 cycle. Fig. 2(c) shows the integral hysteresis of heat production. The integral value of heat production rate from the LTR start to HTR end is consider 100% and then CA50 is defined 50% of heat production timing.

3. Analytical method

3.1 The effect of thermal stratification in pre mixture gas for reducing pressure rise rate

The calculation condition of equal equivalent ratio (Φ=0.25) and initial temperature T0 = 380K(Zone1), T1 = 420K(Zone2) using the DME/air and Methane/air is shown in Fig. 3, 4. The volumetric rate is changed to equalize the heat quantity into the each zone during 1 cycle. Gas pressure in combustion chamber, temperature and heat release rate in each of the zone by using the DME with fuel is shown in Fig. 5. Magnified LTR and HTR shown in

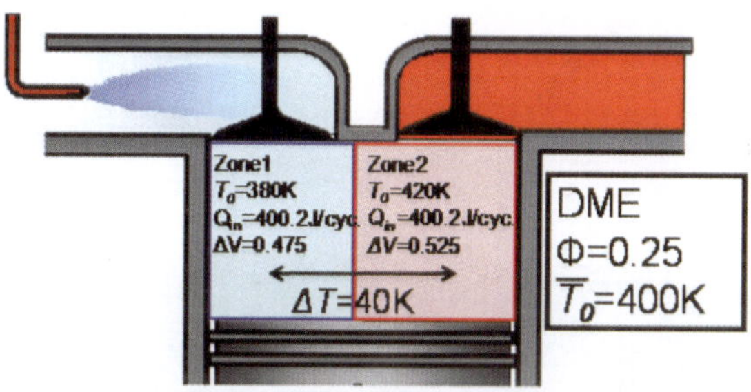

Fig. 3. Calculation condition (DME, Thermal stratification, 2-zones)

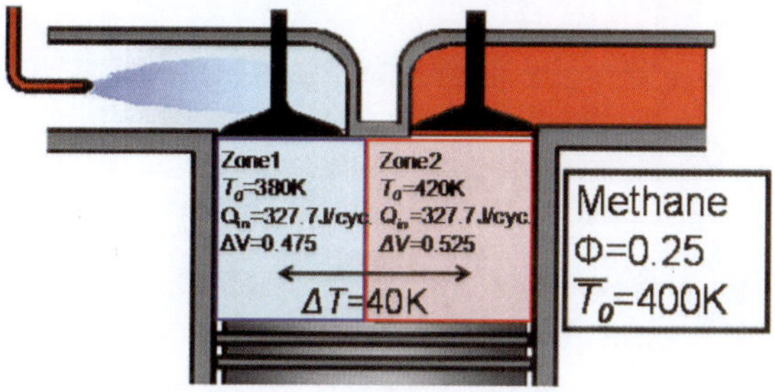

Fig. 4. Calculation condition (Methane, Thermal stratification, 2-zones)

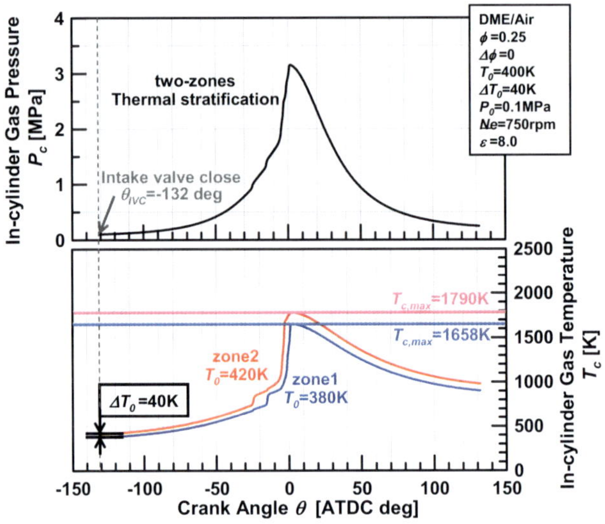

Fig. 5. Histories of in-cylinder gas pressure, in-cylinder gas temperature

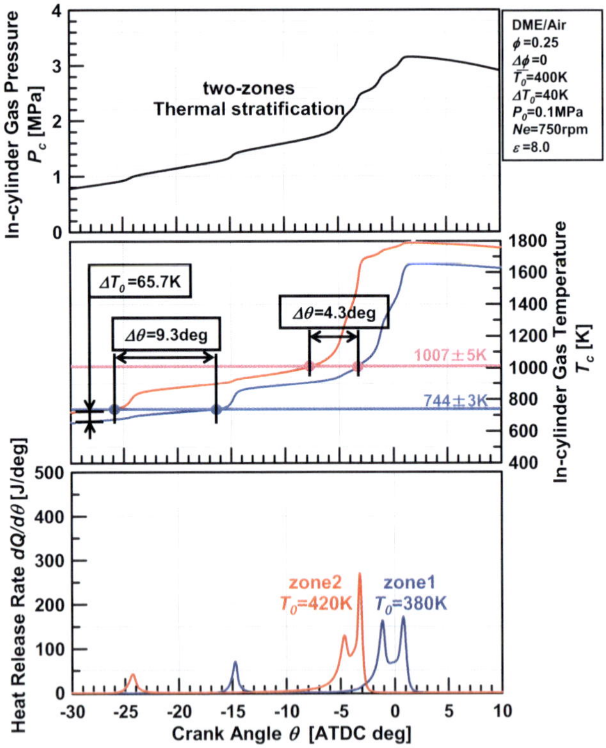

Fig. 6. Histories of in-cylinder gas pressure, in-cylinder gas temperature and heat release rate (DME, Thermal stratification, 2-zones)

Figure 6. First one is the graph of gas pressure in combustion chamber. Second and third one represent temperature and rat of heat release at each of the zone. LTR start temperature, HTR start temperature is almost constant as 744±3K, 1007±5K. Before LTR start, gas temperature difference in combustion chamber which is almost same as 40K according to piston rising is changed 65.7K before LTR start at zone 2. Because LTR start temperature is almost constant, LTR start is earlier about 9.3 deg at zone 2 than zone 1. Temperature difference between zone1 and zone2 is constant after LTR start so that HTR start is earlier about 4.3 deg than zone1. Also, using the fuel as a Methane, gas pressure in combustion chamber, temperature and heat release rate in each zone is shown in Fig. 7. The temperature of HTR start is 1177± 3K. Zone 2 with higher temperature than zone1, HTR start is earlier about 4.5deg than zone 1 before the compression stroke by using the Methane as a fuel.

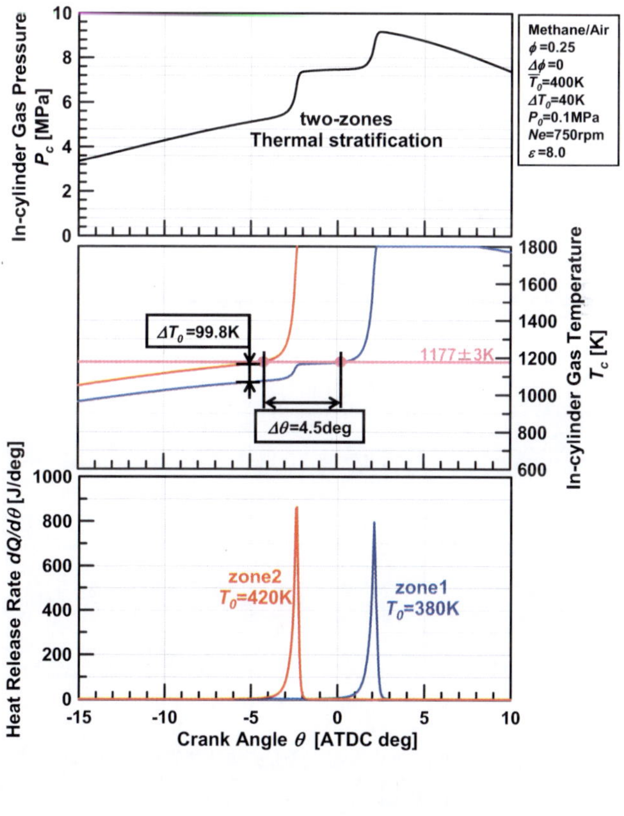

Fig. 7. Histories of in-cylinder gas pressure, in-cylinder gas temperature and heat release rate (Methane, Thermal stratification, 2-zones)

3.2 The effect of fuel stratification in pre mixture gas for reducing pressure rise rate

At the beginning of compression, the average gas temperature (T0 = 400K) is assumed. The calculation condition is shown in Fig. 8, 9 that is Φ = 0.17(zone1) Φ= 0.47(zone2) in each of the zone using the Methane or DME. Gas pressure in combustion chamber, gas temperature and rate of heat release in each of zone are shown in Fig. 10. Magnified graph was shown in Fig. 11. Temperature of LTR start and HTR start is 747±3 K, 1009±1. Temperature difference in combustion chamber is getting bigger according to piston rising before the LTR start due to difference of specific heat caused by equivalent ratio and temperature rising rate. Temperature difference before the compression stroke is changed from 0K to 17.3K before LTR start in zone1. LTR start is earlier at zone 2 about 2.3deg. However, Large amount of heat release during LTR in higher equivalent ration zone make trace of gas temperature be reversed in zone2 when LTR end. Due to gas temperature reversing, HTR start is earlier about 2.3 deg in zone 2 than zone1. Gas pressure in combustion chamber, gas temperature and heat release rate in each of the zone is shown in Fig. 12. HTR start temperature is 1163±11 K. Similar with DME, the Methane gas temperature difference in combustion chamber is getting big according to piston rising. However, Methane doesn't have LTR but 1 stage of heat release. So it can be expected HTR start in zone2 is later than zone 1 about 3.1 because of lean concentration of zone 1.

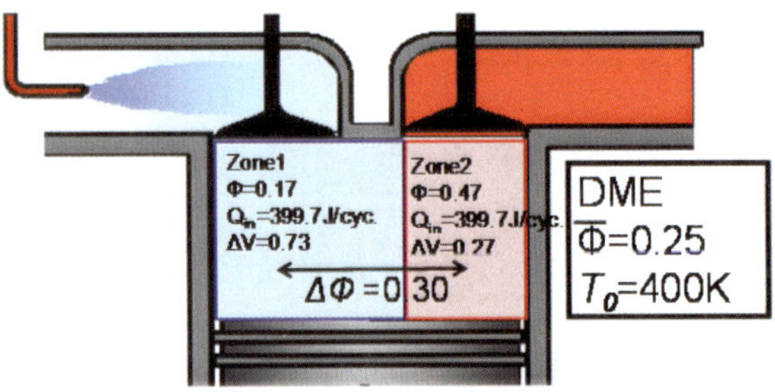

Fig. 8. Calculation condition (DME, Fuel stratification, 2-zones)

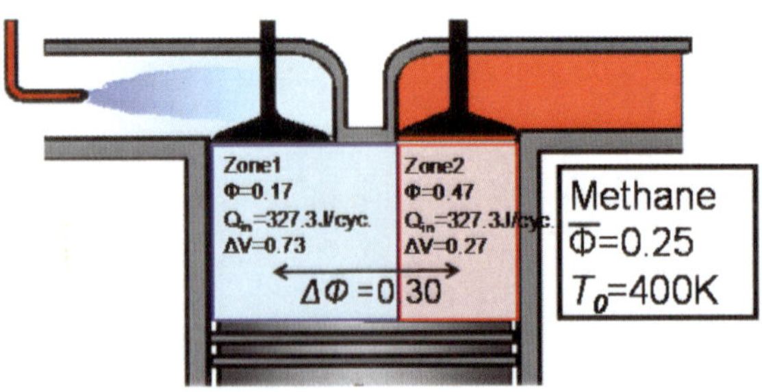

Fig. 9. Calculation condition (Methane, Fuel stratification, 2-zones)

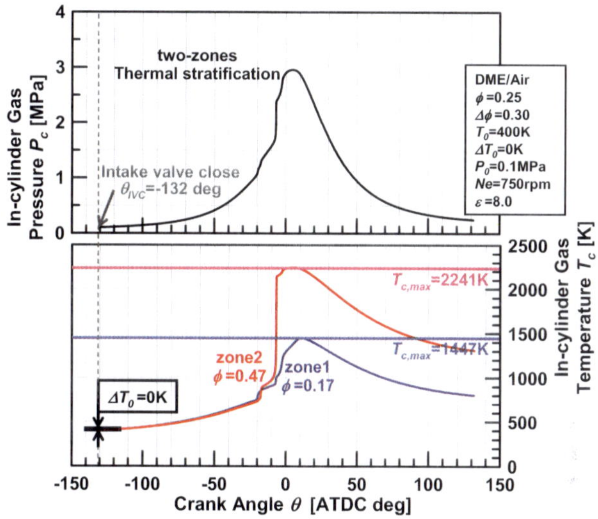

Fig. 10. Histories of in-cylinder gas pressure and in-cylinder gas temperature (DME, Fuel stratification, 2-zones)

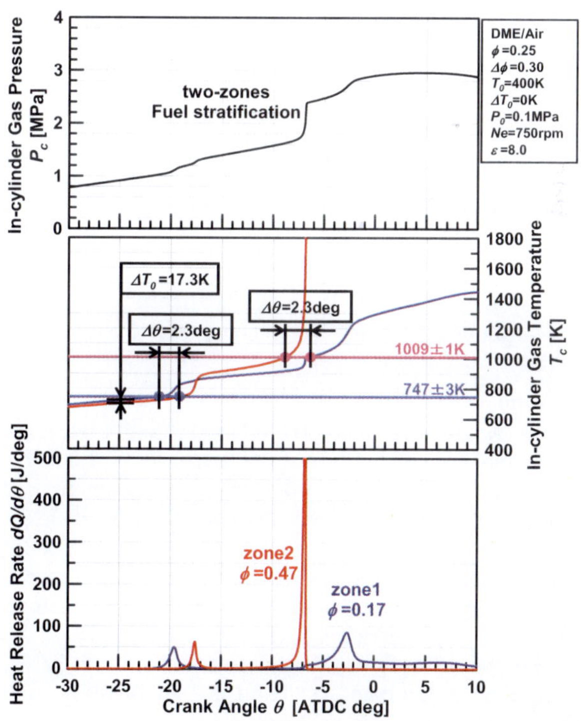

Fig. 11. Histories of in-cylinder gas pressure, in-cylinder gas temperature and heat release rate (DME, Fuel stratification, 2-zones)

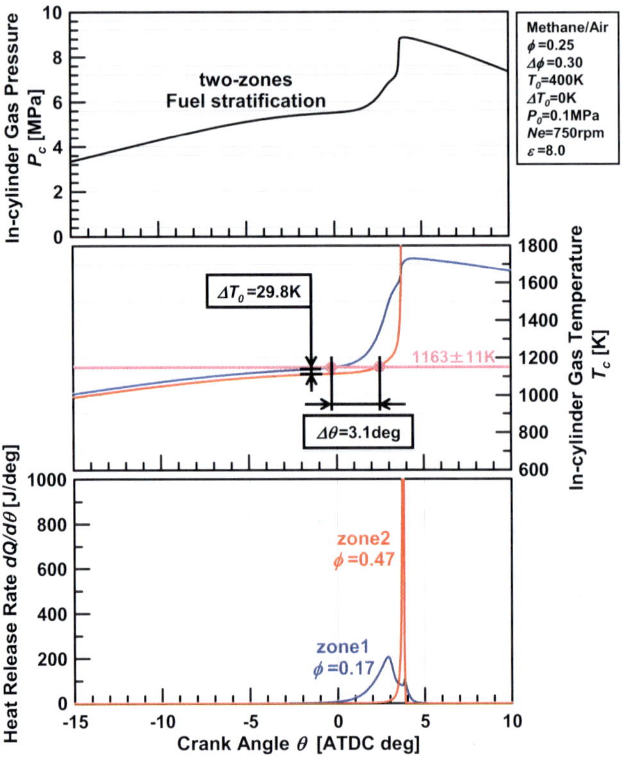

Fig. 12. Histories of in-cylinder gas pressure, in-cylinder gas temperature and heat release rate (Methane, Fuel stratification, 2-zones)

4. Results and discussion

4.1 Analysis of reducing maximum pressure rising rate effect and emission feature by multi-zone

Based on result of 2-zone model, reducing gas pressure rate, heat release and emission is investigated in combustion chamber when there is more temperature and fuel distribution by using the numerical analysis at 5 model-zone to expand and vary the stratification. Using the DME and Methane, the relation between CA50% and maximum pressure rise rate is shown in Fig..13-16 in condition of average equivalent ratio(φ=0,25) and changing the average temperature before the compression from T0=300K to T0=500K. In terms of temperature stratification, 5K average pre mixed gas temperature difference was given between each zone before compression and computation calculation was conducted in condition of T0=20K and T0=40K between highest and lowest zone. On the other hand, in terms of concentration stratification, average equivalent ratio(φ=0.25) is set up and computation calculation was conducted in condition of Δφ=0.10 and Δφ=0.30 between highest and lowest zone. Afterward, this result is compared with condition of equal temperature and concentration of pre-mixture gas. Comparing the result of temperature difference and concentration in pre-mixed gas, without any relation on amount of

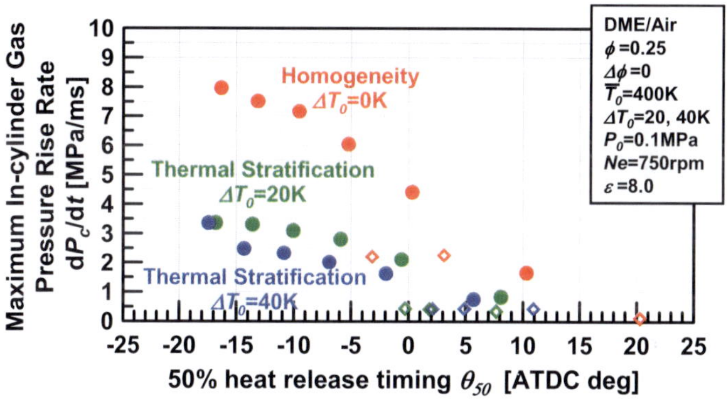

Fig. 13. 50% heat release timing and maximum in-cylinder gas pressure rise rate (DME, Thermal stratification, 5-zone)

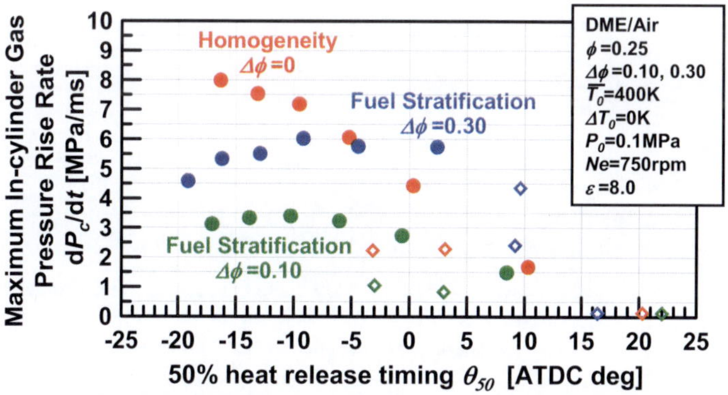

Fig. 14. 50% heat release timing and maximum in-cylinder gas pressure rise rate (DME, Fuel stratification, 5-zone)

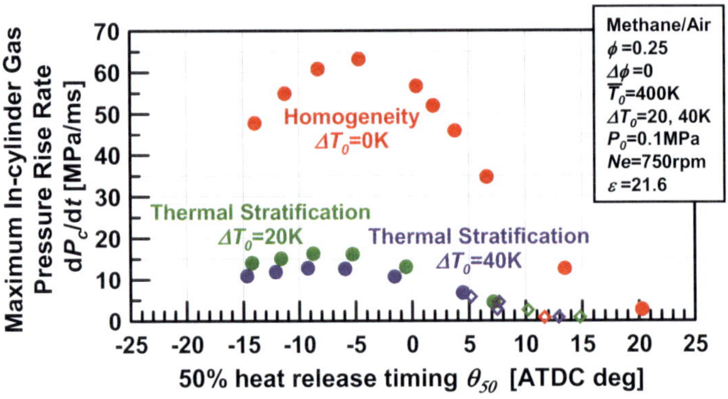

Fig. 15. 50% heat release timing and maximum in-cylinder gas pressure rise rate (Methane, Thermal stratification, 5-zone)

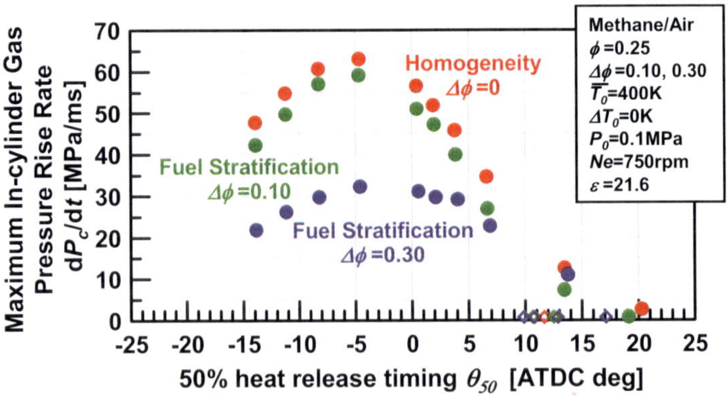

Fig. 16. 50% heat release timing and maximum in-cylinder gas pressure rise rate (Methane, Fuel stratification, 5-zone)

temperature difference, the maximum pressure rise rate is reduced below 50% beside homogeneous pre-mixed gas. The reduce rate is getting big, temperature difference is more. Its decrease rate is changed in a rage of concentration largely although the maximum pressure rise rate is reduced compared with homogenous pre-mixed gas when there is density difference. The rage of concentration which obtained reducing maximum pressure rise rate result is different comparing between DME and Methane. It can be expected that obtained result is different between DME and methane. The reason is that temperature difference by the piston compression before the LTR is disappeared and gas temperature trace is reversed at LTR end due to LTR existing in DME. In condition of 400K gas average temperature before the compression (T0), NOx, CO concentration in emission, combustion efficiency and maximum temperature in combustion chamber is shown in Fig. 17-20. The effect of temperature and concentration stratification on the emission characteristic was discussed by comparing pre-mixed gas with stratified temperature and concentration condition and equal temperature and concentration condition as T0=400K, equivalent ratio=0.25. Concentration of CO is increased bellow 1500K maximum temperature and NOx concentration is increased above 2100K. NOx and CO in emission gas concentration is almost same comparing the equal pre-mixed gas because maximum temperature is between 1500K and 2100K in each zone using DME and Methane existing temperature stratification in pre-mixed gas. NOx, CO concentration is getting big comparing with equal pre-mixed gas in emission gas because maximum temperature is above 2100K with high equivalent ratio in condition of concentration stratification.

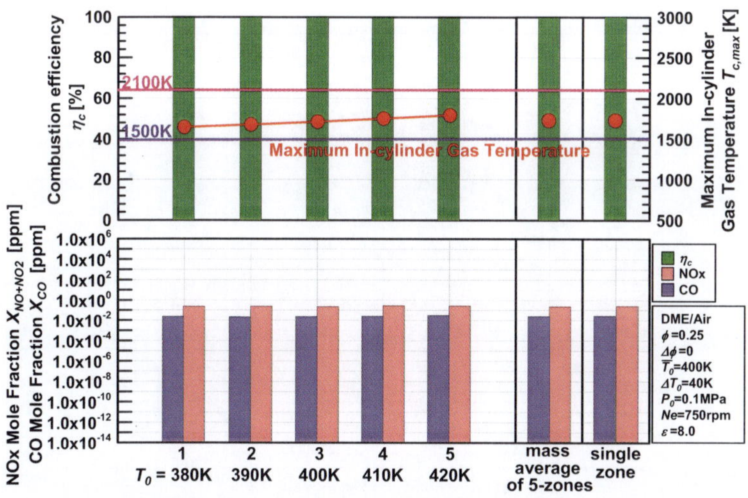

Fig. 17. CO and NOx mole fraction in exhaust gas, combustion efficiency and maximum in-cylinder gas temperature (DME, Thermal stratification, 5-zones)

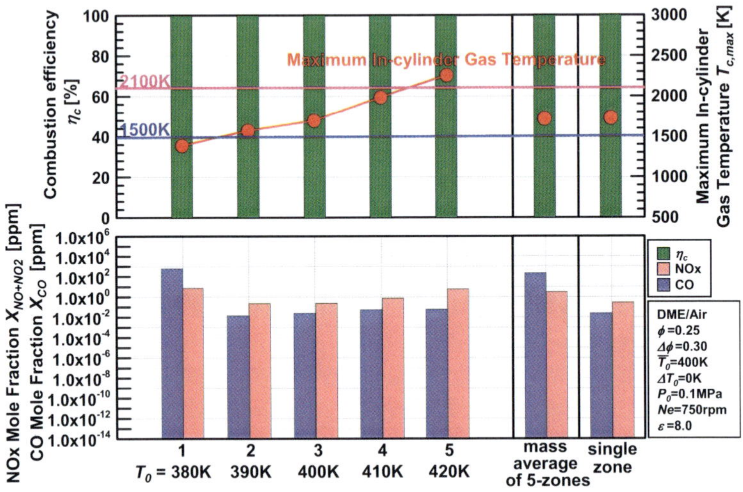

Fig. 18. CO and NOx mole fraction in exhaust gas, combustion efficiency and maximum in-cylinder gas temperature (DME, Fuel stratification, 5-zones)

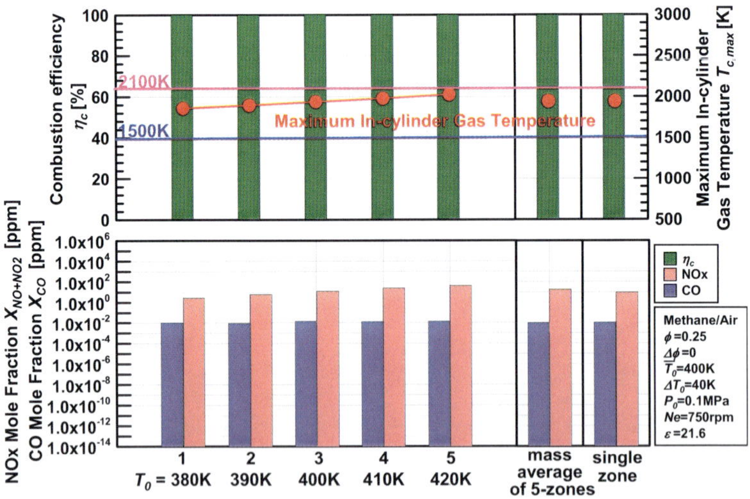

Fig. 19. CO and NOx mole fraction in exhaust gas, combustion efficiency and maximum in-cylinder gas temperature (Methane, Thermal stratification, 5-zones)

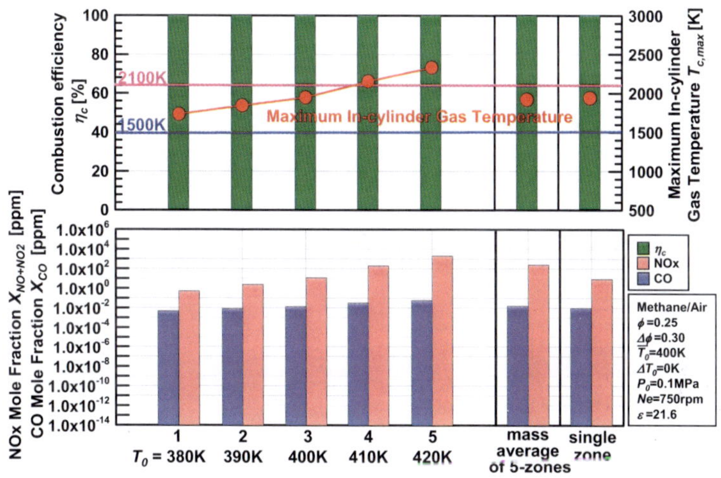

Fig. 20. CO and NOx mole fraction in exhaust gas, combustion efficiency and maximum in-cylinder gas temperature (Methane, Fuel stratification, 5-zones)

5. Conclusion

Chemical reaction numerical computation was conducted by giving a temperature or concentration stratification to pre-mixture. The reducing pressure rise rate effect is investigated by temperature and concentration stratification in pre-mixture. Choosing the DME and Methane that heat release characteristic is different, using the detailed reaction scheme and conducting numerical computation in multi-zone, following knowledge is affordable.

1. In condition of stratified temperature pre-mixture, temperature difference of the combustion chamber is expanded by piston compression. LTR or HTR occur earlier at the zone that gas temperature is higher.
2. In condition of stratified fuel pre-mixture, temperature difference of the combustion chamber is occurred. LTR is occurred earlier in the zone which is lower concentration beside HTR is opposite.
3. In condition of stratified temperature and concentration, maximum pressure rise rate is decreased largely as compared with equal condition. Especially, maximum pressure rise rate is reduced restricting NOx, CO emission amount in condition of stratified temperature which is same as equal condition.
4. Concentrate stratification control is needed to operate the engine between 1500K and 2100K in condition of stratified concentration in pre-mixture.
5. Optimized succeeding investigation what temperature and concentration of stratification is most efficient is needed to reduce both maximum pressure rise rate and emission together efficiently

6. References

Yamashita, D. Kweon, S. Sato, S. & Iida, N. (2005). The Study on Auto-ignition and Combustion Process of the fuel Blended with Methane and DME in HCCI Engines,*Transaction of JSAE*, Vol.36, No.6, pp85-90

Sjoberg, M. John E. D. & Cernansky, N. P. (2005). Potential of Thermal Stratification and Combustion Retard for Reducing Pressure-Rise Rates in HCCI Engines, Basedon Multi-Zone Modeling and Experiments, *SAE,* SAE paper 2005-01-0113

Kwon, O. & Lim O. (2009). Effect of the Boost Pressure on Thermal Stratification on HCCI Engine using multi-zone modeling. *Trans. of the KSME* (B)Vol.33, No.3(accepted)

Kumano K. & Iida, N. (2004). Analysis of the Effect of Charge Inhomogeneity on HCCI Combustion by Chemiluminescence Measurement, SAE paper 2004-01-1902

Luz A.E. Rupley F. & Miller J.A. (1989). CHEMKIN-II:A FORTRAN ChemicalKineticsPacage for the Analysis of Gas-Phase Chemical Kinetics. *Sandia National LaboratoriesReport,* SAND89-8009B

Luz A.E. Kee R.J. & Miller J.A. (1988). SENKIN:A FORTRAN Program for Predicting Homogeneous Gas Phase Chemical Kinetics With Sensitivity Analysis, *Sandia National Laboratories Report*, SAND87-8248

Curran, H.J. Pitz, W.J. Westbrook, C.K. Dagaut, P.B. Boettner, J-C & Cathonnet, M. (1998). AWide Range Modeling Study of Dimethyl Ether Oxidation, *International Journal Chemical Kinetics*, 30-3, 229-241

GRI-Mech3.0, http://www.me.berkeley.edu/gri_mech

Part 3

Chemical Kinetics and Phases

8

The Chemical Kinetics of Shape Determination in Plants

David M. Holloway
Mathematics Department, British Columbia Institute of Technology, Canada

1. Introduction

Plants are integral to our lives, providing food, shelter and the air we breathe. The shapes that plants take are central to their functionality, tailoring each for its particular place in the ecosystem. Given the relatively large and static forms of plants, it may not be immediately apparent that chemical kinetics is involved in, for example, distinguishing the form of a spruce tree from that of a fern. But plants share the common feature that their shapes are continuously being generated, and this largely occurs in localized regions of cell division and expansion, such as the shoot and root apical meristems at either end of a plant's main axis; these regions remain essentially embryonic throughout the life cycle. The final regular structure of a plant, such as the arrangement of leaves along the main stalk, may seem to follow an overall spatial template; but in reality the spatial patterning is occurring at relatively short range, and it is the temporal unfolding of this small scale patterning which generates the plant's form. A key part of understanding plant morphogenesis, or shape generation, therefore, is to understand how the molecular determinants of cell type, cell division and cell expansion are localized to and patterned within the actively growing regions. At this scale, transport processes such as diffusion and convection are obvious components of localization, for moving molecules to the correct places; but the reaction kinetics for molecular creation, destruction and interaction are also critical to maintaining the molecular identity and the size regulation of the active regions.

It was Turing (1952) who first combined the ideas of reaction kinetics with diffusion into a theory of spatial pattern formation - how to establish, and maintain, molecules at specific concentrations in specific locations. The Turing mechanism involves two mutually interacting (activating and inhibiting) intermediates (which he termed 'morphogens'), which diffuse at different rates. While his paper chiefly introduced the kinetics required for pattern formation from homogeneous initial conditions (in particular, finding critical values of rate constants for this to occur), Turing was clearly thinking of the implications in embryonic tissues, as evidenced by his title, "The chemical theory of morphogenesis". In the 1960's, Prigogine and collaborators presented the first specific nonlinear chemical mechanism which could form stable spatial concentration waves (the 'Brusselator'; Prigogine & Lefever, 1968), as well as providing a thermodynamic basis for spontaneous pattern formation (see Nicolis & Prigogine, 1977). In the 1970's, reaction-diffusion (RD) mechanisms were introduced into biology by Meinhardt (see Meinhardt, 1982), Harrison (see Harrison, 1993),

Murray (see Murray, 1989) and many others, through computer simulations of RD mechanisms for particular embryonic phenomena. The Turing mechanism for pattern formation was experimentally confirmed in 1990 with the CIMA redox reaction in gel reactors (Castets et al., 1990; Ouyang & Swinney, 1991). RD is now a broad and mature field (with consistently over 150 citations per year of Turing's paper over the past decade).

This chapter focuses on the development of RD theory in plant morphogenesis, particularly in characterizing the interplay of pattern formation and domain growth (also see Holloway, 2010, for a short review). In contrast to animal embryogenesis, in which pattern formation generally occurs in fixed domains, the continuous growth of plants inextricably links chemical localization (patterning) and growth (shape change). Growth affects patterning: at the least patterns must be generated and maintained in the face of domain growth, since RD mechanisms (like other dynamic mechanisms) have harmonic solutions which depend on domain geometry, size and boundary conditions. But perhaps more importantly, patterning affects growth: plant cells expand through localized wall material addition or wall material relaxation, both chemically dependent processes. The patterning mechanisms which determine where expansion-associated chemicals are localized are therefore critical determinants in the shapes of plant tissues. The complex mechanical properties of plant cells are also important in the deformations leading to final overall shape, and will be discussed below in relation to chemical patterning. However, biochemical processes (interpreted broadly, e.g. genetic regulation, hormone response) generally precede shape change, and how these processes create spatial pattern is central to morphogenesis. (For further discussion on morphogenetic modelling in general, please see the recent reviews of Braybrook & Kuhlemeier, 2010; Grieneisen & Scheres, 2009; Jönsson & Krupinski, 2010; Roeder et al., 2011; and Zwieniecki & Dumais, 2011).

Many developmental phenomena depend on a sequence of patterns, for example from simple extending tip growth to branching. RD theory provides a means for understanding the kinetic constraints involved in such symmetry-breaking transitions. The development of RD theory for growing domains, in conjunction with experimental tests, illuminates how chemical kinetics shape the plants around us, from ferns to spruce trees.

2. The chemical kinetics of spatial pattern formation

The regulation of reaction rates is central to maintaining biological order. At its simplest, kinetics maintain a homeostasis of production and destruction of an organism's component molecules; at the somewhat more complex, nonlinear kinetic mechanisms underlie temporal regulation, such as the heartbeat. But reactions are local, and do not immediately provide a mechanism for establishing the spatial pattern or regulation necessary for forming and maintaining an organism's body plan. For this, Rashevsky (1940) was one of the first to publish the idea of combining simple Fickian diffusion, as a spatially-dependent process, with local reactions to regulate biological spacing. Turing (1952) formulated the first RD theory mathematically, demonstrating the conditions for these processes to spontaneously form pattern (stable concentration waves) from uniform initial conditions, i.e to self-organize pattern. These ideas have been greatly expanded, theoretically and experimentally, into a field of RD pattering. Since Turing, other spatially-dependent processes – such as convection, mechanical stresses and anisotropic diffusion – have been combined with reaction terms to explore the broader dynamics of chemical pattern formation. The dynamics have been most fully explored for simple diffusion, however, and RD has become a very well-characterized means by which to study pattern formation in general.

2.1 Turing's ideas: How activation, inhibition and diffusion create concentration waves

Turing's focus was on how a uniformly distributed chemical could spontaneously form spatial pattern, or 'standing' concentration waves. This transition implies an instability in the uniform equilibrium condition; the final concentration waves exist (and must be held) away from thermodynamic equilibrium. (For further discussion of far-from-equilibrium thermodynamics, see Nicolis & Prigogine, 1977.) To reduce some of the mystique in this symmetry-breaking process, Turing used the analogy of an electrical oscillator – that what appears to be uniform concentration is in fact comprised of the elements of any spatial pattern necessary, as noise at the microscopic scale – and that there is a natural frequency of the oscillator, or the chemical system, such that this frequency can be amplified from the noise to achieve macroscopic proportions. Turing showed that such a chemical amplifier could be devised for two mutually reacting chemicals, X (activator) and Y (inhibitor), which diffuse at different rates. Fig. 1 illustrates the mechanism.

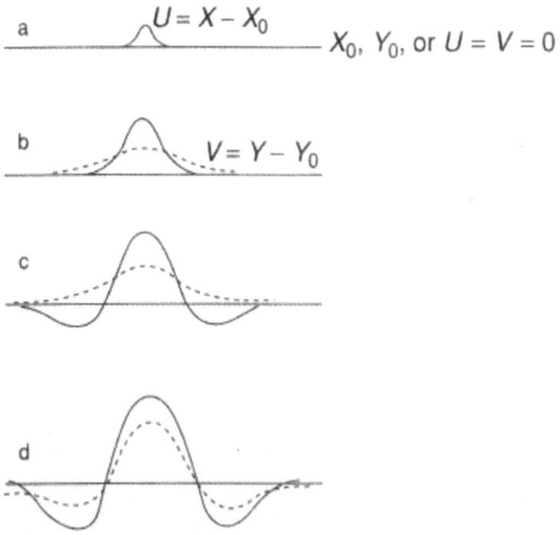

Fig. 1. Growth of perturbations into sinusoidal patterns (vertical – concentration, horizontal – distance). **a**) An initial small positive perturbation of X from its uniform steady-state value of X_0. **b**) If X is autocatalytic (enhances its own production) and cross-catalyzes Y, the initial X perturbation grows and begins to produce a Y peak. Y diffuses faster than X. **c**) If Y inhibits X, it begins to create troughs in X, which **d**) also become troughs in Y (since X activates Y). The pattern achieves a spacing dependent on reaction and diffusion constants. Reproduced from Harrison (1993), redrawn from Maynard Smith (1968), with permission.

Mathematically, for $U=X-X_0$, and $V=Y-Y_0$, the deviations of X and Y from the uniform state, the linear reaction-diffusion equations are:

$$\partial U/\partial t = k_1 U + k_2 V + D_X \Delta U \tag{1a}$$

$$\partial V/\partial t = k_3 U + k_4 V + D_Y \Delta V \quad (1b)$$

with diffusivities D and Laplacian operator Δ (2nd partial derivative with respect to distance, 1 to 3 dimensions). The conditions illustrated in Fig. 1 correspond to k_1, k_3>0, k_2<0, and D_X<D_Y. Solutions for U and V take the form of (1D, for illustration)

$$U = \cos(\omega s)e^{\sigma t} \quad (2)$$

where s is the spatial dimension, t is time, ω^2 is the wavevector of the spatial pattern (for 1D, the spacing between peaks is given by wavelength $\lambda = 2\pi/\omega$), and σ is the eigenvalue or growth constant of the perturbations. In 1D, cos and sin solutions can be viewed as components of the Fourier representation of a pattern (in the uniform initial condition, Fourier components of the microscopic noise). In 2D and 3D, solutions to (1) similarly are harmonics of the Laplacian operator for the given geometry (e.g. Bessel functions on 2D discs; surface spherical harmonics for spherical shells, section **2.4**). Turing derived conditions for which $\sigma > 0$, indicating when pattern modes will amplify (below this 'Turing instability' $\sigma < 0$ and the uniform concentration is stable). The eigenvalue, σ, is a function of the wavevector ω^2; this functionality is a complex expression involving all the parameters in equations (1), but with the general form of $\omega^2 \propto k/D$. In 1D terms, wave*length* is shortened by increasing reaction rates (k's) or decreasing diffusivities (D's). There may be a number of wavevectors with positive σ fitting the particular boundary conditions (e.g. no-flux or fixed concentration); generally the wavevector with largest eigenvalue will grow to dominate the macroscopic pattern, analogous to the natural frequency of an electrical oscillator. For more on the mathematics of the linear Turing equations (1), please see Edelstein-Keshet (1988); Harrison (1993; 2011); or Holloway (1995).

2.2 The Brusselator, a nonlinear kinetic patterning mechanism

The linear rate equations (1) are an approximation from real chemical dynamics. In real chemical mechanisms, the reactions giving Turing dynamics are nonlinear; for example, autocatalysis gives a rate law for X which is greater than 1st order in X. Linear analysis is accurate for growth rates and wavevectors at the Turing instability, i.e. for conditions just supporting positive eigenvalues. For conditions with many growing wavevectors and for long times (beyond the exponential growth phase described by equation (2)), linear analysis is not as good a predictor of observed pattern. In these cases, numerical simulation or nonlinear analysis of the chemical mechanism is needed. Prigogine & Lefever (1968) devised the first chemical mechanism (the 'Brusselator') with Turing pattern-forming dynamics:

$$A \xrightarrow{a} X \quad (3a)$$

$$B + X \xrightarrow{b} Y + D \quad (3b)$$

$$Y + 2X \xrightarrow{c} 3X \quad (3c)$$

$$X \xrightarrow{d} E \quad (3d)$$

in which the X and Y morphogens are reactive intermediates in the creation of D and E from precursors A and B. Prigogine and Lefever commented that the termolecular step in equation (3c) could be unlikely in gas phase; but such conditions would be common in multi-step enzyme kinetics. Since X depletes Y in this 3rd step, X and Y waves form out-of-phase, in contrast to Fig. 1. The Brusselator has a strong tendency to form regular patterns which follow linear predictions (e.g. Lacalli, 1981; Holloway & Harrison, 1995), and we have found it very appropriate for modelling regular events in plant development, such as branching (Harrison et al., 1981; Harrison & Kolář, 1988; Holloway & Harrison, 1999; Harrison et al., 2001; Holloway & Harrison, 2008).

2.3 Early biological applications

Computer simulation of nonlinear RD mechanisms expanded greatly in the 1970's and 1980's, accompanied by an increase in applying RD to biological development. Gierer & Meinhardt (1972) derived an RD pattern-forming mechanism independent of knowledge of prior work in the 1960's and 1970's, but which has Turing dynamics. They used this mechanism and variants to successfully model numerous phenomena in animal and plant development (e.g. Meinhardt, 1982; 1984; 1986; 1988; 1995). A chief contrast with the Brusselator dynamics is the tendency for the Gierer-Meinhardt model to form 'spike', or isolated, peaks (Lacalli, 1981; Holloway & Harrison, 1995; Iron et al., 2001). This can be very appropriate for modelling localized structures, such as single organs (heads, hearts), and the dynamics can be derived from multi-step activation in enzyme kinetics (Holloway et al., 1994). In animal development, Murray (1981ab) developed RD models for animal coat markings; Kauffman and co-workers (Kauffman 1977; 1981; Kauffman et al., 1978; Hunding et al., 1990) began RD modelling of fruit fly segmentation, which was greatly expanded by many workers (e.g. Nagorcka, 1988; Lacalli et al., 1988; Lacalli, 1990; Lyons et al., 1990); and Nagorcka & Mooney (1982; 1985) developed an RD model for hair follicle patterning. Many of these early directions continue as active areas of research. Early work on RD modelling of plants, with the intrinsic challenge of coupling growth and patterning, will be presented in more detail in section **3**.

2.4 Geometry and pattern selection in 3D

As introduced in **2.1**, solutions to RD equations are harmonics of the Laplacian, dependent on boundary conditions (e.g. no-flux or fixed concentration) and geometry. In 1D, this dependence can be studied as the fit of the linear wavelength $\lambda = 2\pi/\omega$ to the system length. Many patterning forming events in plants tend to occur on growing tips, which are roughly dome shaped. In these cases, the geometry can be approximated by a hemisphere, and RD pattern formation understood in terms of the surface spherical harmonics, polynomials designated by Y_l^m. These functions are familiar as the hydrogen-like atomic orbitals, where l is the index denoting s, p, d, f, etc. orbitals, and m denotes different patterns within each of the l levels. For these harmonics, $\omega^2 = l(l+1)/r^2$: the wavevector depends on index l and the radius of the hemisphere. Linear analysis predicts that any patterns of the same l should grow at the same rate (i.e. equal eigenvalues). This has bearing on pattern selection in plants: at l=3, m=0 gives a circularly-symmetric annular pattern; $m = \pm 2$ gives 'quartered' patterns; and the equal mix of these modes gives a dichotomous branch pattern (Fig. 2). Linear analysis would predict the annular and quartered patterns to grow equally, and therefore to mix and always produce dichotomous branches. But both annular patterns (underlying tip flattening) and dichotomous branches occur in plant development. Harrison et al. (2001) and Nagata et al. (2003) showed, through simulation and nonlinear analysis respectively, that RD dynamics can produce both types of patterns (i.e. linear analysis does not provide the full picture). Intriguingly, the Brusselator model shows about an 80:20 preference for dichotomous branching over annuli, and such proportional selection can be seen experimentally in conifer development (von Aderkas, 2002). Current work (Nagata, Zangeneh and Holloway, unpublished results) is addressing how pattern selection changes as a hemisphere is deformed into a disc (where Bessel functions are the natural harmonics), representing a tip-flattening sequence common to many plants.

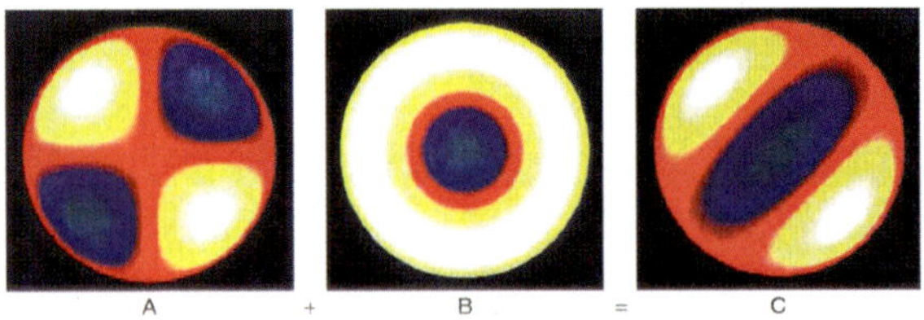

Fig. 2. Pattern selection on a hemisphere (approximating the growing tip of a plant). Surface spherical harmonics for index l=3: (A) $m = \pm 2$; (B) m=0; (C) equal mix of (A) and (B) produces a dichotomous branch pattern. Linear analysis predicts (A) and (B) patterns would grow equally, therefore always producing (C). Plant development shows both (B) and (C) patterns. Simulation and nonlinear analysis show that the full RD dynamics (Brusselator model) do have the capacity to produce both (B) and (C) patterns. From Holloway & Harrison (2008), with permission.

3. Plant morphogenesis and reaction-diffusion: The challenge of growth-patterning feedback

RD theory is well-established for pattern formation on fixed-size domains. Understanding plant development, however, requires consideration of the interaction between pattern formation and growth, since plants grow throughout their life cycles. The interaction between patterning and growth can be considered at many levels. First, as discussed above, RD patterns (like other dynamic mechanisms) develop according to boundary conditions, system size and system geometry (as well as reaction and diffusion parameters). It must be understood, therefore, how patterns are formed, maintained, and respond to changes in size and geometry stemming from growth (Fig. 3, top arrow). I.e., how do the biochemicals (e.g. hormones, gene regulators) responsible for the differentiation of particular tissue types form and stay in the correct regions of the plant during growth? Or, moving beyond simple maintenance of pattern, do developmental changes in tissue size or location originate from the response of the dynamic mechanism (RD) to growth? As shown in Fig. 3, however, there is also a return arrow in the growth-patterning interaction to consider: the response of growth to patterning. Plant cell growth itself involves localized chemicals, for the localized relaxation of walls or the localized delivery of new wall materials. These patterns of growth catalysts can therefore shape the plant, and be, to use Turing's title, 'the chemical basis of morphogenesis'. This section addresses some of the dynamic issues involved in the full feedback cycle of Fig. 3.

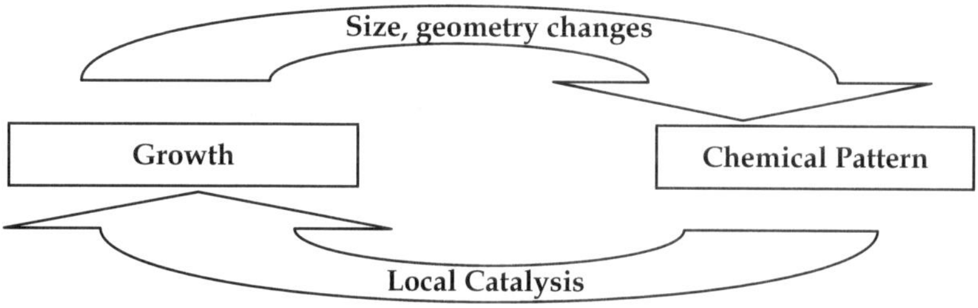

Fig. 3. The patterning-growth feedback involved in plant morphogenesis: Growth affects the types of chemical patterns which form; if the patterns are of growth catalysts, the pattern in turn affects growth.

3.1 RD response to uniform growth

The potential for RD spacing (e.g. the 1D wavelength) to produce pattern changes in response to growth has been recognized for some time. Lacalli & Harrison (1978) quantified how the fit of dominant wavelength to system size can produce increasingly complex pattern (additional morphogen peaks) as system size increases. This was developed for hemispherical surfaces in Harrison et al. (1981): Fig. 4A shows a succession of (circularly-symmetric) morphogen patterns caused by uniform growth of the hemisphere. If X were associated with growth, this sequence would correspond to successive cycles of tip extension followed by tip flattening; such cycles are seen in many events in plant

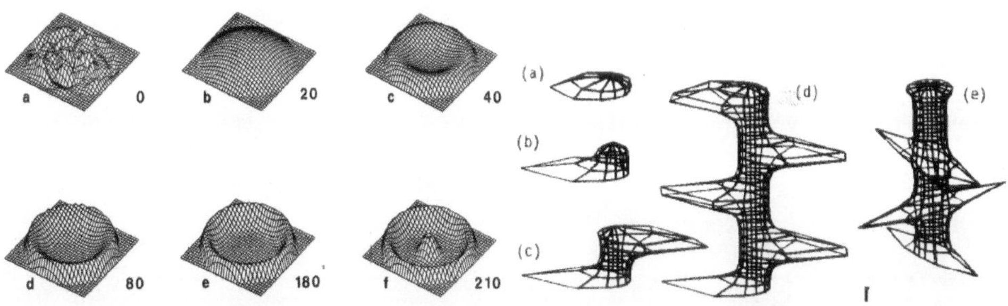

Fig. 4. RD pattern successions with uniform system growth. **A**) Brusselator computation from Harrison et al. (1981), with permission; planar projection of hemispherical shape (distance from centre is distance along a meridian). Vertical relief represents X morphogen concentration; numbers indicate computational time. As the hemisphere radius increases linearly in time, pattern forms first as a dome (b), then an annulus (c-e), then forms a new peak in the centre (f). **B**) Meinhardt's (1982) model for formation of lateral structures in a plant stalk. Computations are on a cylinder, with uniform growth produced by doubling the top cells at regular intervals. Morphogen (X) concentration is represented as lateral displacement. Inhibition (Y) flowing from established morphogen peaks (X, Y in-phase, as in Fig. 1) causes new peaks to form on opposite sides of the cylinder (a-d; 'distichous' branching). For larger cylinder radius or slower inhibitor diffusion, peaks can form at 90° angles (e; 'decussate' branching). From Meinhardt (1982), with permission.

development. Meinhardt (1982) computed RD patterning on a uniformly growing cylinder (Fig. 4B) to model different modes of lateral organ formation in plants. Both of these projects began to demonstrate the degree to which RD patterns could respond to growth and, to the degree morphogens are associated with cell growth or differentiation, for RD to determine events in plant development. But this and subsequent related work represents only the forward arrow of Fig. 3.

3.2 Full feedback: Driving growth with RD patterns

To investigate the degree to which RD pattern can determine plant shape, RD models needed to be developed in which morphogens explicitly cause localized growth (backward arrow, Fig. 3).

3.2.1 RD mechanism control of growth-rate boundaries required for morphogenesis

Harrison & Kolář (1988) first directly coupled RD and growth, with a Brusselator model for the morphogenesis of single-celled desmid algae of the genus *Micrasterias*. These cells develop elaborate stellate forms via repeated dichotomous branching (Fig. 5 H-N). Computations started with a circular initial shape in 2D, discretized into several hundred line segments. Growth per unit time was computed in proportion to the amount of X morphogen on the segment. The RD wave forming on the initial circle caused ripples of outgrowth in the shape; as system length increased, additional peaks (for the given wavelength) could fit in, leading to branching in pattern and shape. However, it was found that the branching morphology was transitory, due to the re-adjustment of peak positions following branching. In a sense, the RD wavelength is too good at spacing, and will erase old growth trajectories as it readjusts to the overall system length. In general terms, plant growth patterns need to be compartmentalized, such that separate structures (separate branches) develop relatively independently. Patterning may occur over the whole structure of the plant at early stages, but at later, larger stages patterning occurs in multiple active centres which are minimally coordinated. Plant shapes are composed of the integrated growth rates of the different regions of the whole organism, with shape critically depending on the placement and regulation of the boundaries between fast- and slow-growing regions. Chemical morphogenetic mechanisms, therefore, need both the symmetry-breaking power of RD, for example to account for branching phenomena, and the ability to segregate pattern-forming regions following a symmetry-breaking. To add this critical aspect to their model, Harrison and Kolář added an aging mechanism to the precursor A in the Brusselator. Where growth is rapid at high X, the cell surface is continually rejuvenated; at low X, growth is low and A decreases below a critical threshold, shutting off the pattern-forming mechanism. X peaks can in this way become segregated from one another, producing multiple active regions on the cell surface, each of which retains its own Turing dynamics. This mechanism succeeded in transforming RD branching patterns into branching shapes, the critical piece being a means by which the RD mechanism could control its own system boundaries; i.e. for each fast-growing X peak region to be able to control the size of said region.

3.2.2 Fast boundary control needed for acute branching

The Harrison-Kolář mechanism created branching morphologies, but all branches were obtuse-angled. The stellate shapes of *Micrasterias* are generated chiefly by acute branching,

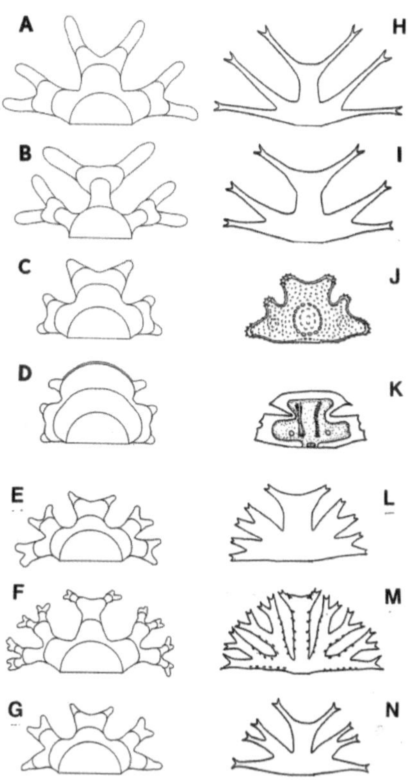

Fig. 5. RD driven growth in 2D: cellular morphogenesis of desmid algae. H-N) observed semicell outlines for six species of *Micrasterias* and one related *Euastrum* species (J). Whole *Micrasterias* are two semicells joined at their bases (bottom centre, as drawn). With mitosis, new semicells start as small 'bubbles' attached to the mature semicells; the new semicells then undergo repeated dichotomous branching to achieve the mature shape. A-G) corresponding outlines computed with a Brusselator-driven growth mechanism (Holloway & Harrison, 1999). Computations start from an initial semicircle shape (post-mitotic new semicell); outward growth occurs in proportion to local X morphogen concentration, with growth boundaries controlled by the X_{th} mechanism (see text). Outlines are shown at successive times during development of the shape, and correspond to experimentally observed developmental sequences. Differences between shapes are due to differences in X_{th} values. From Harrison (2011), with permission.

however (and acute branching is common in many other developmental phenomena as well). We approached this problem in Holloway & Harrison (1999), finding that new branches in a Brusselator would tend to spread apart, adjusting to their Turing wavelength, unless the boundary-specifying mechanism was fast enough to prevent this. The Harrison-Kolář aging mechanism was too slow. Instead of an aging threshold, we used a more direct X threshold (X_{th}), below which RD patterning shut off. This produced growth rate boundaries lateral to established X peaks, isolating fast-growing domains from one another;

but most importantly, it allowed for fast boundary creation at just-formed troughs following an X peak splitting, critical for acutely branched morphologies. With this mechanism, we were able to generate many of the diverse shapes seen across species of *Micrasterias* (Fig. 5 A-G). X_{th}, the coupling between the RD mechanism and the growth boundaries, was the key parameter for shaping the cells. Some shapes required shifting of the X_{th} over the course of development, a process which could be controlled by the cell's physiology.

More recently, there have been several mathematical studies further characterizing the dynamics of growth-patterning feedback in RD models (Neville et al., 2006; Crampin et al. 2002), including morphogen-driven growth (in 1D, without shape change). Also, see Baker & Maini (2007) for an application of 1D morphogen-driven expansion in insect wing development.

3.2.3 Pattern selection with 3D growth, a finite-element RD model

Micrasterias cells are relatively flat, with growth occurring along an edge, making them well suited to 2D modelling. Many cases of plant development, however, occur fully in 3D. What is a dichotomous branch in 2D could, in 3D, still be a dichotomous branch. But it could also be a planar section through a flattened tip or through a multiply-branched whorl structure (e.g. a flower). There are many more pattern modes available in 3D: how do RD dynamics select among them? Section **2.4** introduced some of the issues of pattern selection on fixed hemispheres. To address patterning questions for RD-growth mechanisms in 3D, we developed a finite-element model to solve RD systems on surfaces (i.e. no thickness) of arbitrary shape in 3D (Harrison et al., 2001), with growth (normal to the surface) catalyzed in proportion to local *X* concentration.

One of the first questions we addressed was how clefts are maintained between growing tips. In 2D, an arbitrary rule was needed to keep clefts in position and not be pulled up by fast growth in the tips. In 3D, computations demonstrated that geometry is sufficient: clefts are saddles, with a fast-growing plane through the tips orthogonally intersecting a slow-growing plane in the cleft (Harrison et al., 2001).

The finite-element model (with the X_{th} Brusselator mechanism) has allowed us to map pattern selection for large RD-driven deformations, and characterize the degree to which RD patterns can produce some of the fundamental morphogenetic sequences seen in plants. These results (Holloway & Harrison, 2008) are summarized in Fig. 6. Tip extension is one of the fundamental modes of growth seen in plants: Fig. 6A shows a computation in which an initial hemisphere has extended over ten times its original height. Tip growth depends on a balance between the X_{th} value and the *X*-catalyzed growth rate: X_{th} relatively too high kills off the tip; X_{th} relatively too low forms 'bubble' tips. Neither case extends. Large deformations in the computations require a continual relatticing of the finite element mesh specifying the surface. Local relatticing results in an irregular mesh (Fig. 6B), but does not affect shape or RD solution accuracy. Dichotomous branching occurs with decreased diffusivity (Fig. 6C) or increased reaction rates, selecting a higher order harmonic (c.f. higher *l* for hemispheres). The X_{th} mechanism is more effective at creating acute angles in 3D than in 2D; branching angles of nearly zero can be generated in 3D. Higher order branching, creating whorled structures, can be achieved with further decreased diffusivity (Fig. 6D) or increased reaction rates.

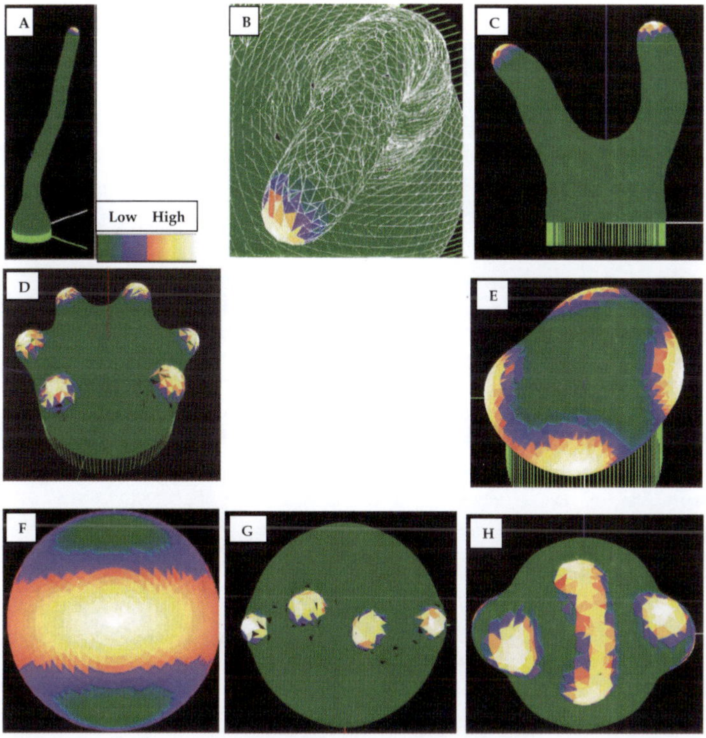

Fig. 6. Finite element computations of RD-driven growth in 3D. All shapes start from a hemisphere, growth is catalyzed according to local *X* morphogen concentration (colour-coded yellow, high - green, low). A) extending tip growth, over 10 times increase in height from original shape. B) shows the computational mesh used, and the mesh (but not shape or pattern) irregularity that develops from the local relatticing procedure. C, D) branching events of increasing complexity can be produced by decreasing diffusivity or increasing reaction rate constants (i.e. selecting higher order harmonics). E) RD patterns tend to produce successive branches in alternating planes. A chemical gradient in precursor *A* (F) can maintain a single branching plane (G), though this is more effective in wing lobes than in the polar lobe (H), as seen in real *Micrasterias* cells. Adapted from Holloway & Harrison (2008), with permission.

The flatness of *Micrasterias* allowed us to model them to good approximation in 2D. However, a deeper question might be why they are so flat. I.e. what keeps successive dichotomous branches in the same plane, when the natural tendency of RD patterns is to branch orthogonally (Fig. 6E; new peaks tend to avoid the inhibition of the old peaks; also note the orthogonal extension of the surface spherical harmonic in Fig. 2C). Lacalli (1976) discussed the idea of a 'morphogenetic template' affecting inheritance of the branching plane from the older semicell. This template could either be geometric, from the asymmetric (elliptical) shape of the isthmus between the semicells, or of a chemical nature. We tested the geometric hypothesis by running computations on ellipsoidal initial shapes (rather than hemispherical). Even with axial ratios up to 6:1 (far greater than experimentally observed), secondary branches are orthogonal: geometry is unlikely to define the branching plane for chemical patterning. We then tested the ability for a chemical prepattern to specify and maintain a branching plane. A harmonic in the precursor *A* (the negative of Fig. 2C) is a natural way to define the plane (Fig. 6F). Subsequent branching events are successfully kept in this plane (Fig. 6G). The branching plane is more dominant in the wing (i.e. lower latitude) lobes than in the polar lobe (Fig. 6H). This reflects the lack of directionality of the harmonic (Fig. 6F) at the pole, and its strong gradient at lower latitudes. The polar lobe in real *Micrasterias* cells is generally the only branch which is out-of-plane; our computations indicate this may reflect the harmonics of a chemical pattern defining the branching plane.

3.3 A self-contained chemical mechanism for creating growth boundaries

Use of the X_{th} mechanism allowed us to study the interplay between patterning rates (the RD mechanism), growth rates (the rate of X catalysis of surface expansion), and the movement of patterning boundaries to either maintain pattern or break symmetry. However, though concentration thresholds are commonly invoked in developmental biology, the X_{th} mechanism does not explain where this threshold comes from: the change in pattern dynamics at the X_{th} is specified by instructions in computer code rather than by chemical dynamics.

More recently, we have devised a self-contained chemical mechanism which is capable of controlling boundary formation and movement (Harrison, Adams and Holloway, in preparation). The X_{th} mechanism defined the edges of the active Turing patterning region; our new mechanism uses a kinetic mechanism (2nd RD model) to perform this function. The full mechanism involves two coupled Brusselators, with the 1st Brusselator defining the region in which the 2nd Brusselator (which has the growth catalyst) can form pattern. I.e. Brusselator 1 controls the position of the Turing instability for Brusselator 2. Fig. 7 shows schematically how the double Brusselator mechanism operates.

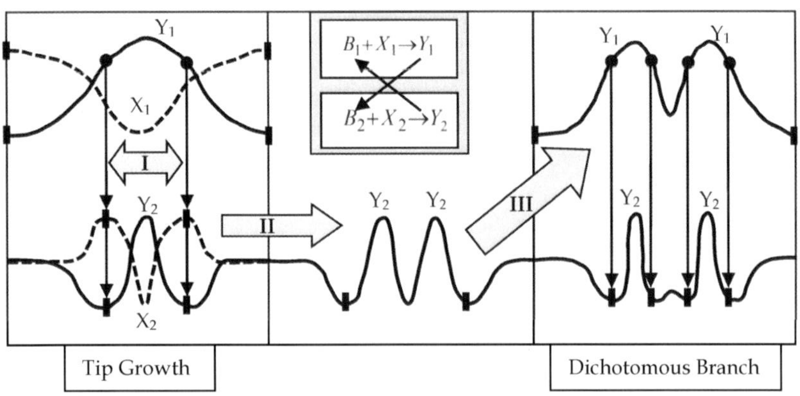

Fig. 7. Two coupled Brusselators provide a self-contained mechanism for the pattern formation, growth, and growth-boundary formation necessary for morphogenesis. Coupling occurs through the 2nd steps of the Brusselators, with Y_2 forming B_1, and Y_1 forming B_2 (grey box; top, centre). Left, Brusselator 1 (X_1, Y_1) is initiated with a single wave pattern. Vertical bars represent pattern formation boundaries. **I**) Y_1 controls threshold B_2 levels which define pattern formation boundaries for Brusselator 2 (X_2, Y_2), vertical arrows. Y_2 is the growth catalyst (*Y* used rather than *X*, since *B* directly controls its equilibrium value). Extending tip growth

occurs with a proper balance of Brusselator 1,2 wavelengths and rate of growth catalysis; or **II**) growth rate and wavelengths can allow peak splitting in Brusselator 2, centre (only Y_2 shown). **III**) Peak splitting in Brusselator 2 is transmitted to Brusselator 1, via $Y_2 \rightarrow B_1$ (only Y_1 shown). The two Y_1 peaks form 4 patterning boundaries for Brusselator 2 (via B_2), vertical arrows, isolating each new peak and forming a permanent dichotomous branch.

Having RD patterning ability in both stages is key to being able to complete transitions from one pattern to another (symmetry breaking): the model can stably propagate initial patterns over several-fold change in length (1D), but its key feature is that pattern changes in Brusselator 2 (due to its catalysis of growth) feed back and induce pattern changes in Brusselator 1. Since Brusselator 1 controls where Brusselator 2 operates, this defines the new growth boundaries necessary for transforming pattern into shape. Computations with this model have successfully simulated the growth patterns necessary for extending tips and for transforming tips into branches.

4. RD experiments in plants

So far, discussion has been on the development of RD theory for patterning and growth in plants, focusing on the particular kinetic issues that arise for regulating morphogenesis. Theories need experimental confirmation, however, and a number of efforts have been conducted over the years. Laboratory confirmation of Turing dynamics in the CIMA reaction (Castets et al., 1990; Ouyang & Swinney, 1991) was a major step for the RD field, but highlighted the subtleties in establishing that a particular dynamic mechanism is operating in a particular case. The CIMA reaction involves inorganic reagents in a small reactor vessel; establishing Turing dynamics in a biochemical system in vivo is a far greater challenge. But, circumstantial evidence from classical physical chemical experimental techniques can provide strong indications about the chemical dynamics underlying morphogenetic phenomena. And more recently the ability to visualize particular reactants via molecular biology techniques has allowed RD mechanisms to be identified for several cases in plant development.

4.1 Physical chemistry on algae

Beginning in the late 1970's, Harrison and co-workers began experiments on morphogenesis in the unicellular alga *Acetabularia*. Whorls of vegetative hairs (Fig. 8A) form every few weeks over a several month lifespan (in which the cells grow up to 5 cm long). Harrison et al. (1981) found that these hairs are evenly spaced. Spacing (λ) decreases with increasing temperature; this can be expected for an RD driven pattern, in which $\lambda \propto \sqrt{D/k}$ (section **2.1**), with exponential temperature dependence for rate constants (Arrhenius relation) and linear temperature dependence for diffusivities (Einstein relation). Plotting $\ln\lambda$ against $1/T$ does show a good fit to the Arrhenius relation (Fig. 8B), indicating that spacing is largely determined by reaction rates. Spacing was also found to increase for decreasing Ca^{2+} concentration (Fig. 8C; Harrison & Hillier, 1985). If spacing is proportional to the reciprocal of a rate constant and Ca^{2+} is considered as a substrate, the slope of a Lineweaver-Burk plot ($1/k$ vs. $1/$[substrate]; Fig. 8C; commonly used to characterize enzyme kinetics) can be used to calculate the Ca^{2+} binding constant. The temperature dependence of the binding constants (van't Hoff plot) can be used to calculate the entropy and enthalpy for Ca^{2+} binding. The

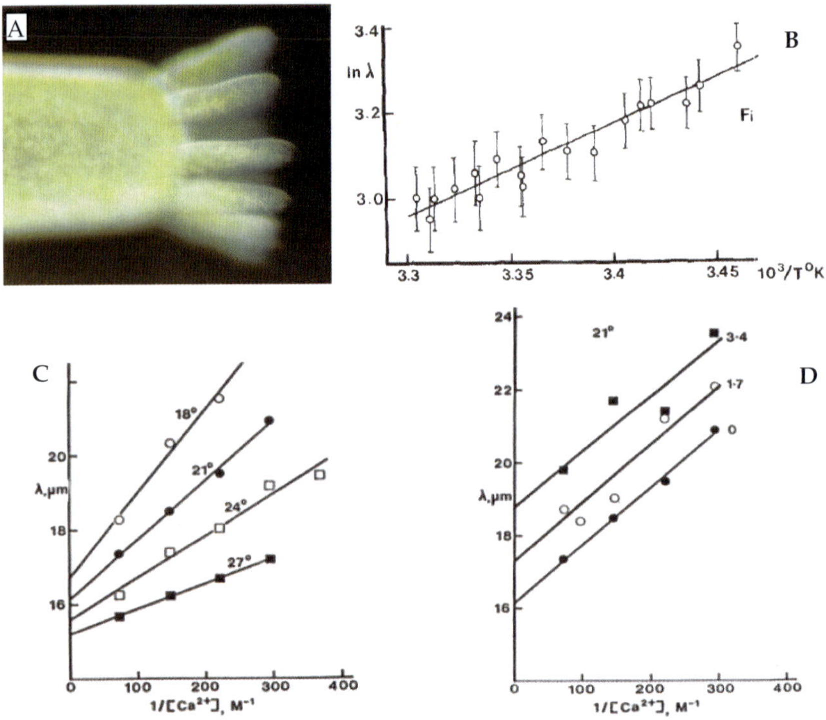

Fig. 8. Physical chemistry on algae: temperature and Ca^{2+} effects on hair spacing in *Acetabularia*. **A**) growing tip of an *Acetabularia* cell, showing a whorl of vegetative hairs. These hairs are evenly spaced, consistent with a wavelength from a pattern-forming process. **B)** The temperature dependence of the spacing (λ) follows an Arrhenius relation, suggesting the control of spacing is dominated by reaction rates (from Harrison et al., 1981, with permission). **C)** Linear plots of λ vs. $1/[Ca^{2+}]$ indicate that spacing is inversely proportional to a rate constant and Ca^{2+} activates the spacing process (reproduced from Harrison, 2011, with permission). Ca^{2+} binding constants and thermodynamics can be calculated from these slopes. **D)** EGTA (mM concentrations shown to right of lines) uncompetitively inhibits the Ca^{2+} activation (reproduced from Harrison, 2011, with permission). These relations indicate chemical kinetic control of hair morphogenesis in *Acetabularia*, consistent with the hypothesis that a membrane-bound Ca^{2+}-activated protein is a Turing morphogen.

Ca^{2+} hair-spacing effect can be inhibited with the chelate EGTA (Fig. 8D), with a concentration and temperature dependence indicating uncompetitive inhibition (Harrison et al., 1997). Harrison et al. (1988) were able to visualize membrane-bound Ca^{2+} patterns preceding tip flattening and hair morphogenesis with fluorescence microscopy. The thermodynamics and kinetics found in these studies are consistent with the hypothesis (e.g. see discussion in Harrison, 2011, Ch. 3) that a Turing morphogen controls hair spacing, and that this morphogen is a membrane bound protein activated by Ca^{2+} binding. Using classic physical chemical techniques, this series of experiments provided circumstantial evidence that a macroscopic observable such as hair spacing was due to kinetics in the underlying chemistry, and was consistent with an RD mechanism.

4.2 Patterning of multicellular whorls: Conifer embryogenesis

Are these spacing effects seen in higher plants? von Aderkas (2002) found that embryos in a clonal population of conifer trees (larch; Fig. 9A) showed variable numbers of 'seed leaves', or cotyledons. This is a first indication of a constant spacing phenomenon (i.e., with a wavelength); Harrison & von Aderkas (2004) showed that indeed this number variability was due to embryo diameter variability, with cotyledons being evenly spaced on the tip of the embryo. Further, their data indicated that radial positioning of the cotyledons varied with the circumferential spacing, suggesting that a single pattern forming mechanism controlled both aspects of spacing. Their data is consistent with RD patterning on a flattened disc (Bessel function solutions); embryogenesis in conifers does proceed from dome-shaped to a flattened tip before cotyledons form. These patterning trends have now been corroborated in Douglas fir and spruce (Holloway et al., unpublished results), and experiments are under way, in the spirit of the *Acetabularia* experiments, to test the temperature dependence of cotyledon spacing and to find chemical reagents which can directly alter spacing, likely through hormonal growth control pathways.

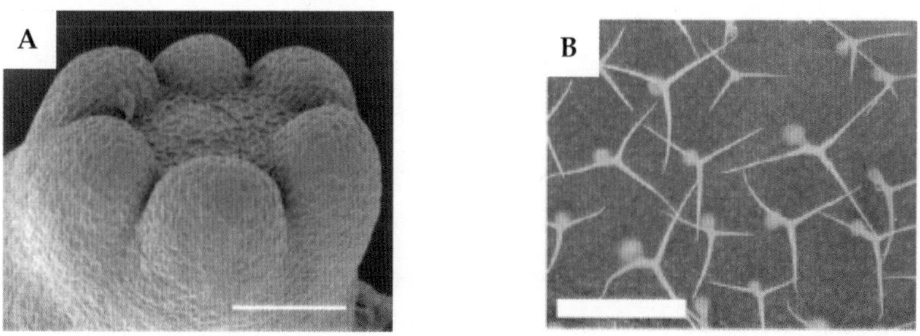

Fig. 9. RD in higher plants. **A)** Scanning electron micrograph (SEM) of the growing tip of a conifer tree embryo (larch). The cotyledons (bumps) are the first 'seed' leaves of the embryo. Harrison & von Aderkas (2004) found the cotyledons to be spaced, radially and circumferentially, by a single pattern-forming mechanism (from Harrison & von Aderkas, 2004, with permission). Work continues, to characterize whether RD acts at this developmental stage in some of the world's largest plants. **B)** SEM of trichomes (protective hairs) on the underside of a leaf of *Arabidopsis*; image from Deeks et al. (2007), with permission. Digiuni et al. (2008) found that trichomes are patterned by an RD mechanism, by quantitatively matching experimental manipulations of specific trichome genes with a dynamic (RD) model of trichome gene interactions.

4.3 RD in plant genetics

Knowledge of the genetic underpinnings of developmental phenomena have increased vastly in recent decades, with enormous strides in understanding not only the complete genomes of model organisms, but also the complex pathways regulating gene expression and tissue formation in development. With more complete sets of data on the molecules involved in development, and the tools to manipulate these molecules, it is becoming increasingly possible to investigate the kinetics of pattern formation at the molecular level. *Arabidopsis thaliana* is the major model organism in higher plants, with the largest toolkit for genetic manipulation. Several groups have recently published work on RD mechanisms in specific genetic pathways in *Arabidopsis* development, identifying specific known molecules as Turing morphogens.

Digiuni et al. (2008) determined that trichomes, protective hairs on the undersides of *Arabidopsis* leaves (Fig. 9B), are patterned by an RD mechanism. They developed a dynamic model of the GLABRA/TRIPTYCHON reaction network known to underlie trichome formation. The network dynamics are RD, with activation occurring through catalyzed formation of an 'active complex', and inhibition occurring through several possible pairwise interactions of the constituent gene products. Matching model results to experiments allowed the authors to select a particular one of these inhibition pathways (interaction between GLABRA3 and TRIPTYCHON). This study not only investigated normal, wild-type trichome patterns, but used targeted manipulations (overexpression) of particular genes in the network to narrow down the kinetic possibilities.

As discussed in the Introduction, much of the shaping of higher plants occurs in localized zones, with the shoot apical meristem (SAM) at the top of a plant chief among these. For *Arabidopsis* and a selection of other plants, the genes expressed in the SAM and the interactions between them are very well characterized. The response of the SAM to perturbations can be very complex, however. A recent paper by Fujita et al. (2011) presents an RD model of the SAM gene network, identifying the activator as the *WUSCHEL* (*WUS*) product (i.e. protein) and the inhibitor as the *CLAVATA* (*CLV*) gene product. They invoked a 3rd morphogen for RD patterning to control the spatial extent of the SAM in the face of cell divisions, a means of approaching the growth-patterning issues discussed in prior sections. The authors were able to successfully model the complex patterning responses seen for a series of genetic knockdown and overexpression experiments, as well as for physical cell ablation and incision experiments. (Also see Jönsson et al., 2005, for an earlier RD model of SAM patterning.)

Finding RD mechanisms through detailed study of gene network dynamics is being paralleled in animal development, where for example Turing morphogens have been identified in skin patterning (e.g. Sick et al., 2006; Jung et al., 1998; Jiang et al., 1999). The molecular work in plants is reaching a point where we can begin to discuss the theoretical growth-patterning issues (section **3**) in terms of known molecules.

5. Other factors in plant morphogenesis

This chapter has focused on the development of RD theory, particularly with respect to the patterning-growth dynamics seen in plant development. RD mechanisms allow the chemical kinetic underpinnings of growth control to be explored, and experimental work is beginning to illuminate how RD operates in particular developmental phenomena. Something as complex as plant shape, however, has numerous aspects and can be approached from a number of complementary directions. Here, we will discuss newer developments in transport in plants, and the relation of chemical patterning to the mechanical properties of plant tissues in determining morphology.

5.1 Auxin transport

Auxin is a small organic molecule which has long been known to have powerful effects on plant growth. Mitchison (1981) developed a model for auxin's role in vein formation in leaves, in which the flow of auxin is autocatalytic: auxin flow in a particular direction will reinforce flow in that direction, leading to a 'canalization' and formation of veins. In more recent years, discovery of the auxin-transporter PIN genes has filled in much of the molecular biology of auxin transport (Friml, 2003). PIN genes are involved in cellular intake and efflux of auxin, and have been found to be active from embryogenesis to apical meristem activity. PIN localization is positively related to auxin. Models exist for this relation being proportional to either auxin concentration or to auxin flux (as in Mitchison's model), but the result of either is to create auxin flows *up* a gradient, as opposed to diffusion (down a gradient). A number of models have been developed for pattern formation via auxin transport in apical meristems, which have had a high degree of success in describing the morphogenesis of lateral structures (e.g. leaves) from the SAM (i.e. phyllotaxis; de Reuille et al., 2006; Jönsson et al., 2006; Smith et al., 2006) and growth patterns in the root apical meristem (Grieneisen et al., 2007; Laskowski et al., 2008). For further discussion, see Braybrook & Kuhlemeier, 2010, and references therein (e.g. Heisler & Jönsson, 2007; Kramer, 2008; Smith & Bayer, 2009). Auxin modelling and its close matching to newly discovered molecular biology has had a great impact on the use of mathematics to understand patterning and growth in plant development. In terms of pattern formation, while auxin flux and diffusion are different, they serve a similar purpose in introducing a spatial dependence to the dynamics. Mathematical analysis is far more developed for RD models at this point, though it is likely that pattern-forming dynamics in auxin transport models will be found to be similar. Due to the maturity of the RD mathematics, it is immediately more promising for elucidating the growth-patterning-boundary formation dynamic issues discussed in section 3. But the auxin work shows that a diversity of transport mechanisms are likely significant in plant development, and the mathematics must keep abreast of differences and commonalities between the various types of transport.

5.2 Plant mechanical properties

While the focus of this chapter, and of genetic research into morphogenesis, is on the chemical pattern formation underlying growth, plants have unique mechanical characteristics which can also affect form.

5.2.1 Mechanical approaches to morphogenesis

Mechanically, plant cell shapes balance a high internal turgor pressure against the complex macromolecular structure of the cell walls. At relatively low turgor, the wall can act approximately elastically; at high pressure, deformation can be described as a viscoplastic flow (Dumais et al., 2006). Mechanical theories have been developed mathematically for rotationally symmetric shapes such as growing tips (Dumais et al., 2006; Ben Amar & Goriely, 2005), but the treatment of non-axisymmetric shapes, such as clefts and branches, remains unsolved and very challenging. The cell wall macromolecular structure also creates anisotropic mechanical properties, with, for example microtubule 'hooping' causing far greater extensibility in one direction than another (e.g. Green and Lang, 1981; Green et al.,

1998). The complex interplay between microtubule arrangements and cellulose wall structure has been explored in depth in recent years (e.g. see Paredez et al., 2008), for instance illuminating how microtubule arrangements dynamically control cell division planes (Besson & Dumais, 2011), which can affect growth directions. A recent growth model involving cellular-scale microtubule orientation successfully modelled the response of the apical surface to localized laser ablation experiments (Hamant et al., 2008). This is a very active area and the interested reader is directed to the present references for further exploration of the mechanical aspects of morphogenesis.

5.2.2 Combining mechanics and chemistry

Chemical models, involving genes or other biomolecules - whether RD, auxin-transport, or other - have largely been studied apart from mechanics, or the consideration of forces. This is generally justified since gene expression and pattern formation frequently precede shape change. At the same time, many purely mechanical models have had success describing a range of morphogenetic phenomena (e.g. Green & Poethig, 1982; Linthilac, 1984). It is likely that most phenomena in plant morphogenesis have contributions from both mechanical and chemical dynamics. Modelling needs to proceed in this direction, though not at the expense of fully understanding the dynamics of purely chemical or purely mechanical mechanisms. Chemistry can affect mechanics, through the local catalysis of wall changes (softening, addition of new material) which affect extensibility and allow internal turgor to push surface out (for instance see Zerzour et al., 2009, on wall softening preceding tip growth). But mechanics can also affect chemistry, for example stretch-activated Ca^{2+} channels have been found in tip growth (e.g. Kroeger et al., 2008), and there is evidence that stress can activate genes (e.g. Desprat et al., 2008, in animals). More complete models of morphogenesis will need to combine chemical dynamics with mechanics (see, for example, the recent synthesis for the SAM in Besnard et al., 2011); in the first instance to predict correct deformations for chemically catalyzed growth, but ultimately to account for mechanical effects on chemistry. Spontaneous pattern formation in mechanochemical dynamics should also be considered; Oster and co-workers developed and analyzed such a model in which Ca^{2+} effects on cytoskeleton were autocatalytic, but the spatial dependence of the patterning was through mechanical stress (Oster, 1983; Oster et al., 1983). See Howard et al. (2011) for a recent discussion of mechanical stress as the spatially dependent component of reaction-based patterning. Vast amounts are now known about the interplay between cytoskeleton chemistry and plant cell morphogenesis, with scope for extensive development of appropriate mathematical mechanochemical models (e.g. see review by Szymanski & Cosgrove, 2009; model of Jilkine et al., 2007). At a continuum level, focusing on tissue-wide interactions between patterning and deformation, recent morphogenetic models have combined chemical gradients with accurate mechanical representations of plant tissues (Kennaway et al., 2011; Matthews, 2002). With mathematical analysis of a combined mechanochemical model, Shipman & Newell (2005) have been able to provide an explanation for phyllotactic patterns, for example in sunflower heads. Such work opens the way for a more complete exploration of the pattern forming dynamics of integrated mechanochemical systems; i.e. can we proceed from a theoretical understanding of patterning via RD kinetics, combine this with continuum mechanics, and begin to understand how these interact in real plant morphogenesis?

6. Conclusion

This chapter has explored the development of RD theory and the role of RD dynamics in plant development. RD is a well-developed kinetic theory for spontaneous spatial pattern formation, and as such provides a framework for understanding how the biochemical patterns underlying embryonic development may be established. The theoretical challenge for applying RD to plant development is to understand how RD patterning operates in growing systems, and, if the localized growth catalysis responsible for morphogenesis is patterned by RD, what dynamics arise in the full feedback of RD-driven growth. A critical part of transforming chemical pattern into shape is the control of boundaries between fast- and slow-growing regions. Sections **3.2** and **3.3** presented potential mechanisms by which this can occur. Because their pattern-selection can be well-characterized in terms of reaction and transport rates, size and geometry, RD-growth models are particularly well-suited to describing and understanding developmental sequences which involve symmetry-breaking, for instance the tip growth to branching transition.

In addition to providing a theoretical framework for problems in patterning and growth, experimental evidence is accumulating for RD mechanisms in specific cases of plant development, with the molecular identification of Turing morphogens. Plant shapes are also affected by the unique mechanical properties of their cell walls. Ultimately, more complete understanding of how shapes are determined will require a synthesis of chemical and mechanical theories, but this synthesis will only be clear if both theories are fully characterized, so that the contributions of each, and the properties emergent from their interaction, are properly understood.

7. Acknowledgments

Thanks to T.C. Lacalli for comments on the manuscript, and to BCIT and NSERC Canada for financial support.

8. References

Baker, R.E., & Maini, P.K. (2007). A mechanism for morphogen-controlled domain growth. *Journal of Mathematical Biology*, Vol.54, pp. 597-622.

Ben Amar, M., & Goriely, A. (2005). Growth and instability in elastic tissues. *Journal of the Mechanics and Physics of Solids*, Vol.53, pp. 2284-2319.

Besnard, F., Vernoux, T., & Hamant, O. (2011). Organogenesis from stem cells in planta: multiple feedback loops integrating molecular and mechanical signals. *Cellular and Molecular Life Sciences*, Vol.68, pp. 2885-2906.

Besson, S., & Dumais, J. (2011). Universal rule for the symmetric division of plant cells. *Proceedings of the National Academy of Sciences USA*, Vol.108, pp. 6294-6299.

Braybrook, S.A. & Kuhlemeier, C. (2010). How a plant builds leaves. *Plant Cell*, Vol.22, pp. 1006-1018.

Castets, V., Dulos, E., Boissonade, J. & De Kepper, P. (1990). Experimental evidence of a sustained standing Turing-type nonequilibrium chemical pattern. *Physical Review Letters*. Vol.64, pp. 2953-2956.

Crampin E.J., Hackborn W.W., & Maini P.K. (2002). Pattern formation in reaction-diffusion models with nonuniform domain growth. *Bulletin of Mathematical Biology*, Vol.64, pp. 747-769.

Deeks, M.J., Rodrigues, C., Dimmock, S., Ketelaar, T. Maciver, S.K., Malhó, R., & Hussey, P.J. (2007). *Arabidopsis* CAP1 – a key regulator of actin organisation and development. *Journal of Cell Science*, Vol. 120, pp. 2609-2618.

Desprat, N., Supatto, W., Pouille, P.A., Beaurepaire, E., & Farge, E. (2008). Tissue deformation modulates twist expression to determine anterior midgut differentiation in *Drosophila* embryos. *Developmental Cell*, Vol.15, pp. 470-477.

de Reuille, P.B., Bohn-Courseau, I., Ljung, K., Morin, H., Carraro, N., Godin, C. & Traas J. (2006). Computer simulations reveal properties of the cell-cell signalling network at the shoot apex in *Arabidopsis*. *Proceedings of the National Academy of Sciences USA*, Vol.103, pp. 1627-1632.

Digiuni, S., Schellmann, S., Geier, F., Greese, B., Pesch, M., Wester, K., Dartan, B., Mach, V., Srinivas, B.P., Timmer, J., Fleck, C. & Hülskamp M. (2008). A competitive complex formation mechanism underlies trichome patterning in *Arabidopsis* leaves. *Molecular Systems Biology*, Vol.4, Article 217.

Dumais, J., Shaw, S.L., Steele, C.R., Long, S.R., & Ray, P.M. (2006). An anisotropic-viscoplastic model of plant cell morphogenesis by tip growth. *International Journal of Developmental Biology*, Vol.50, pp. 209-222.

Edelstein-Keshet, L. (1988). *Mathematical Models in Biology*. Random House, New York.

Friml, J. (2003). Auxin transport – shaping the plant. *Current Opinion in Plant Biology*, Vol.6, pp. 7-12.

Fujita H., Toyokura, K., Okada, K., & Kawaguchi, M. (2011). Reaction-diffusion mechanism in shoot apical meristem of plants. *Public Library of Science One*, Vol.6, Article e18243.

Gierer, A. & Meinhardt, H. (1972) A theory of biological pattern formation. *Kybernetik*, Vol.12, pp. 30-39.

Green, P.B., & Lang, J.M. (1981). Toward a biophysical theory of organogenesis: birefringence observations on regenerating leaves in the succulent, *Graptopetalum paraguayense* E. Walther. *Planta*, Vol.151, pp. 413-426.

Green, P.B., & Poethig, R.S. (1982). Biophysics of the extension and initiation of plant organs. In: *Developmental Order: Its Origin and Regulation*, S. Subtelny (Ed.), pp. 485-509. Alan R. Liss, New York.

Green, P.B., Steele, C.S. and Rennich, S.C. (1998) How plants produce pattern. A review and proposal that undulating field behavior is the mechanism. In Symmetry in Plants (Jean, R. V. and Barabé, D., eds), pp. 359-392, World Scientific, Singapore.

Grieneisen, V.A., Xu, J., Maree, A.F.M., Hogeweg, P., & Scheres, B. (2007). Auxin transport is sufficient to generate a maximum and gradient guiding root growth. *Nature*, Vol.449, pp. 1008-1013.

Grieneisen, V.A. & Scheres, B. (2009). Back to the future: evolution of computational models in plant morphogenesis. *Current Opinion in Plant Biology*, Vol.12, pp. 606-614.

Hamant, O., Heisler, M.G., Jönsson, H., Krupinski, P., Uyttewaal, M., Bokov, P., Corson, F., Sahlin, P., Boudaoud, A., Meyerowitz, E.M., Couder, Y., & Traas, J. (2008). Developmental patterning by mechanical signals in *Arabidopsis*. *Science*, Vol.322, pp. 1650-1655.

Harrison, L.G, Snell, J., Verdi, R., Vogt, D.E., Zeiss, G.D. & Green, B.R. (1981) Hair morphogenesis in *Acetabularia mediterranea*: temperature-dependent spacing and models of morphogen waves. *Protoplasma*, Vol.106, pp. 211-221.

Harrison, L.G. & Hillier, N.A. (1985). Quantitative control of *Acetabularia* morphogenesis by extracellular calcium: a test of kinetic theory. *Journal of Theoretical Biology*, Vol. 114, pp. 177-192.

Harrison, L.G. and Kolář, M. (1988). Coupling between reaction-diffusion prepattern and expressed morphogenesis, applied to desmids and dasyclads. *Journal of Theoretical Biology*, Vol.130, pp. 493-515.

Harrison, L.G., Graham, K.T., & Lakowski, B.C. (1988). Calcium localization during *Acetabularia* whorl formation: evidence supporting a two-stage hierarchical mechanism. *Development*, Vol.104, pp. 255-262.

Harrison, L.G. (1993). *Kinetic Theory of Living Pattern*. Cambridge University Press.

Harrison, L.G., Donaldson, G., Lau, W., Lee, M., Lin, B.P., Lohachitranont, S., Setyawati, I., & Yue, J. (1997). CaEGTA uncompetitively inhibits calcium activation of whorl morphogenesis in *Acetabularia*. *Protoplasma*, Vol.196, pp. 190-196.

Harrison, L.G., Wehner, S. & Holloway, D.M. (2001) Complex morphogenesis of surfaces: theory and experiment on coupling of reaction-diffusion to growth. *Faraday Discussions*, Vol.120, pp. 277-294.

Harrison, L.G., & von Aderkas, P. (2004) Spatially quantitative control of the number of cotyledons in a clonal population of somatic embryos of hybrid larch *Larix* x *leptoeuropaea*. *Annals of Botany*, Vol.93, pp. 423-434.

Harrison, L.G. (2011). *The Shaping of Life: the Generation of Biological Pattern*. Cambridge University Press.

Heisler, M.G., & Jönsson, H. (2007). Modelling meristem development in plants. *Current Opinion in Plant Biology*, Vol.10, pp. 92-97.

Holloway, D.M., Harrison, L.G. & Armstrong, J.B. (1994). Computations of post-inductive dynamics in axolotl heart formation. *Developmental Dynamics*, Vol.200, pp. 242-256.

Holloway, D.M. (1995). *Reaction-Diffusion Theory of Localized Structures with Application to Vertebrate Organogenesis*. PhD Thesis, University of British Columbia, Canada.

Holloway, D.M. & Harrison, L.G. (1995). Order and localization in reaction-diffusion pattern. *Physica A*, Vol.222, pp. 210-233.

Holloway, D.M. & Harrison, L.G. (1999) Algal morphogenesis: modelling interspecific variation in *Micrasterias* with reaction-diffusion patterned catalysis of cell surface growth. *Philosophical Transactions of the Royal Society, London, series B*, Vol.354, pp. 417-433.

Holloway, D.M. & Harrison, L.G. (2008) Pattern selection in plants: coupling chemical dynamics to surface growth in three dimensions. *Annals of Botany*, Vol.101, pp. 361-374.

Holloway, D.M. (2010). The role of chemical dynamics in plant morphogenesis. *Biochemical Society Transactions*, Vol.38, pp. 645-650.

Howard, J., Grill, S., & Bois, J.S. (2011). Turing's next steps: the mechanochemical basis of morphogenesis. *Nature Reviews Molecular Cell Biology*, Vol. 12, pp. 392-398.

Hunding, A., Kauffman, S.A., & Goodwin, B.C. (1990). *Drosophila* segmentation: supercomputer simulations of prepattern hierarchy. *Journal of Theoretical Biology*, Vol.145, pp. 369-384.

Iron, D., Ward, M.J., & Wei, J.C. (2001). The stability of spike solutions to the one-dimensional Gierer-Meinhardt model. *Physica D*, Vol.150, pp. 25-62.

Jiang, T-X., Jung, H-S., Widelitz, R.B., & Chuong, C-M. (1999). Self-organization of periodic patterns by dissociated feather mesenchymal cells and the regulation of size, number and spacing of primordial. *Development*, Vol.126, pp. 4997-5009.

Jilkine, A., Maree, A.F., & Edelstein-Keshet, L. (2007). Mathematical model for spatial segregation of the Rho-family GTPases based on inhibitory crosstalk. *Bulletin of Mathematical Biology*, Vol.69, pp. 1943-1978.

Jönsson, H., Heisler, M., Reddy, G.V., Agrawal, V., Gor, V., Shapiro, B.E., Mjolsness, E., & Meyerowitz, E.M. (2005). Modeling the organization of the WUSCHEL expression domain in the shoot apical meristem. *Bioinformatics*, Vol. 21 *[Suppl.]*, pp. i232–i240.

Jönsson, H., Heisler, M.G., Shapiro, B.E., Mjolsness, E., & Meyerowitz, E.M. (2006). An auxin-driven polarized transport model for phyllotaxis. *Proceedings of the National Academy of Sciences USA*, Vol.103, pp. 1633-1638.

Jönsson, H. & Krupinski, P. (2010). Modeling plant growth and pattern formation. *Current Opinion in Plant Biology*, Vol.13, pp. 5-11.

Jung, H-S., Francis-West, P.H., Widelitz, R.B., Jiang, T-X., Ting-Berreth, S., Tickle, C., Wolpert, L., & Chuong, C-M. (1998). Local inhibitory action of BMPs and their relationships with activators in feather formation: implications for periodic patterning. *Developmental Biology*, Vol.196, pp. 11-23.

Kauffman, S. A. (1977). Chemical patterns, compartments, and a binary epigenetic code in *Drosophila*. *American Zoologist*, Vol.17, pp. 631-648.

Kauffman, S.A., Shymko, R.M., & Trabert, K. (1978). Control of sequential compartment formation in *Drosophila*. *Science*, Vol.199, pp. 259-270.

Kauffman, S.A. (1981). Pattern formation in the *Drosophila* embryo. *Philosophical Transactions of the Royal Society, London, series B*, Vol. 295, pp. 567-594.

Kennaway, R., Coen, E., Green, A., & Bangham, A. (2011). Generation of diverse biological forms through combinatorial interactions between tissue polarity and growth. *Public Library of Science Computational Biology*, Vol.7, Article e1002071.

Kramer, E.M. (2008). Computer models of auxin transport: a review and commentary. *Journal of Experimental Botany*, Vol.59, pp. 45-53.

Kroeger, J.H., Geitmann, A., & Grant, M. (2008). Model for calcium dependent oscillatory growth in pollen tubes. *Journal of Theoretical Biology*, Vol.253, pp. 363-374.

Lacalli, T.C. (1976). Morphogenesis in *Micrasterias*. III. The morphogenetic template. *Protoplasma*, Vol. 88, pp. 133-146.

Lacalli, T.C., & Harrison, L.G. (1978). The regulatory capacity of Turing's model for morphogenesis, with application to slime moulds. *Journal of Theoretical Biology*, Vol. 70, pp. 273-295.

Lacalli, T.C. (1981). Dissipative structures and morphogenetic pattern in unicellular algae. *Philosophical Transactions of the Royal Society, London, series B*, Vol.294, pp. 547-588.

Lacalli, T.C., Wilkinson, D.A., & Harrison, L.G. (1988). Theoretical aspects of stripe formation in relation to *Drosophila* segmentation. *Development*, Vol.104, pp. 105-113.

Lacalli, T.C. (1990). Modeling the *Drosophila* pair-rule pattern by reaction-diffusion: gap input and pattern control in a 4-morphogen system. *Journal of Theoretical Biology*, Vol.144, pp. 171-194.

Laskowski, M., Grieneisen, V.A., Hofhuis, H., ten Hove, C.A., Hogeweg, P., Maree, A.F.M., & Scheres, B. (2008). Root system architecture from coupling cell shape to auxin transport. *Public Library of Science Biology*, Vol. 6, Article e307.

Lintilhac, P.M. (1984). Positional controls in meristem development: a caveat and an alternative. In: *Positional Controls in Plant Development*, P.W. Barlow & D.J. Carr, (Eds.), Chap. 4, Cambridge University Press.

Lyons, M.J., Harrison, L.G., Lakowski, B.C., & Lacalli, T.C. (1990). Reaction diffusion modelling of biological pattern formation: application to the embryogenesis of *Drosophila melanogaster. Canadian Journal of Physics*, Vol.68, pp. 772-777.

Matthews, M.J. (2002). Physically based simulation of growing surfaces. M.Sc. thesis, University of Calgary, Canada.

Maynard Smith, J. (1968). *Mathematical Ideas in Biology.* Cambridge University Press.

Meinhardt, H. (1982). *Models of Biological Pattern Formation.* Academic Press, London available at:
http://www.eb.tuebingen.mpg.de/departments/former-departments/h-meinhardt/82-book/Bur82.htm.

Meinhardt, H. (1984). Models of pattern formation and their application to plant development. In: *Positional Controls in Plant Development*, P.W. Barlow & D.J. Carr, (Eds.), Chap. 1. Cambridge University Press.

Meinhardt, H. (1986). Hierarchical induction of cell states: a model for segmentation in *Drosophila. Journal of Cell Science [Suppl.]*, Vol.4, pp. 357-381.

Meinhardt, H. (1988). Models for maternally supplied positional information and the activation of segmentation genes in *Drosophila* embryogenesis. *Development [Suppl.]*, Vol.104, pp. 95-110.

Meinhardt, H. (1995). *The Algorithmic Beauty of Seashells.* 1st edition, Springer-Verlag, Berlin. (2nd edition, 1998; 3rd edition, 2003).

Mitchison, G.J. (1981). The polar transport of auxin and vein patterns in plants. *Philosophical Transactions of the Royal Society, London, series B*, Vol.295, pp. 461-471.

Murray, J.D. (1981a). A pre-pattern formation mechanism for animal coat markings. *Journal of Theoretical Biology*, Vol.88, pp. 161-199.

Murray, J.D. (1981b). On pattern formation mechanisms for lepidopteran wing patterns and mammalian coat markings. *Philosophical Transactions of the Royal Society, London, series B*, Vol.295, pp. 473-496.

Murray, J.D. (1989). *Mathematical Biology*. Springer-Verlag, Berlin.

Nicolis, G. & Prigogine, I. (1977). *Self-Organization in Nonequilibrium Systems.* Wiley-Interscience, New York.

Nagata, W., Harrison, L.G., & Wehner, S. (2003). Reaction-diffusion models of growing plant tips: bifurcations on hemispheres. *Bulletin of Mathematical Biology*, Vol.65, pp. 571-607.

Nagorcka, B.N. (1988). A pattern formation mechanism to control spatial organization in the embryo of *Drosophila melanogaster. Journal of Theoretical Biology*, Vol. 132, pp. 277-306.

Nagorcka, B.N., & Mooney, J.R. (1982). The role of a reaction-diffusion system in the formation of hair fibres. *Journal of Theoretical Biology*, Vol.98, pp. 575-607.

Nagorcka, B.N. & Mooney, J.R. (1985). The role of a reaction-diffusion system in the initiation of primary hair follicles. *Journal of Theoretical Biology*, Vol.114, pp. 243-272.

Neville A.A., Matthews P.C. & Byrne H.M. (2006). Interactions between pattern formation and domain growth. *Bulletin of Mathematical Biology*, Vol.68, pp. 1975-2003.

Nicolis, G., & Prigogine, I. (1977). *Self-Organization in Nonequilibrium Systems*. Wiley Interscience, New York.

Oster, G.F. (1983). Mechanochemistry and morphogenesis. In: *Biological Structures and Coupled Flows*, A. Oplatka & M. Balaban, (Eds.), pp. 417-443. Academic Press, New York.

Oster, G.F., Murray, J.D., & Harris, A.K. (1983). Mechanical aspects of mesenchymal morphogenesis. *Journal of Embryology and Experimental Morphology*, Vol.78, pp. 83-125.

Ouyang, Q. & Swinney, H.L. (1991). Transition from a uniform state to hexagonal and striped Turing patterns. *Nature*, Vol.352, pp. 610-611.

Paredez, A.R., Persson, S., Ehrhardt, D.W., & Somerville, C. (2008). Genetic evidence that cellulose synthase activity influences microtubule cortical array organization. *Plant Physiology*, Vol.147, pp. 1723–1734.

Prigogine, I. & Lefever, R. (1968). Symmetry-breaking instabilities in dissipative systems. II. *Journal of Chemical Physics*, Vol.48, pp. 1695-1700.

Rashevsky, N. (1940). An approach to the mathematical biophysics of biological self-regulation and of cell polarity. *Bulletin of Mathematical Biophysics*, Vol.2, pp. 15-25.

Roeder, A.H.K., Tarr, P.T., Tobin, C., Zhang, X., Chickarmane, V., Cunha, A., & Meyerowitz, E.M. (2010). Computational morphodynamics of plants: integrating development over space and time. *Nature Reviews Molecular Cell Biology*, Vol.12, pp. 265-273.

Shipman, P.D., & Newell, A.C. (2005). Polygonal planforms and phyllotaxis on plants. *Journal of Theoretical Biology*, Vol.236, pp. 154-197.

Sick, S., Reinker, S., Timmer, J., & Schlake, T. (2006). WNT and DKK determine hair follicle spacing through a reaction-diffusion mechanism. *Science*, Vol.314, pp. 1447-1450.

Smith, R.S., Guyomarc'h, S., Mandel, T., Reinhardt, D., Kuhlemeier, C. and Prusinkiewicz P. (2006) A plausible model of phyllotaxis. *Proceedings of the National Academy of Sciences USA*, Vol.103, pp. 1301-1306.

Smith, R.S., & Bayer, E.M. (2009). Auxin transport-feedback models of patterning in plants. *Plant Cell Environment*, Vol.32, pp. 1258-1271.

Szymanski, D.B., & Cosgrove, D.J. (2009). Dynamic coordination of cytoskeletal and cell wall systems during plant cell morphogenesis. *Current Biology*, Vol.19, pp. R800-R811.

Turing, A.M. (1952). The chemical basis of morphogenesis. *Philosophical Transactions of the Royal Society, London, series B*, Vol.237, pp. 37-72.

von Aderkas, P. (2002). In vitro phenotypic variation in larch cotyledon number. *International Journal of Plant Science*, Vol.163, pp. 301-307.

Zerzour, R., Kroeger, J., & Geitmann, A. (2009). Polar growth in pollen tubes is associated with spatially confined dynamic changes in cell mechanical properties. *Developmental Biology*, Vol.334, pp. 437-446.

Zwieniecki, M.A. & Dumais, J. (2011). Quantifying *green life*: grand challenges in plant biophysics and modeling. *Frontiers in Plant Science*, Vol.2, Article 31.

9

Chemical Kinetics in Cold Plasmas

Ruggero Barni and Claudia Riccardi
Department of Physics G. Occhialini,
University of Milano-Bicocca, Milan,
Italy

1. Introduction

The chapter deals with the chemical kinetics in the gas-phase of cold plasmas. After a section concerning cold plasmas and the modeling scheme of the chemical kinetics happening in their gas-phases, the text will focus on hydrocarbon plasma chemistry. After a general review of the chemical kinetic pattern, we discuss several features presenting applications to two main fields, carbon film deposition by radiofrequency low pressure plasmas (discussing a typical Plasma Enhanced Chemical Vapour Deposition process) and hydrogen reforming by atmospheric pressure plasmas.

As for the first topic, methane and other light hydrocarbon plasmas are of great interest in industrial applications, in particular in the chemical vapor deposition processes. Amorphous carbon and diamond-like thin films, suitable for mechanical and electronic applications can be prepared using low pressure discharges of hydrocarbon gases . The research in this field is mainly devoted to the understanding of the nature of the film growing mechanism but in spite of intense experimental and theoretical work it is not yet fully understood which species are responsible for the deposition process.

New data concerning the interaction of ions and hydrocarbon radicals allow to have a quite complete mapping of the relevant reaction rates in an Ar/CH_4 plasma by now and it is possible to investigate the effect of the chemical kinetics in such a system and eventually to identify the gaseous precursor of the chemical species incorporated in the deposited film. We have modeled the gas-phase chemistry of a typical radio frequency CH_4/Ar plasma used for the deposition of diamond and diamond-like carbon films, with the aim of understanding the effects of the chemical kinetics of argon ions and metastables.

As for the second topic, hydrogen reforming from methane is up to now the most viable source for large scale as well as localized production of hydrogen for fuel cell systems. Conventional reforming is carried out thermally in oven with oxygen and steam or using catalytic beds, but the development of more compact devices is actively pursued too. Plasma reformers based on different kind of discharges, as arcs, microwave plasmas and dielectric barrier discharges have been investigated so far. We present recent results concerning the viability of a hydrocarbon plasma reforming process to produce a hydrogen enriched gas-mixture based on atmospheric pressure discharges operating in the spark regime.

2. Plasma chemical kinetics

Plasmas are gas phase systems where a consistent fraction of molecules is ionised and free electrons move around interacting under electromagnetic forces in a collective fashion (Raizer, 1991). Considerable energy could be delivered to the charged components through their electric interactions. Part of this energy could be used also to promote chemical reactions between neutral molecules in the gas phase. Then plasmas could become interesting gas chemical reactors. The specificity of the gas and plasma dynamics makes them suitable for material processing and atomic chemistry (Lieberman, 1994). Besides a few examples, mostly in natural environment, plasmas are systems far from thermodynamic equilibrium. Then different energy content is normally found in electrons, charged and neutral components. In particular, when only electrons have energies far exceeding set temperature, plasma could be named cold, since its heat capacity is usually very low and thermal load is limited (Raizer, 1991). Chemical kinetics in such systems and their modelization are a fascinating field of applied research, crossing the borders of plasma, atomic physics and chemical engineering.

2.1 Modeling of the gas-phase evolution in cold plasmas

In a plasma reactor fed with a gas mixture several different processes are at work, as summarized in the scheme of fig.1 for the argon/methane system (Riccardi, 2001). In a cold plasma the characteristic discharge chemistry processes are mainly driven by free electrons which are by far the most energetic particles in the reactor, and include (Mc Daniel, 1993):

a. ionization reactions producing further free electrons and positive ions;
b. electronic transitions to excited energy levels responsible for the rich light emission spectra of the discharges, molecular excitations of reactive vibrational and rotational states;
c. molecular dissociation with production of highly reactive free radicals;
d. electron attachment, particularly important in electronegative gases.

The gas mixture composition in the reactor is determined by the chemical reactions between the reactive species and by the transport processes. The transport depends on the hydrodynamical flow driven by the pumping system, by the diffusion of the neutral and charged species towards reactor walls and by the surface interactions at gaseous-solid interface. The last process includes adsorption of gaseous species, which eventually react with the surface atoms, desorption of volatile species generated in the solid lattice and sputtering due to energetic particles, mainly ions impinging onto the surface after being accelerated by the sheath at the walls. A detailed simulation of the reactor performances requires the knowledge of several molecular mechanisms. Some of them are only poorly known such as the ones crucially depending on the surface structure and composition (physical and chemical adsorption, sputtering yields). Moreover the active processes are each characterized by its own times and magnitude, thus implying a considerable degree of complexity. Therefore in order to keep the problem manageable some approximations are badly needed. As far as it concerns the plasma, we point out that the characteristic times ruling the discharge development are very short (for instance, when radiofrequency is employed as discharge supply unit using 13.56 MHz commercial frequency, the RF cycle period is 74 ns, the confinement time for electrons drifting to the walls is about a few μs) compared to the ones governing the radical species transport and the gas-phase reactions:

therefore the plasma produced in the reactor can be considered in a quasi-stationary state determined by the external working parameters (pressure P, flowrate Q and discharge electric power W) and slowly adapting to the changements in the neutral species concentration.

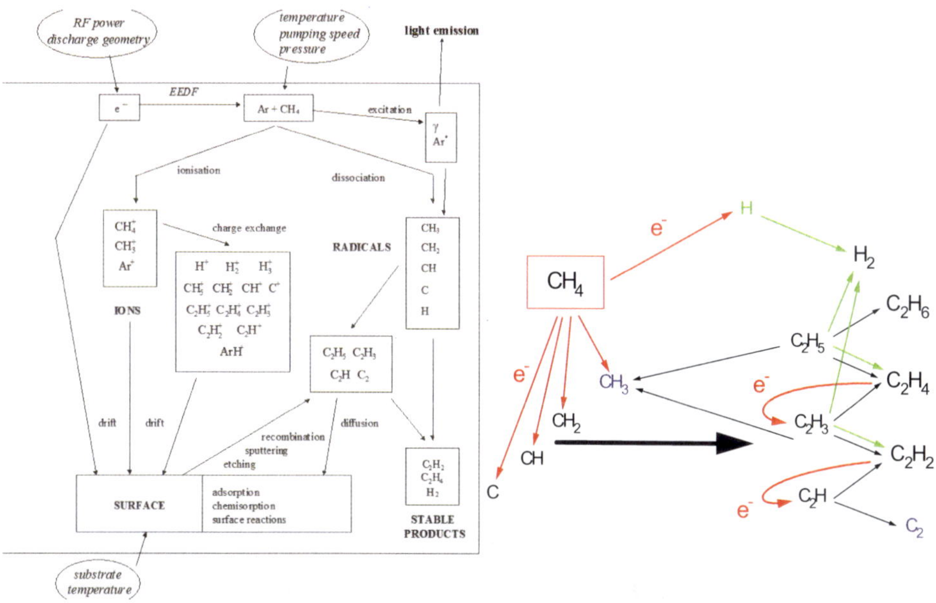

Fig. 1. Chemical kinetics in a CH_4-Ar plasma, main chemical species and processes.

Therefore the plasma evolution decouples almost completely from gas kinetics. The chemical kinetics of plasma driven processes to be considered in the model can be then fully characterized by prescribing the correct plasma state as an external condition, setting as parameters the electron density $n_e(r,z,t)$ and their energy distribution function EEDF $f_E(r,z,t)$. Despite several processes are involved in the electron energy losses, due to the rich molecular structure of the gas, the measured EEDFs appear in most of the cases approximately Maxwellian and therefore can be parameterized simply by an electron temperature $T_e(r,z,t)$ making easier the comparison and the analysis (Raizer, 1991). Outside of this scheme remains the connection between such microscopic parameters and the external operative ones, which should be assured by the analysis of the experimental data or by a dedicated plasma discharge modeling. However, in general, phenomenological relations hold. For instance, at fixed pressure, the electron density n_e comes out to be nearly proportional to the electric power feeding the discharge, while the electron temperature T_e is almost independent of it (Rhallabi, 1991).

The problem of determining the evolution of the concentration of the different n chemical species (neutral and charged) can be managed by writing the balance equation for each density $n_k(r,z,t)$ of the k-th species:

$$\frac{dn_k}{dt} = \Pi(n_k) - \Delta(n_k) \quad (1)$$

where at the left hand side there is the total time derivative. The first term Π (k) consists of the sum of all production processes of the k-th species, due to both chemical reactions, in the gas phase or at the reactor surface, and to the external gas fed, and it can be written as

$$\Pi(n_k) = \sum_{i<j=1}^{N} K(i+j \rightarrow k)n_i n_j + \sum_{l=1}^{N} K(l \rightarrow l(w) \rightarrow k)n_l + Q(k(in) \rightarrow k) \quad (2)$$

where K are the reaction rates for the gas phase reactions and the effective rate for the surface ones (consisting of the chain process: adsorption of species l, reaction at the surface and desorption of species k) and Q is the flowrate. In the same way the contributions to the loss term of the k-th species are the destruction of k in a gas phase reaction, the diffusion followed by adsorption at the reactor surface and the pumping outside.

$$\Delta(n_k) = \sum_{i,j=1}^{N} K(k+i \rightarrow j)n_k n_i + D(k \rightarrow k(w))\nabla^2 n_k + Q(k \rightarrow k(out))\frac{n_k}{n_{tot}} \quad (3)$$

where D is the diffusion coefficient of the k_{th} species. In parallel a simulation of the hydrodynamical flow should also be performed, so that the right velocity field can be inserted in the total derivative in order to close the system of differential equations. For the sake of simplicity, in a preliminary stage where the focus is mainly on the chemical kinetics effects, some other approximation is worthy.

Since in normal operative conditions (for instance in a low pressure gas flow, P=0.1 mbar, Q=50 sccm (Rhallabi, 1991)) the Reynolds number is small, a simple laminar flow in a cylindrical tube is an adequate representation of the reference reactor hydrodynamics. Moreover it is in general appropriate to distinguish between cases where the flow velocity exceeds the diffusion one from the opposite. From a chemical engineering point of view, indeed it means that the model can be formulated as a plug-flow or a well-mixed reactor (Benson, 1982; Smith, 1987). The gas-phase composition in the reactor is then determined only by the chemical reactions among the reactive species and the transport processes to the walls. In low pressure cold plasmas the former is more common. As a reference, the flow velocity V in a 10 cm diameter tube, at P=0.1 mbar and Q=50 sccm, is about 1 m/s and exceeds the diffusion one ($V_{diff} \sim D/2R$ where R is the vacuum chamber radius). Indeed the so-called Peclet number Pe is about 5. So, it is implied that a plug-flow approximation, that is neglecting diffusion in the flow direction is appropriate. As a result the geometry is slab and the total derivative simply reduces to a single derivative along the streamline z. The equations can be further simplified treating the diffusion process according to a scheme discussed in literature (Chantry, 1987). It implies, in short words, in approximating the transverse (in a cylinder, radial) profile of the concentration as the first normal mode dictated by the reactor chamber geometry (in our cylindrical geometry, this leads to the use of the Bessel function $J_0(kr)$). Within this approximation diffusion should be considered only for species that can be absorbed at the surface (for which the so called sticking coefficient S is not zero) and its contribution to the loss term becomes

$$D(k \rightarrow k(w))\nabla^2 n_k(r,z) \approx \frac{D}{\Lambda^2} n_k(z) \quad (4)$$

where the coefficient Λ depends only on geometrical factors and on the sticking coefficient S of each chemical species (Chantry, 1987). This formulation leads to the substitution of the Laplacian operator with an effective diffusion length and makes the system of balance equations only dependent from a single independent variable, here the distance along the streamline, or time in a well mixed formulation. So linearized this differential equations system can be integrated by means of standard numerical techniques, for instance using an adaptive Kutta-Runge routine, or other finite elements methods (Press, 1985). Additional computing time can be saved, especially in the early steps, by using as variables the logarithm of density and of time, thus effectively smoothing the system. As a result a complete mapping of the gas-phase composition and of the flows towards the surfaces could be obtained. The bulk of the modelization then stays in the collection of the relevant reaction rates at the low pressure conditions of the experiments. The most critical are ions and electrons interactions, since coherence with the underlying plasma state could not be taken for granted. Electron detachment should be added for completeness, even if it comes out that it plays a minor role in negative ion kinetics. Diffusion coefficient for ions can be extracted from mobility studies and as far as concerns the sticking coefficients S, the value S=1 is appropriate for charged particles. The introduction of a dedicated charge balance equation avoids the unphysical violation of the quasi neutrality of the bulk plasma affecting many existing and published simulations (Kline, 1989). This is badly needed whether one would take properly into account the ion recombination on the surface. It turns out that this is an important source of radicals since new data indicate that the electron recombination of molecular ions can be a strongly dissociative process (Semaniak, 1998; Riccardi, 2000). Even in the case of ion diffusion to surfaces, ions recombine with electrons on the wall, so that neutrals are back injected in the plasma.

2.2 Low pressure radiofrequency plasmas

Simulation of the chemical kinetics of a CH_4/Ar radiofrequency (RF) discharge at low pressure, is a typical case study of cold plasmas modelling. As a reference we consider, having in mind the actual experiments performed in literature, a cylindrical vacuum chamber. The gas flows along the cylinder axis and enters the plasma region through a grid electrode. There an uniform plasma (for the sake of simplicity, however it is straightforward to include in the simulation any longitudinal profile) is present. After reaching the second electrode, the neutral gas exits the plasma region. Downstream only neutral reactions could happen. The discharge balance is supposed to be assured by the compensation of the bulk ionization rate and the radial (ambipolar) diffusion of charged particles towards the walls. For the sake of simplicity it was assumed that the steady plasma condition can be described by an uniform electron density and temperature in the discharge region. The characteristic plasma chemistry processes, which are mainly driven by high energy electrons, include ionization, dissociation with production of highly reactive free radicals and transition to excited states. Besides the rich emission spectra of the discharge, these processes produce highly reactive metastable (i.e. long lived) species. In particular argon could trigger very interesting chemical kinetics effects due to its metastables (Tosi, 1995). Such processes can be taken into account by prescribing the correct plasma state as an external condition, by setting the electron density n_e and temperature T_e as parameters. The model discharge parameters could be related to external operating parameters in order to make comparison with existing experiments. For instance, an electron temperature of 4 eV has been estimated from the solution of the Boltzmann equation in pure methane for radiofrequency plasmas at a power level of 50 W, a value that agrees with experimental data (Rhallabi, 1991). A change in this parameter will affect mainly the different weight of electron impact reaction channels, at first the balance of ionization and neutral dissociation. As for the estimate of the electron density, one could solve the global energy balance equation (Rhallabi, 1991). A change in this parameter will affect mainly the dissociation degree reached by the end of the plasma region. In general, during experiments it is preferred to have moderately high flow velocity and short residence times. This assures that a uniform and steady flow of precursors is delivered to the downstream target, which is mandatory whether steady deposition is needed and uniform growth of the thin film is to be assured. As discussed above the model will be formulated as a plug-flow reactor model (Benson, 1982).

2.3 Spark discharges at atmospheric pressure

The second cold plasma system whose chemical kinetics we would like to discuss is the so called spark discharge (Raizer, 1991). This kind of intermittent discharge is produced by means of a d.c. high voltage supply when it is applied between two facing metal electrodes and it is controlled with a suitable external circuitry. Sparks are rapidly quenched inhibiting transition to arc, while the produced plasma state lasts enough to efficiently process a gas flow. Below we will discuss application to hydrogen reforming using an hydrocarbon flow.

As a reference we consider a setup where the two electrodes are coaxial cylinders, the external hollow, and in the space between them the gas flows and the discharge takes place. Due to the limitation in the output current provided by the generator and the external circuit impedance, which inhibits the development of a burning d.c. arc (Raizer, 1991) the discharge assumes an intermittent character, consisting of individual events of electrical current flow of limited amplitude and time, the sparks. The system shows intense current bursts with a limited duration, separated by dead times, corresponding to a sequence of spark discharges. Although not exactly constant, both the shape, the amplitude, the duration and the repetition rate of bursts are comparable and fairly cyclic. The spatio-temporal structure of such discharge events is displayed in fig. 2, where a frame recorded by a commercial CCD camera (Nikon Coolpix-4500, 30 fps, exposure time 2 ms) is compared with the time series of the discharge current, in a spark device developed at the laboratory of the authors (Barni, 2009). While the pattern of the single discharge is somewhat fuzzy, it appears that most of the flow cross-section is affected by the discharge and emits light. This is obtained with the insertion of a high external circuitry resistance. This opens the way for a simulation of the gas phase evolution using monodimensional approximations, extending the low pressure modelling to the new situation. From the geometrical point of view, the model formulation used treats the spark channel as a rectangular prism with the axis parallel to the electric field and a square cross-section, aligned with the gas streamlines. The actual value of the spark size l is treated as a free parameter of the simulation. Here the value was fixed to the experimentally estimated spark diameter, l = 500 μm. The contribution of the electrons to the discharge chemical kinetics depends on their local density and energy distribution. Both can be linked to the local amplitude of the electric field E_S. Although it is possible to predict the shape of the electric field in a given electrode setup and this could depend also on the position along the spark path, the differences are not large, and we chose to neglect them, assuming uniformity along the spark path. This implies that simulations assume a constant value for both the electron density and their mean energy. In the simulations, both parameters were varied in an extended range, which easily includes realistic values of the local electric field. In particular it includes density scaled electric field strength E_s/N in the range 0–200 Td (1 Td = 10^{-21} V m^2). In order to estimate the average electron density in the spark channel, we have neglected the contribution of ions to the measured discharge current. Under such approximation the current is determined by the size of the discharge section and the electron mobility as a function of the electric field, which was taken from literature for pure methane (Davies, 1989). This should be approximately right also for argon/methane mixtures, since mobility at the same electric field increases by a merely 10% even in pure argon. The other parameter which affects the chemical kinetics is the mean electron energy distribution function (EEDF) in the spark channel. We have assumed a Maxwellian EEDF, described by a single parameter, the electron temperature T_e. This can be easily connected with the mean electron energy, which is determined by the local electric field through the Boltzmann equation (Raizer, 1991).

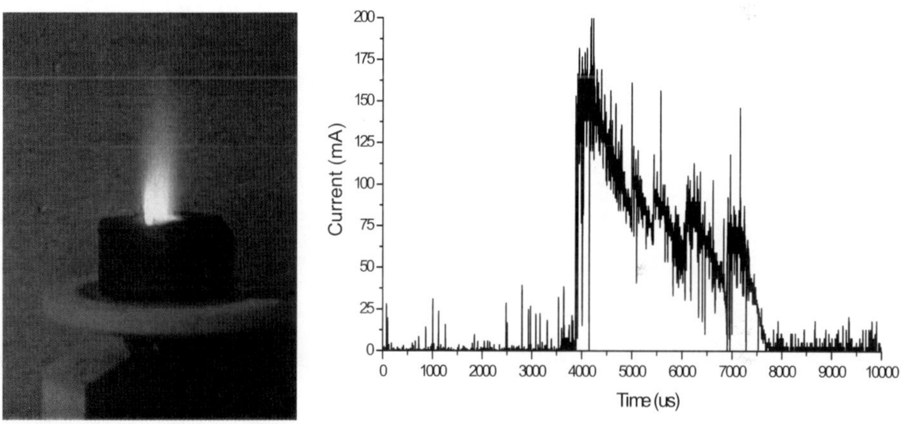

Fig. 2. Spark discharge in a hollow cathode setup, with the time evolution of the current.

3. Hydrocarbon plasma chemical kinetics

Methane and other light hydrocarbon plasmas are of great interest in industrial applications, in particular in the chemical vapor deposition processes (CVD) and specifically in plasma enhanced deposition (PECVD). Amorphous carbon and diamond-like thin films, suitable for mechanical and electronic applications can be prepared using low pressure discharges of hydrocarbon gases (Angus, 1988). The research in this field is mainly devoted to the understanding of the nature of the film growing mechanism but in spite of intense experimental and theoretical work it is not yet fully understood which species are responsible for the deposition process. Different growth species have been proposed, such as CH_3, C_2H_2, C, C_2, and CH, depending on the chemical kinetics pattern in the discharges. As an example we discuss the topic of the doping of CH_4 with Argon. Doping with Ar or Ne shows marked changes in the film properties (Gruen, 1995). This means that rare gases can significantly affect the plasma composition, opening new possibilities through their additional ion or metastable excited atom chemical reactions. This makes largely interesting the study of the chemical kinetics in such plasmas. A significant advance was made possible after a rather complete survey of the charge exchange cross-section and its branching ratios between argon ions and methane have also been performed. As a result, a quite complete mapping of the relevant reaction rates in an Ar – CH_4 plasma now exists and it is possible to investigate the effect of the chemical kinetics in such a system and eventually to identify the gaseous precursor of the chemical species incorporated in the deposited film.

3.1 Radiofrequency plasmas in argon/methane mixtures

We have then modeled the gas-phase chemistry of a typical radio frequency CH_4/Ar plasma used for the deposition of diamond and diamond-like carbon films, with the aim of understanding the effects of the chemical kinetics of argon ions and metastable (Riccardi, 2000). Moreover, since the role of the walls and in particular of the ion transport processes is generally neglected, we have also tried to quantify its contribution to the plasma composition and to the formation of the radical species of interest. We find that the most abundant carbon containing radical is CH_3 in pure methane discharges, but it is the carbon dimer C_2 in discharges of methane highly diluted by argon. Thus we propose that the gaseous precursor of the film is CH_3 in methane plasmas, and C_2 in CH_4/Ar plasmas. This proposal resolves outstanding discrepancies between experimental observations, that can now be rationalized by considering two different growth species (Shih, 1993). The analysis is performed through the implementation of the theoretical (numerical) model for the chemical kinetics simulation of the Ar/CH_4 plasmas, discussed above. The model is able to predict the neutral and charged species densities along the vacuum chamber as a function of several parameters, like operating pressure, flowrate, feeding mixture composition, RF power. We have solved the balance equations for the density of 16 neutral species and 15 ionic species by considering 194 chemical reactions and 15 electron-ion surface recombination processes. A cylindrical vacuum chamber (22 cm-diameter) was modeled. The gas flows along the cylinder axis (z) and enters the plasma region through a grounded grid, which acts as reference electrode for the discharge. After reaching the driving electrode (located downstream and 4.5 cm apart from the grid), the neutral gas exits the plasma region, pulled by the pumping system. An uniform flowrate is then supposed everywhere. As already discussed plasma chemical kinetics is mainly determined after prescribing the correct plasma state as an external condition, by setting the electron density n_e and temperature T_e as parameters. The discharge parameters considered here lie in the range 10^8 -10^{10} cm^{-3} for the electron density and 3–6 eV for the electron temperature. Here we consider an electron temperature of 4 eV as a reference. Such a temperature was used also in the simulation of Ar/CH_4 mixtures unchanged. Such a choice allows to identify pure chemical effects and to distinguish them from those simply arising from the different dissociation degree. For the sake of a realistic physical picture, we cannot neglect however that it is expected that T_e should increase with the Ar fraction due to the higher ionization potential of argon. The conditions imagined in our setup are consistent with moderately high flow velocity (Vflow ~ 30 cm/s for a flow rate of 120 sccm) and short residence times, of about 0.2 s. Then the plug-flow reactor model is a realistic choice for the simulations. In fact, in the low pressure range here considered (actually P = 0.2 mbar was used), the flow velocity exceeds the diffusion one, making negligible the mixing along the flow direction, as assumed in the model. The evolution of the concentration of the different N species in the gas phase is then determined by integrating each balance equation for the density n_k of the k-th species, along the cylindrical axis z. Densities of the most abundant neutral species in a pure CH_4 plasma are shown in figure. As could be expected the result is the finding that starting from pure methane the most abundant species at the end of the plasma region, are CH_4, H, CH_3, H_2, C_2H_2, and C_2H_4. Methyl radical is the most important reactive species that gets involved in the film deposition and growth. Atomic hydrogen will intervene mainly as an etching agent, controlling the H content in the film. The chemical kinetics pattern appears completely different when highly diluted mixtures of methane in argon are considered. Densities of the most abundant neutral species in CH_4 and 1% CH_4/Ar plasmas are shown in figure.

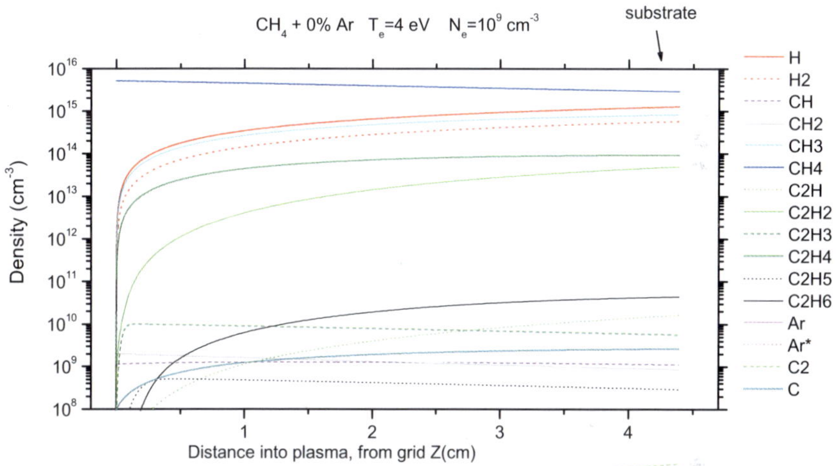

Fig. 3. Evolution of the neutral gas-phase in a pure methane plasma

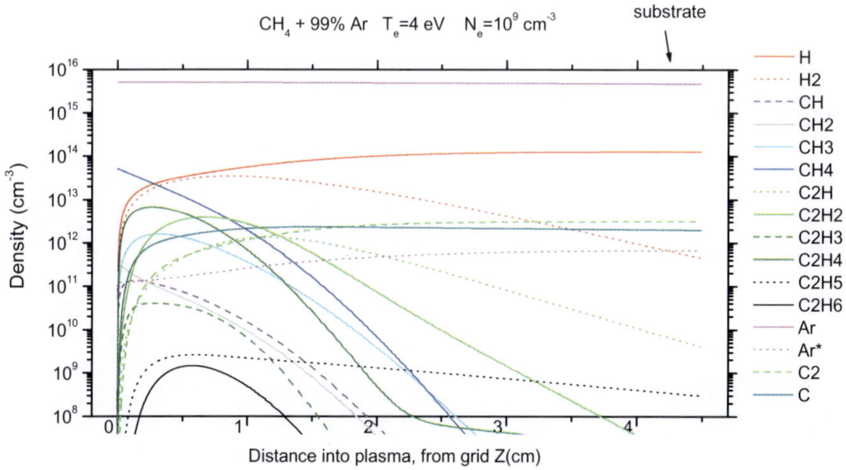

Fig. 4. Evolution of the neutral gas-phase in a 1% methane in argon plasma

The most striking result is the finding that while starting from pure methane the most abundant species at the end of the plasma region, are CH_4, H, CH_3, H_2, C_2H_2, and C_2H_4, in the case of an initial composition given by 1% CH_4 diluted in Ar, the most abundant species in the plasma are Ar, H, C_2, and H_2. Reactions responsible for such behavior are mainly those of metastable argon. In fact Ar* increases significantly the dissociation of methane, producing CH_x radicals. The chemistry of these species eventually produces C_2H_2 and C_2H_4, thus forming the strong C-C bond. Successive dissociative processes involving C_2H_x species finally result in the production of C_2. This kinetic chain is inhibited by CH_4 and therefore proceeds only if most of methane has been dissociated. This finding is coherent with recent experimental observations indicating that high fractions of argon in H_2/Ar/CH_4 plasmas result in an increase in the C_2 concentration (Riccardi, 2000). Above results have been obtained by considering ion recombination and subsequent neutral species desorption from the surface.

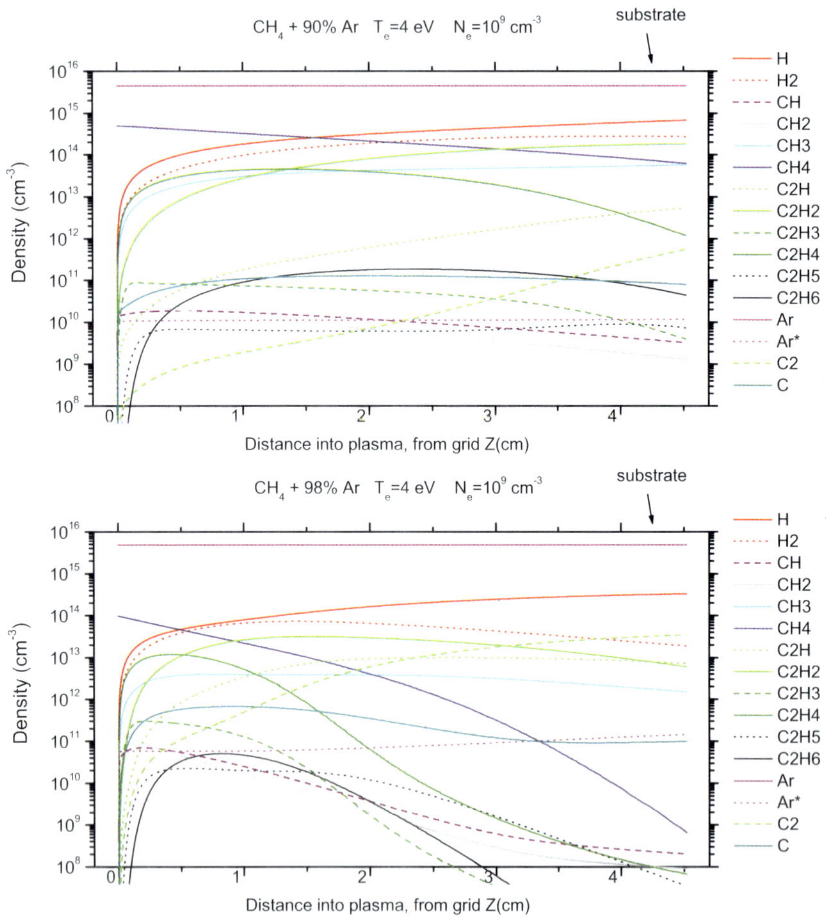

Fig. 5. Evolution of the neutral gas-phase in different methane/argon plasmas.

The transition between a CH_3 to a C_2 dominated gas-phase happens at increasing dilution in the initial gas mixture, as it can be seen by figures above. The kinetic chain inhibition by methane could be appreciated by enlarging the horizonthal axis, using a log scale. In this way the fast evolution in the initial steps could be appreciated. The formation of C_2H_x radicals proceeds indeed only after most of methane has been dissociated. The development of the discharge gas-phase in the early times can be appreciated in figure.

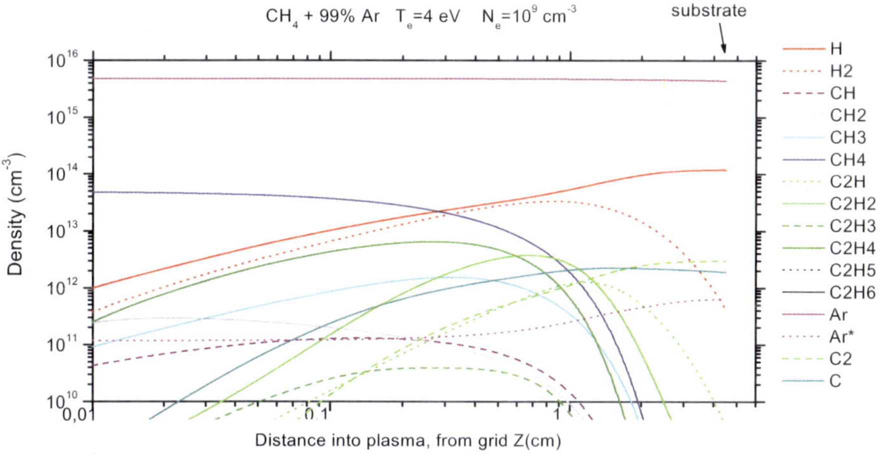

Fig. 6. Expanded evolution of the neutral gas-phase in a 1% methane in argon plasma

As for the charged species in the plasma gas-phase, they show interesting trends too. Our simulations indicate that, in pure methane, the most abundant ion species are CH_3^+, CH_4^+, $C_2H_4^+$ and $C_2H_5^+$.

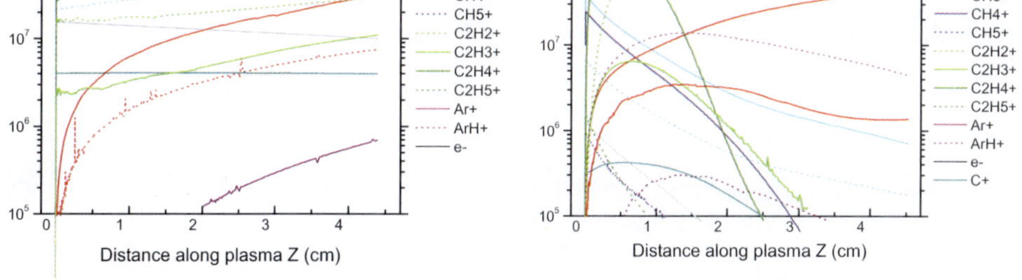

Fig. 7. Charged species in plasmas of methane and argon diluted methane.

The CH_5^+ ion, whose density initially appears to be comparable to that of these other ions, decreases along the flow, being quickly removed by ethylene and atomic hydrogen. This picture closely resembles the findings obtained by direct mass spectrometric analysis (Matsukura, 1996). Another important aspect concerns the ion contribution to the chemical kinetics pattern. Common wisdom favours a minor effect of ion chemistry due to very small concentrations of charged species respect to the neutral ones. Results discussed so far have been obtained by considering a null ion sticking coefficient, so that the ion recombination is taken into account and the proper neutral species are desorbed from the surface for each ion impinging on the walls. For comparison, next figures show the corresponding results obtained by assuming complete ion absorption. It is clear that ion recombination processes on the surface contribute significantly to the density number of a few species, in particular in pure methane about 20% of the CH_3 comes from the walls.

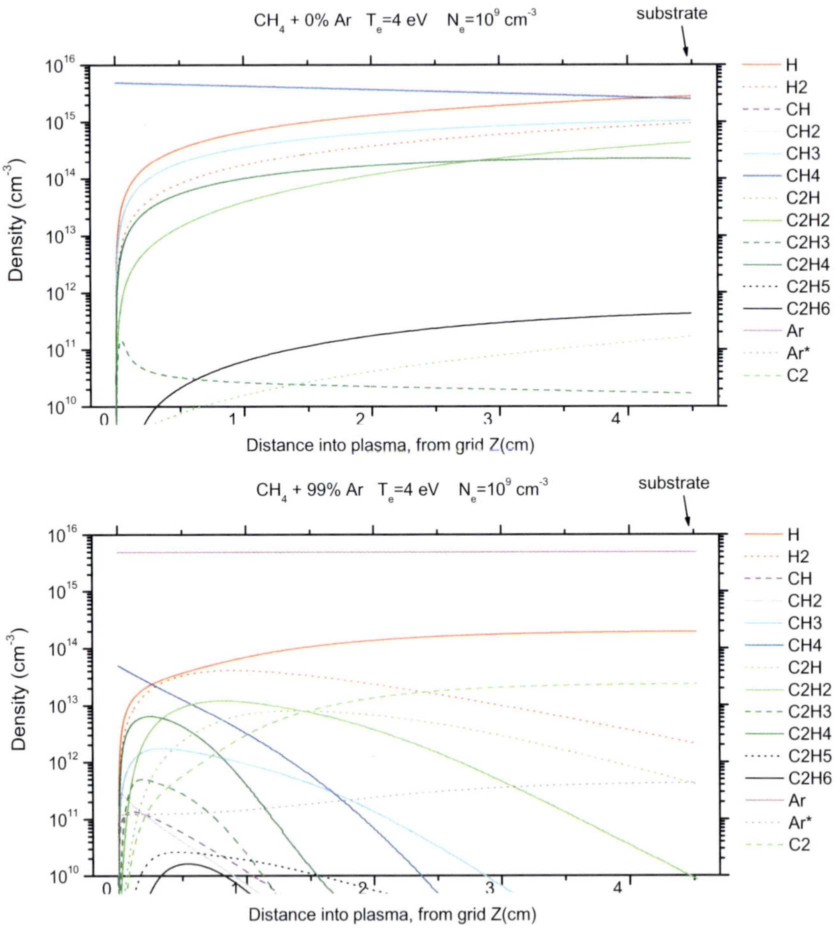

Fig. 8. Evolution of the neutral gas-phase in different methane/argon plasmas when complete ion sticking is considered.

Even more striking is the effect in the Ar/CH_4 plasma where the C_2 density is reduced by about one order of magnitude in the case of unitary sticking coefficient and the majority of carbon atoms, initially fed through CH_4 molecules, are adsorbed as ionic species on the walls. This is clearly at variance with the common belief that ion chemistry can be neglected as ion densities are typically lower than those of neutrals by many orders of magnitude. On the contrary, though ions are much less abundant than neutrals, the cumulative effect of the ambipolar diffusion transport cannot be neglected in those cases where the interaction with the walls is expected to play a role. At each plasma condition there is a dilution level at which a sharp transition in the final gas-phase composition happens. For our conditions it could be appreciated from the data at different Ar concentrations, reported in figure. In the end we show also the effects of physical parameters of the discharge, that is the electron density and temperature on the evolution of the gas phase. The first has only a rescaling effect, increasing the velocity of the dissociation, without affecting the transition concentration. The latter affects also the transition since the relative levels of CH_3 and CH_4 depend on the electron temperature, as it could be grasped from figure.

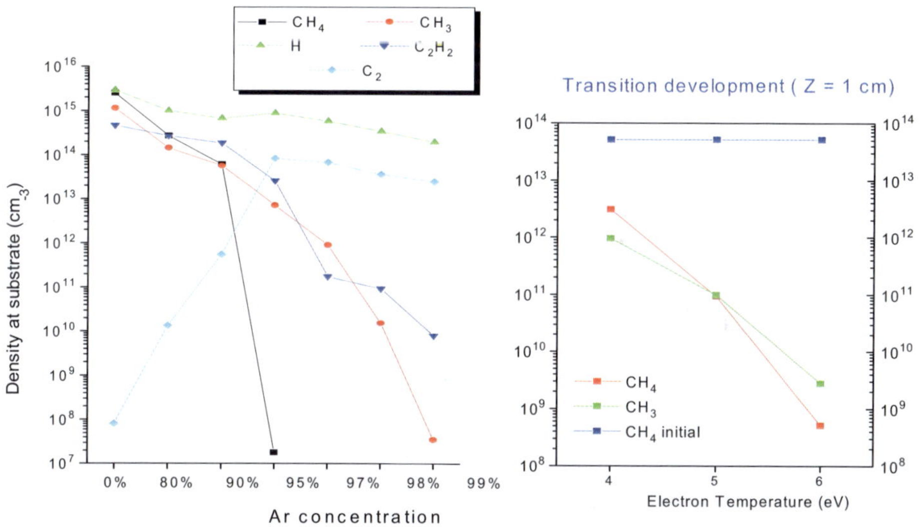

Fig. 9. Evolution of the neutral gas-phase as a function of the electron density and temperature

3.2 Hydrogen reformer based on spark discharges

Hydrogen reforming from methane is up to now the most viable source for large scale as well as localized production of hydrogen for fuel cell systems. Conventional reforming is carried out thermally in oven with oxygen and steam or using catalytic beds but the development of more compact devices is actively pursued too. Electrical discharges at atmospheric pressure are widely used in applied research for instance in material surface processing and pollutant waste disposal. Their application for the promotion of chemical reactions as alternative to conventional process has emerged too. In particular atmospheric pressure plasmas have been suggested as hydrogen reforming devices, based on arc discharges, microwave plasmas and dielectric barrier discharges (Paulmier, 2005).

Here we present a discussion of hydrogen reforming using a pulsed spark discharge in an air/methane mixture (Barni, 2006). The simulations have been developed to help in the experimental research, using an already existing electrode setup, which was designed for burning a continous arc discharge. It consists of a cathode, an hollow pin of copper ending with a tungsten tip, and an anode, a block of copper with a shrinking cylindrical cavity surrounding coaxially the cathode (Barni, 2009). Details of the setup relevant for the model build-up are discussed briefly here. The anode is mantained fixed at a distance from the cathode which is 1.2 mm at the closest location. A gas flow passes through the electrode gap, entering from three small holes at the beginning of the cathode. Technical (dry) air and high purity methane, were used to prepare the controlled air/methane mixtures employed. High purity methane and technical air (80% N_2, 20% O_2) have been used, to avoid contamination from impurities and water vapour in the environment atmosphere. A termocouple was inserted downstream in order to measure the temperature of the outgoing gas. No effort was made to fix the electrodes temperature, although this was technically feasible, partly because heating should increase methane decomposition and partly in order to maintain the system setup simple. Light emitted from the discharge is collected and analysed in a low resolution spectrometer. This allows to measure integrated emission spectra of the discharge, which give access to information about the composition of the produced gas-phase in the discharge. Initially the simulation targeted only argon/methane mixtures which were much simpler to simulate. Results of the modeling will be discussed here. The parameters were: a gas mixture of 4% CH_4 in argon, a flowrate Q = 2600 sccm, an electron density of 5.6×10^{15} cm^{-3} and an electron temperature Te = 2.6 eV (Barni, 2006). At such dilution a complete transformation of methane in hydrogen and carbon is obtained. Recombination of neutral radicals happens quickly downstream the discharge region, producing an outgoing flow composed of hydrogen with less than 10% of heavy hydrocarbons. The transition in the gas-phase composition is very fast (in the first 81 nm corresponding to 87 ns).

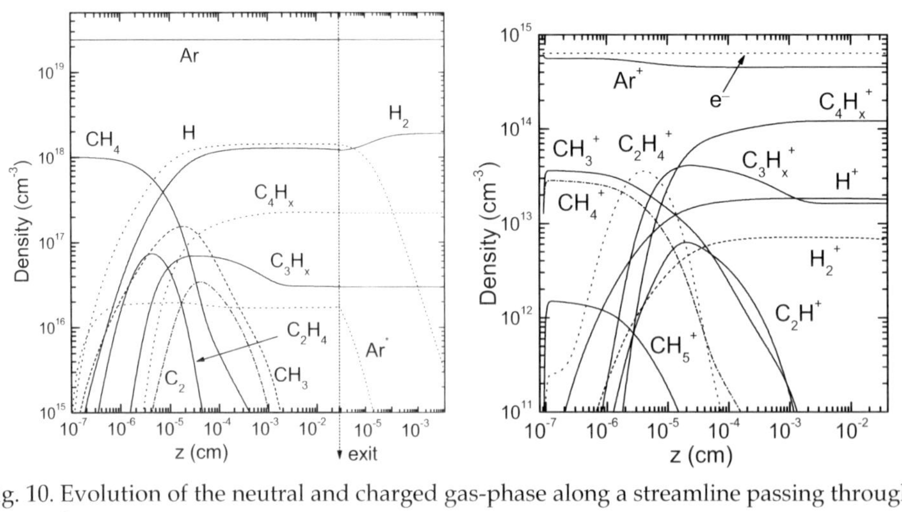

Fig. 10. Evolution of the neutral and charged gas-phase along a streamline passing through the spark.

For the discharge simulation described above the conversion factor C was 94.61%. However the predicted efficiency of the device is only 0.14% which depends on to the very small duty cycle of these discharges. It is interesting to notice that the chemical kinetics in the neutral gas-phase favours the polymerization of heavier hydrocarbons, here included all as C_4H_x radicals, with a small hydrogen content. This is driven by a trade off between the hydrocarbon radicals reactions, which favours the formation of C-C bonds (for instance the fast $CH + CH \rightarrow C_2H + H$) and the dissociation processes, which preferentially leads to hydrogen abstraction rather then to C-C bond breaking. In next figure the conversion factor as a function of the plasma parameters is shown. The conversion factor C reaches a maximum (~98%) and then decreases slightly, as electron density rises. A sharp drop in the conversion is observed for lower density. Indeed at a relatively low density the chemical kinetics is slowed down and complete transition cannot be accomplished before the flow exits outside the discharge region. A similar trend is reported by changing the electron temperature. Again the conversion factor is almost independent on the effective value of Te in a wide range (more than 90% for Te between 2 and 5 eV). However, for low temperatures, the conversion factor drops, reaching a mere 16.7% at 1.5 eV.

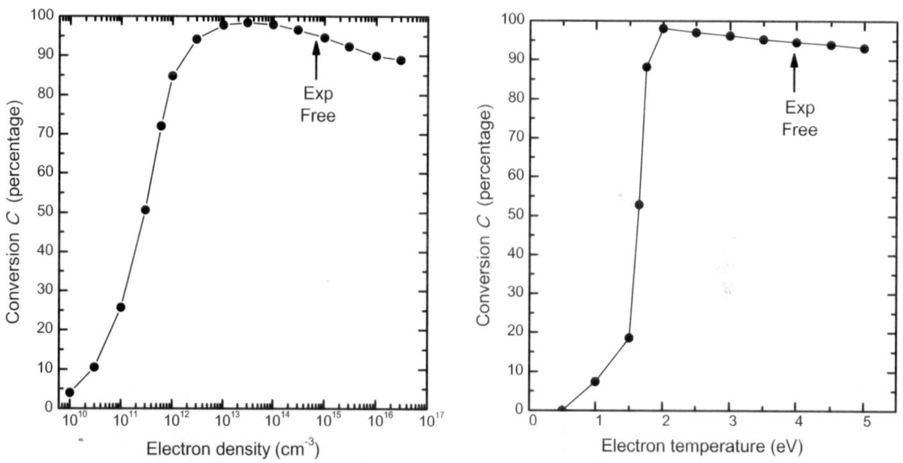

Fig. 11. Conversion efficiency of spark discharges depending on plasma parameters.

4. Conclusions

A chemical kinetics modeling scheme suitable for cold plasmas simulations has been presented. The model was used to study the chemical kinetics of hydrocarbon plasmas in particular the effect of argon dilution. The results obtained have been used to discuss the composition of the gas phase and the possible precursors for carbon thin film growth. The model was then used for atmospheric pressure spark discharges as a system for hydrogen reforming with plasmas. These examples show that important and significant aspects determined by the chemical kinetics effects could be investigated through simulations. Then they could prove worthy in order to study the applications of plasmas as processing reactors.

5. Acknowledgment

The authors are deeply grateful to all their collaborators and students that over the years have partecipated in their research studies, contributing to the success of the enterprise, or more poetically adventure, of the PlasmaPrometeo Center of Excellence. We could enlist M.Piselli, S.Zanini, P.Tosi, A.Quintini, F.Picciolo, C.Broggi, R.Benocci, M.Orlandi, A.Brandirali just to mention only a few involved in the topics of this chapter.

6. References

Angus, J.C. & Hayman, C.C. (1988). *Science,* Vol. 241, pp. 913

Barni, R.; Broggi, C. ; Benocci, R. & Riccardi, C. (2006). Chemical kinetics of an argon/methane plasma in a hydrogen reforming reactor, *European Physical Journal - Applied. Physics,* Vol. 35, pp. 135-143

Barni, R.; Quintini, A. ; Piselli, M. & Riccardi, C. (2009). Experimental study of hydrogen plasma reforming by intermittent spark discharges, *Journal of Applied. Physics,* Vol. 103, pp. 063302.1-9

Barni, R. & Riccardi, C. (2009). Hydrocarbon plasma reforming through intermittent spark discharges, *High Temperature Material Processes,* Vol. 13, pp. 119-127

Benson, S.W. (1982). *Thermochemical Kinetics,* Wiley, New York US

Chantry, P.J. (1987). *Journal of Applied. Physics,* Vol. 62, pp. 1141

Davies, D.K. ; Kline, L.E. & Bies, W.E. (1989) *Journal of Applied. Physics,* Vol. 65, pp. 3311

Kline, L.E. ; Partlow, W.D. & Bies, W.E. (1989) *Journal of Applied. Physics,* Vol. 65, pp. 70-77

Gruen, D.M. ; Zuiker, C.D. ; Krauss, A.R. & Pan, X. (1995). *Journal of Vacuum Science & Technology A,* Vol. 13, pp. 1628

Kline, L.E. ; Partlow, W.D. & Bies, W.E. (1988) *Journal of Applied. Physics,* Vol. 65, pp. 70-77

Li, H.Q. ; Zou, J.J. & Lin, C.J. (2005) *Progress in Chemistry,* Vol. 17, pp. 69

Lieberman, M.A. & Lichtenberg, A.J. (1994). *Principles of Plasma Discharges and Materials Processing,* J.Wiley & Sons, New York US

Mutsukura, N. & Yoshida, K. (1996). *Diamond Related Materials,* Vol. 5, pp. 919

Mc Daniel,E.W. (1993). *Atomic Collisions,* Wiley, New York US

Paulmier, T. & Fulcheri, L. (2005). *Chemical Engineering Journal,* Vol. 106, pp. 59

Press, W.H. (1985). *Numerical Recipes,* Cambridge University Press, Cambridge UK

Raizer, Y.P. (1991). *Gas Discharge Physics,* Springer-Verlag, Heidelberg Germany

Rhallabi, A. & Catherine, Y. (1991) *IEEE Transactions on Plasma Science,* Vol. 19, pp. 270

Riccardi, C. ; Barni, R. & Fontanesi, M. (2001). *Journal of Applied. Physics,* Vol. 90, pp. 3735

Riccardi, C. ; Barni, R. ; Fontanesi, M. & Tosi, P . (2000). Gaseous precursors of diamond-like Carbon films in CH4/Ar plasmas, *Chemical Physics Letters,* Vol. 392, pp. 66-70

Riccardi, C. ; Barni, R. ; Sindoni, E.; Fontanesi, M. & Tosi, P. (2001). *Vacuum,* Vol. 61, pp. 211

Semaniak, J.; Andfersen, L.H.; Heber, O.; Kella, D., Pedersen, H.B., Schmidt, H.T. & Zajfman, D. (1998). *Astrophysical Journal,* Vol 498, pp. 886-895

Shih, H.C. (1993). *Diamond Related Materials,* Vol. 2, pp. 531

Smith, J.M. (1987). *Introduction to Chemical Engineering Thermodynamics,* McGraw-Hill, New York US

Tosi, P. ; Bassi D. ; Brunetti, B. & Vecchiocattivi, F. (1995). *International Journal of Mass Spectrometry and Ion Processes,* Vol. 149/150, pp. 345-353

10

Chemical Kinetics in Air Plasmas at Atmospheric Pressure

Claudia Riccardi and Ruggero Barni
Department of Physics G. Occhialini,
University of Milano-Bicocca, Milan,
Italy

1. Introduction

The chapter, after a general introduction concerning plasmas produced in air at atmospheric pressure, describes the chemical kinetics happening in the plasma gas-phase, focusing on the nitrogen oxides mechanism of formation and elimination. After a general review of the chemical kinetic pattern, we discuss dielectric barrier discharges and their use for NOx remediation. In fact, research concerning the use of plasmas for the promotion of chemical reactions has emerged as one of the most prominent application field. Gas treatment aimed to toxic waste disposal or to pollutant emission reduction is an important field where plasma processing can prove to be a very effective technology. We have studied the characteristics of plasma reactors based on dielectric barrier discharges (DBD) operating in a streamer regime, as well as those based on high voltage electrical discharges operated in an intermittent spark regime. Both kind of discharges have been considered for the promotion of chemical reactions aimed to nitrogen oxides removal form a diluted gas flow. Detailed modeling of the chemical kinetics happening in an air plasma gas-phase has been investigated in our previous research. The evolution of the gas-phase composition during and after the interaction in the discharge region was calculated under different operating conditions. The results have been used to predict the NOx reduction achievable and to study the role played by the different discharge parameters in order to determine the optimal interaction between plasma and gas mixture. Comparison between streamer and spark discharges could be performed too.

2. Discharges at atmospheric pressure

Let's consider a system where at least two electrodes (conductive, in general metal surfaces) are separated by a gap filled with air at atmospheric pressure. Then one of the electrode electrical potential is increased respect to the second, which we could suppose, without any lack of generality to be grounded. An electric field arises in the gas gap, whose magnitude and space distribution depend on the potential applied and the geometry of the system. At large enough values of the field a discharge could spark in the gas. When an electrical breakdown happens in atmospheric pressure air the discharge quickly evolves towards to a condition allowing large electric current flows and strong heating of the gas. Self-sustaining discharges at such high pressure could not develop as the usual glow regime, since heating and ionization instability leads to the contraction of the discharge electrical current channel and, if the system could sustain it, the discharge evolves to a so called arc. Under such conditions the air in the gap becomes very hot, reaching a few thousands of K and electrical current could exceed hundreds Ampers (Raizer, 1991).

These kinds of discharges have interesting chemical kinetics in their own, being almost thermal equilibrium systems, but their behaviour as chemical kinetics reactors bears more resemblances with that of a hot gas than of a plasma. Moreover such devices require very large power and the high temperatures imply a considerable stress of the materials used, which somewhat limits their use as processing tools in material chemistry.

2.1 Corona and radiofrequency discharges

More interesting from the point of view of plasma chemical kinetics is another kind of discharge, the so called corona. However corona discharges occur only whether the electric field is sharply non-uniform in space, which means that the electrode setup should reflect such condition. The easiest way to accomplish this is when one of the electrode size is much smaller than the inter-electrode or gap distance. Point or wire electrodes are the best instances of that. Corona are self-sustaining discharges, producing plasmas in steady conditions and burning in a stable manner for quite long periods (Raizer, 1991) . Then chemical kinetics have time to evolve and an interesting pattern of radical formation and oxidation could develop in the air of the gap. On the other hand, corona discharges are inherently disuniform in space, requiring geometry to be taken into account and complicating the task of modeling. The result is, in a sense, to obscure partially the true chemical kinetics effects. Corona discharges draw relatively small electrical currents and plasma density is usually small too, making their reactivity quite low. Then their use in material processing is somewhat limited, even if, mainly in non specialized literature, the term corona is often employed and abused for other kind of discharges and setups. In the following sections we will discuss briefly the chemical kinetics associated with their plasmas. Although the use of an oscillating voltage as supply could make several differences in the gas breakdown and in the discharge formation, there are striking similarities in the plasma state which is produced. Indeed at the somewhat large density of an atmospheric pressure gas the oscillation frequency is order of magnitude smaller than the elastic collision frequency (in air at STP this is about 3 THz or 3×10^{12} Hz). Under such conditions averaging

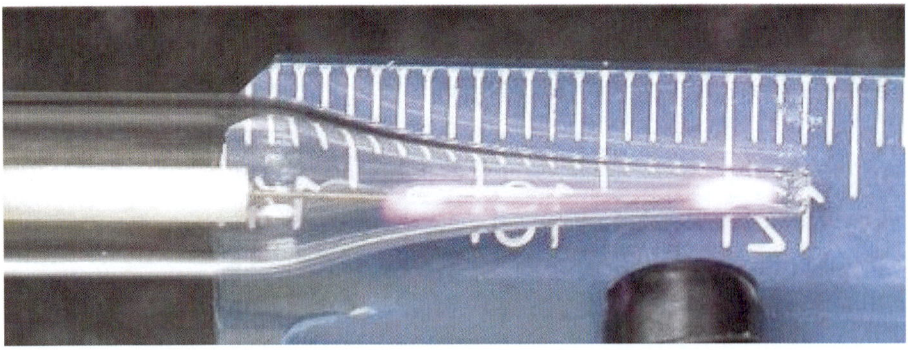

Fig. 2.1.1. A radiofrequency atmospheric pressure air plasma produced by a plasma needle.

occurs and a steady plasma state is formed, independent on time and, in first approximation, determined only by the effective, i.e. rms, electric field value and not from the wave frequency (Raizer, 1991). Then modeling as well as the pattern of the chemical kinetics associated with these plasmas could be grasped from the trends observed in d.c. corona discharges. The oscillating electric field however prevent most of the charges to be lost at the walls or the electrodes by drifts alone and the plasma state is less influenced by badly known parameters linked to electrode surface and material properties as in general it happens in d.c. configurations. This make the realization of suitable plasma sources in form of plasma jets, pencils or needles much easier and user-friendly (Mariotti, 2010).

2.2 Dielectric barrier discharges

The main characteristic of a Dielectric Barrier Discharge (DBD) device lays in the setup of the electrodes. In particular the setup includes the presence of a dielectric layer within the discharge gap distance d (in general in the 0.1-5 mm range for an atmospheric plasma) insulating at least one of the electrodes. The dielectric presence forbids the flow of a direct current in the gap, preventing the formation of arcs or sparks, as well as of a steady plasma state. To sustain the discharge an a.c. voltage or a pulsed one is applied to the electrodes at a frequency ranging from several hundreds of hertz to a few hundreds of kHz. While many different kinds of DBD exist, in general, for a such high value of the product pd of gas pressure p and the electrode gap width d, the discharge operates in a streamer regime (Raizer, 1991). Just to make a little example, let's consider a discharge gap d of 1 mm supplied by an HV voltage of 5 kV, which makes an electric field of 5 MV/m whether it would be uniform. Using the data reported in Fig. 2.2.1 it easy to see that the ionization length is well below 0.1 mm. Actually the product $\alpha \cdot d$ turns out 21.3 exceeding the threshold value of 18-20 , known as the Meek criterion, for streamer discharge onset (Raizer, 1991).

But what characterises most the steamer regime? These discharges are built up of many repeated microdischarges, each leading to the formation of narrow discharge filament (with an electron density in the range 10^{12}-10^{17} cm^{-3}) of some nanoseconds duration (Kogelschatz, 2003). In particular a plane electrode DBD at near atmospheric pressure which operates in streamer regime, under an a.c.voltage supply displays an uniform glow filling the gap. At a closer inspection the glow reveals itself as built up with a large number of current filaments appearing through the gap at seemingly random locations and not exactly at the same time during an active phase which happens each voltage half-cycle (Kogelschatz, 2003). The uniformity is just brought in by the high rate of repetition and superposition of such microdischarges. Depending on the operating conditions, at each half-cycle a new streamer head could propagate in the opposite direction starting from the same location when the voltage is reversed. On the other hand, during the active phase, the streamers cannot propagate on the same path, being inhibited by the space charge accumulated on the dielectric surfaces. This has important consequences on the chemical kinetics and its modeling since streamers can be considered as isolated and repeating at frequency which is the double of the a.c. voltage frequency. Another key feature is that, at least in small gaps like the one we are considering, they appear to be very thin (radius R ~ 100 μm) while their average distance is much larger (a few mm, of the order of the gap width) as discussed in literature (Raizer, 1991). So, as a first approximation one could chose to simulate the chemical kinetics induced in a single isolated streamer and its repetition at a fixed frequency. The results of this approach are examined in the following.

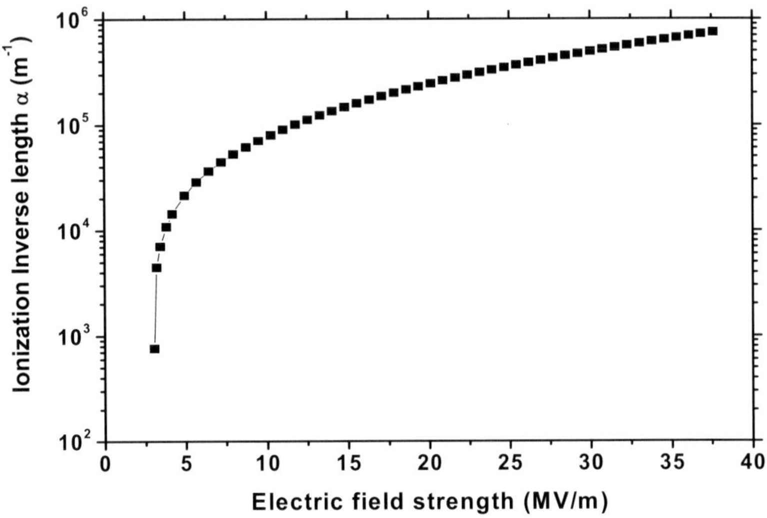

Fig. 2.2.1. The ionization inverse length coefficient in atmosperic pressure air

Several models (see for instance Kulikovsky, 1997-1998) and a few experimental observations (Malik, 2008) of streamer development and propagation exist by now. Despite many differences, the overall picture appears to be the same in all kind of DBDs. The microdischarges develops in three steps. After a phase of charge accumulation in the head, coming from previously deposited charges or from electron multiplication (Raizer 1991), the stremer head starts moving towards cathode. Streamer propagation is very fast (v ~ 10^5 - 10^6 m/s) and is sustained by the electron avalanche multiplication in the strong field ahead of the streamer (E_{max} ~ 5-15 MV/m). After the head has reached the cathode, spreading its charge on the dielectric surface, in the gap a discharge filament is left. The streamer body consists of a thin channel of weakly ionized gas, almost quasi-neutral (n+ ~ n- ~ 10^{13}-10^{16} cm^{-3}) and driven by a small or just vanishing electric field. After the streamer head reaches the dielectric barrier insulating the cathode, the channel allows the flow of a limited discharge current, which is rapidly quenched by the space charge accumulating at the dielectric surface. At high pressures electrons moves along the electric field at the drift velocity and almost instantaneously (the corresponding relaxation times for velocity and energy, dictated by collisions with neutrals, are τ ~ 0.3 ps, τ_E ~ 50 ps) reach a mean energy determined by the local amplitude of the field. On the other hand ions inertia keeps them almost frozen and substantially cold, that is at the set temperature. At a fixed position along the streamer path, the electric field rises quickly as the streamer head is approaching and then decay almost as fast to the much smaller value it assumes in the streamer channel. This has important consequences on the chemical kinetics and its modeling too. Indeed the high energy bond-dissociation and ionization processes happens only through electron impact interactions, since neutral and ions are mostly cold. Then a simple cold plasma approximation is valuable. Moreover tha active phase happens only in a very short time when the streamer head is propagating. Since propagation is so fast, chemical kinetics could be considered freezed and happening independently at each position along the streamer channel (Siliprandi, 2008).

3. Chemical kinetics in atmospheric pressure air plasmas

In numerous problems of plasma chemistry, electro-physics, gas lasers physics and atmospheric physics a detailed consideration of the kinetics of non-equilibrium plasma-chemical processes in nitrogen-oxygen mixtures is essential (Raffaele-Addamo, 2003; Esena, 2005). Another relevant topic concerns the need to examine the ecological consequences of projects involving a prolonged use of powerful electromagnetic radiation in the atmosphere. Channels determining the balance of neutral and charged particles in a non-equilibrium plasma are highly diverse, making plasma chemical kinetics vastly different from that of an ordinary hot gas. In plasmas, the main chemical processes proceed on the basis of reactions with nitrogen and oxygen atoms being formed by electron impact dissociation of the initial molecules. In some cases, electronically excited molecules play an important role, as for instance, the influence of oxygen molecules in the state a' on the process of ozone formation. This makes relevant any work undertaken in an attempt to form a kinetic scheme of non-equilibrium discharge in nitrogen-oxygen mixtures (Kossyi, 1992).

3.1 Modeling of the air kinetics in dielectric barrier discharges

As discussed above, a sensible starting point to simulate the chemical kinetics induced in a DBD is to study what happens in a single isolated streamer and its repetition at a fixed frequency. For the sake of simplicity we choose to discuss dry air. However the validity of the model can be extended to general electrodes configuration and more extensively to any plasma devices operating in a streamer discharge mode. The inherent difficulty encountered in developing a model for air discharges at high pressure is that one must solve a highly nonlinear coupled set of differential equations which may be both spatially and temporally dependent. In DBDs, moreover, the time scales involved span many order of magnitude, from the very fast connected with streamer formation and propagation to the very slow connected with ion recombination, chemical kinetics of neutral species and diffusion. So several approximation are worthy in order to make tractable the problem. From the chemical kinetics point of view, the process can be seen as consisting of an almost instantaneous phase during which energetic electrons produce mostly ions and atomic radicals, followed by a phase in which electrons cool down almost instantaneously and reach the set temperature or a temperature so low, that further dissociations are stopped. In the latter phase, slow chemical reactions between neutral and charged species happen in the gas phase, while they diffuse outside the streamer channel. Although existing models do predict that the shape as well as the peak value of the electric field pulse depends on the position along the streamer path, the differences are not large, apart from the region near the dielectric surfaces (Kulikovsky, 1997). As a first approximation, one could neglect such differences and thus let's suppose uniformity along the streamer path. From the mathematical point of view, then the model formulation used treats the streamer channel as a cylinder, with a circular cross-section. The radial profile is determined by diffusion and the only parameter describing evolution is time. The actual value of the streamer radius is treated as a free parameter of the simulation. We assume also a square pulse shape for the time evolution of the electric field ahead of the streamer. The pulse is therefore characterized by the time length (here 2 ns, based on the model in (Kulikovsky, 1998)) and by the peak electric field E_{max}. Although it appears as a very rough approximation, it embodies all the relevant dynamics for our aims.

In building our model and performing numerical simulations we have found more sensible to employ two different parameters, which are related to those describing the electric field ahead of the streamer. The first one, arises naturally when we have observed that since the electron density rises almost exponentially as the streamer develops, the total amount of radicals produced by electron impact does not depend strongly on the time length of the pulse or on the initial electron density but only on the actual value reached by the electron density at the end of the pulse. We have treated the value reached by the electron density ne at the end of the streamer passing as the relevant parameter of the simulation. As reference we consider a density of 10^{15} cm^{-3} (Braun, 1991; Kulikovsky, 1998). However we have varied n_e in a broad range in order to investigate how it can affect the gas-phase chemical kinetics.

After imposing that the electron density reached in the streamer channel after its formation were the same, we also checked that the length of the electric field pulse does not make any significant difference in a broad range from 0.2 to 5 ns. This range is enough to cover the different streamer head velocities reported in DBDs (Raizer, 1991). As it could be guessed, most of the chemical kinetics is simply frozen during such fast times and the total production of species through electron impact reactions during the pulse depends on the electron reaction rates (influenced by the electric field amplitude) and on the electron density which is reached at the end of the pulse rather than on the pulse length.

As for the second parameters, the electric field strength E_{max}, we have found more sensible to employ the electron temperature instead. In fact it was simpler to express the electron rate constants, calculated from their cross-sections and evaluated assuming a Maxwellian energy distribution function for electrons, described by a single parameter, their temperature T_e.

Then it was possible to collect reaction rates in form of simple functions of a single parameters with Arrhenius formulas, which are quite common in literature and databases of chemical kinetics and reaction rates. The use of electron temperature as a parameter does not prevent the capability to make comparison with other existing models, since it could be related, in a one to one correspondence, with experimental informations on the streamer electric field. Indeed electron temperature is trivially connected with the mean electron energy, which is determined by the local electric field in the Boltzmann equation (Raizer, 1991). This is sufficient to make straightforward a direct comparison between this simulation and other existing ones or experimental data. In the following we considered as reference an electron temperature value of 4 eV (Kulikovsky, 1998).

Under such simplified description of the streamer development, we could model the subsequent evolution of the gas phase in a standard way, using the continuity equations for each chemical species and solving a system of mono-dimensional first-order differential equations easily and quickly tackled by numerical integration (Riccardi, 2000). From a chemical engineering point of view, indeed it means that the model can be formulated as a well-mixed reactor (Benson, 1982). The gas-phase composition in the reactor is determined by the chemical reactions among the reactive species and the transport processes. The time evolution of the concentration of the different N species in the gas phase is determined by integrating each balance equation for the density n_k of the kth species:

$$\frac{dn_k}{dt} = \sum_{i<j=1}^{N} K(i+j \rightarrow k)\, n_i n_j - \sum_{i,j=1}^{N} K(k+i \rightarrow j)\, n_k n_i + D_k \nabla^2 n_k \qquad (1)$$

where K are the reaction rates for the gas phase reactions and D is the diffusion coefficient. Due to the supposed uniformity, diffusion along the streamer axis is neglected. Adsorption on the dielectric barrier is included but, because of the much smaller extension of the streamer radius respect to the discharge gap, it turns out to be negligible. The choice of species included in the model was based on existing experimental information based on emission spectroscopy or mass spectroscopy. A sub-set of 8 neutral and 9 charged species was included in a preliminary study. Then the code was updated to include 20 neutral and excited and 12 ionic states.

As already discussed, to simulate DBD plasmas a cold plasma approximation is suitable. So reaction rates for ion as well as neutral species are evaluated at the set temperature, that is 300 K. The effect of larger temperatures is addressed below. Since thermal energy is much smaller than the molecular bond energy, the initial step in the decomposition is presumed to involve mainly electron-impact dissociation. Electron-impact cross-sections used in this study were obtained from literature collected in (Riccardi, 2001; Barni, 2005), apart from attachment rates which are taken from recent experiments. Rate constants have been evaluated assuming a Maxwellian energy distribution function for electron, described by a single parameter, their temperature Te. Rate constants for neutral gas-phase, charge exchange and ion recombination reactions have been taken from literature referenced in (Riccardi, 2001; Guerra 1997) or estimated based on approximating techniques (Benson, 1982). In this report we assume a substantial vibrational excitation of nitrogen molecules, which allows direct dissociation from atomic O radicals (Guerra, 1997). A total of 121 reactions have been taken into account in the simulation. The diffusion loss rates are estimated by using a formulation due to (Chantry, 1987) in cylindrical coordinates. The radial density profile of the streamer is approximated in term of the lowest order normal mode and is integrated away. This formulation allows substituting the Laplacian operator with an effective diffusion length and makes the system of balance equations only time dependent. Diffusion of air from the outside the streamer is also included as a source term. Ion diffusion loss rates was corrected by enforcing the plasma quasi-neutrality, following an approach proposed for low pressure electronegative plasmas (Lichtenberg, 2000). Balance equations containing all the processes described above form a system of coupled differential equations which has been integrated to obtain the time evolution by using an adaptive Runge-Kutta routine. Results from the calculations are discussed below and have been partially presented in literature (Barni, 2005; Barni, 2010).

3.2 Chemical kinetics pattern in air

As a first step we start discussing the temporal evolution of the discharge gas phase using a sort of reference values for the free parameters. That is electron temperature was 4 eV, electron density reached in the microdischarge channel is $2x10^{15}$ cm^{-3} in a time length of 2 ns and the streamer radius was 100 μm. At first, we neglect diffusion losses, in order to look directly the evolution pattern of the chemical kinetics alone. Neutral as well charged species densities are displayed as a function of time respectively in figures on a log-log scale.

As expected, the charged phase shows a very fast increase, almost exponential, in almost all species, as the streamer gets formed. Afterwards, as diffusion is not included, the system evolves under recombination alone, giving the overall decreasing trend as the inverse of time (that is linear in the log-log plot). The composition however displays some important

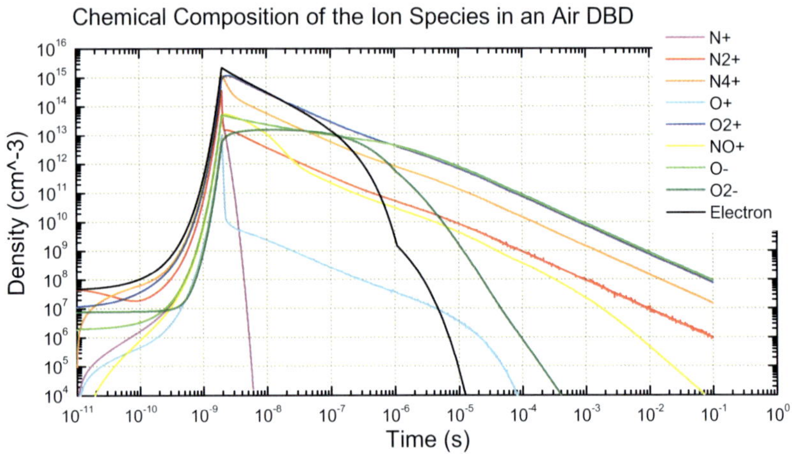

Fig. 3.2.1. Evolution of the charged density in the gas-phase of a streamer in an air DBD.

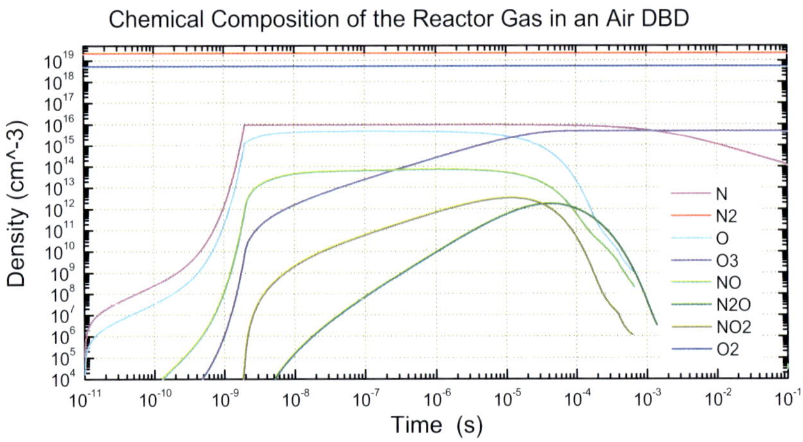

Fig. 3.2.2. Time evolution of the neutral species density in the gas-phase of a streamer in an air DBD. After a brief transient due to streamer formation, the neutral gas-phase reaches an equilibrium with the formation of ozone in a few ms.

changes. First atomic ions are removed immediately due to charge exchange reactions on nitrogen and oxygen molecules. Then electrons are lost, due to prevalence of attachment for cold electrons in the streamer channel. Their evolution reflects the shift between atomic and molecular oxygen negative ions. Later on, a sort of equilibrium in the positive ion composition is reached. It reflects the strength of interactions with main neutral molecules. The major ions are then negative atomic oxygen O^- and positive molecular oxygen ion O_2^+, with traces of nitrogen and nitrogen oxides ions. As for the neutral species, during the time length needed for streamer development mainly atomic N and O species are created, from electron impact-dissociation (the former more than the latter at such an electron temperature). NO production is quite fast, the fastest among other molecules, but even so its density stays under 0.1% by the end of the streamer formation time. Approach to equilibrium is much slower. Between 10 and 100 μs oxygen atoms decline and molecules accumulate, with ozone already dominating. With the disappearance of O, all nitrogen oxides decline, leaving only ozone (besides air) in the gas phase. Nitrogen atoms are much less reactive and are removed only late, in tens ms, mainly through recombination to N_2, as their linear decay in log-log plot clearly reveals. In real world, however such behaviour is difficult to observe. The relative narrow sizes of streamer channel and electrode gap make diffusion enter the game relatively early after only some ms. A more realistic modelization is therefore provided in the following pictures, with a more extended reaction dataset and where again neutral as well charged species densities are displayed as a function of time on a log-log scale. As for the neutral species, during the time length needed for streamer development mainly atomic N and O species are created, from electron impact-dissociation (the former more than the latter at such an electron temperature). NO production is quite fast and its density approaches 0.02% of N atoms one by the end of the pulse. Ozone formation is slower but almost catches up NO. On the other hand NO_2, NO_3 and N_2O production is clearly much slower and become appreciable only on a larger scale time, even more so for N_2O_5. After the pulse end, in the temporal range from 2 to 20 ns, O and NO slowly increase till saturation is reached. N density reaches a value of 9×10^{15} cm^{-3}, whereas O grows to 3×10^{15} cm^{-3} and NO to a value of 4×10^{13} cm^{-3}. The dissociation degree is therefore rather limited, up to 5×10^{-4}. Ozone, on the contrary, keeps increasing eventually reducing O and NO and peaking afterwards. Starting from 0.1 ms, the diffusion term becomes relevant and all species density starts to decrease. The gas phase is practically cleared out after a few ms. Ozone density exceeds atomic oxygen after about 10 μs, at a level of 1.3×10^{15} cm^{-3}, and peaks after 30 μs, at a level of 2×10^{15} cm^{-3} about 100 ppm. The increase is triggered by the partial balancing between production from O + O_2 and loss due to dissociative attachment

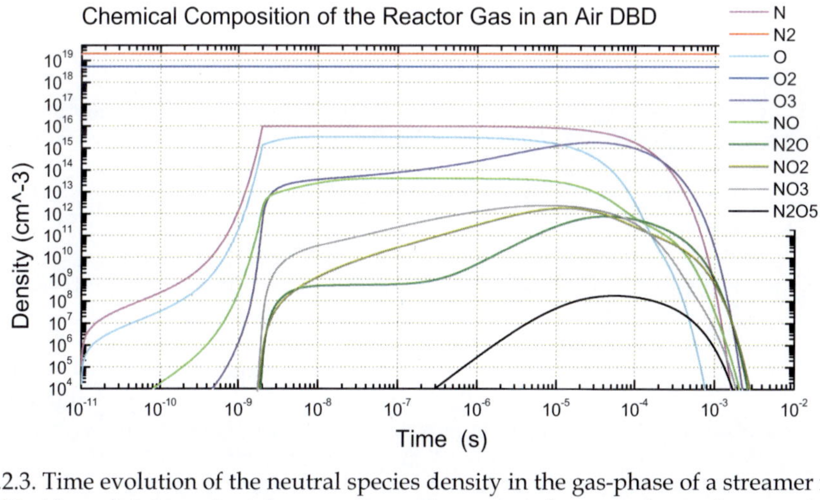

Fig. 3.2.3. Time evolution of the neutral species density in the gas-phase of a streamer in an air DBD. After a brief transient due to streamer formation, the neutral gas-phase reaches a definite composition in about 0.1 ms and it is then dissipated by diffusion in a few ms.

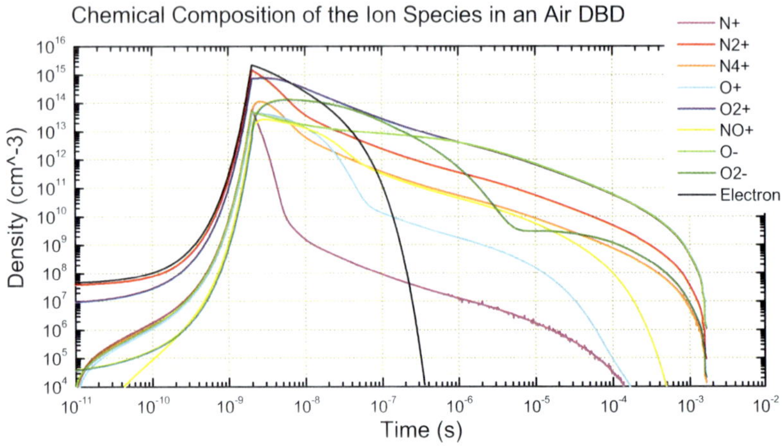

Fig. 3.2.4. Time evolution of the charged species density in the gas-phase of a streamer in an air DBD. After the transient producing an almost exponential increase of charged particles, electrons are quickly removed and an electron-less cold plasma is slowly dissipated due to recombination and then diffusion in about 10 ms.

and charge exchange reactions. Since charged particles are destroyed faster than neutrals due to the high rate of ion-ion recombination, ozone keeps on growing, until atomic O is finished and then declines due to diffusion. NO_2 and NO_3 appear to follow a similar trend, with density three order of magnitude lesser and a peak value after tens of μs, at a level of $2x10^{12}$ cm^{-3}. N_2O_5 also has a similar trend, with much lower density and a slight delay. three order of magnitude lesser and a peak value after tens of μs, at a level of $2x10^{12}$ cm^{-3}. On the other hand, N_2O shows a partial equilibrium within a hundred of ns, then it grows to levels similar to the other nitrogen oxides. Its dynamics is closely controlled by fast dissociative attachment and charge exchange reactions in particular on atomic oxygen ions. So its concentration cannot rise until most of the electrons are removed. N_2O density appears to take over NO_2 after 100 μs and reaches a maximum of $7x10^{11}$ cm^{-3} soon later.

On the other hand, the temporal dynamics of charged species seems to be faster than that of neutrals. This is due to the higher rates of ion-ion recombination and of electron attachment. All the charged species increase almost exponentially during the streamer development time (2 ns) and then the total charge density begins to decrease because of recombination. In presence of oxygen, after the pulse ends, when the electron temperature decreases to less than 2 eV, electrons are quickly removed due to attachment processes. O^- is the majority negative ion, except for a small time window between 10 and 300 ns. This happens because, while at T_e=4 eV the dominant attachment process on oxygen is dissociative to O^-, at set temperature prevails direct attachment to O_2^-. Then electrons disappear and soon after charge exchange reactions on oxygen atoms removes O_2^- and produces again the more stable O^-. Positive charged species composition is mainly determined by charge exchange reactions on N_2 and O_2. They quickly remove atomic ions and leave O_2^+ as the majority ion, with a 10% of N_2^+ and a few % of N_4^+ and NO^+. This situation is reached in about 100 ns. Later on positive charged species density shows the same course: a power-law decrease in time (that is linear on the log-log plot) dictated by the ion-ion recombination process, followed by an exponential decay due to ambipolar diffusion after 0.5 ms. In order to study the influence of the different streamer parameters we have performed several simulations changing their values in a broad range. The overall temporal evolution appears to be similar to the one reported in figures, even if some particulars are affected. In next figures the maximum density of a few neutral species is displayed as a function of the peak electron temperature. We made simulations varying Te from 2 to 4.5 eV with a step of 0.25 eV. We found that a minimum electron temperature of 2.5 eV is needed in order to allow electron density to rise during the streamer formation time. This can be understood since attachment prevails on ionization at small electron temperatures. The general behaviour shows that the maximum density decreases by increasing the electron temperature. This is due to the fact that ionization rate rises faster than the dissociation rate as the electron temperature is increased. Indeed, those simulations were performed keeping the peak electron density constant and since it means that the ionization grade stays constant then the overall dissociation grade should be diminished. The effects are more pronounced for species produced by secondary processes after the streamer formation, such as O_3, NO_2 and N_2O than for atomic radicals such as N and O. We also checked that the length of the electric field pulse does not make any significant difference in a broad range from 0.2 to 5 ns. Indeed most of the chemical kinetics is simply frozen during such fast times and the total production of species through electron impact reactions during the pulse depends on the electron temperature (through the reaction rates) and on the electron density which is reached at the end of the pulse rather than on the pulse length. We have also performed several simulations changing the peak electron density ne from 10^{11} cm^{-3} to 10^{16} cm^{-3}. Again, the temporal dynamics appears to be similar, with the same behavior of nitrogen oxides, ozone and atomic radicals and ions. In figure the maximum density of a few neutral species is displayed as a function of the peak electron density. All the maximum densities appear to increase increasing the electron density. The increase is approximately linear on the log-log scale of the figure. However the effect is much more pronounced for the heavier nitrogen oxides, thus increasing their concentration in the late gas phase, where ozone percentage in excess of 1000 ppm is reported. The strong sensitivity to such a badly known parameter of the discharge is clearly

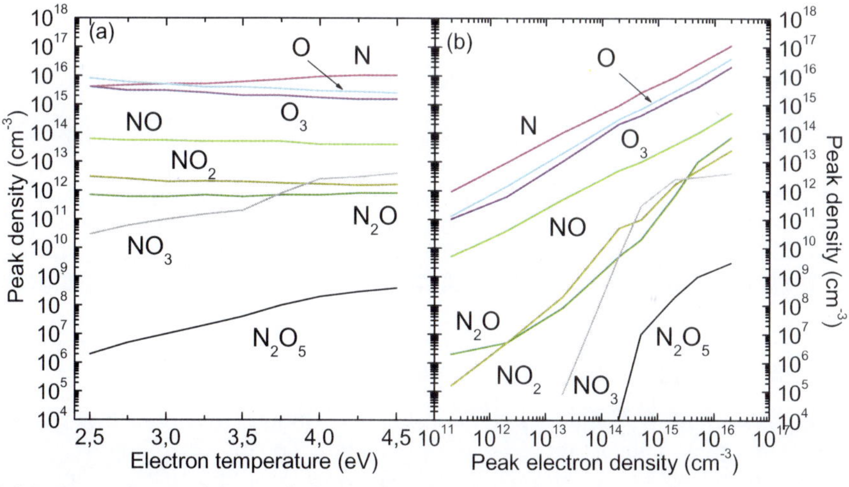

Fig. 3.2.5. Dependence of the peak density reached by different neutral species on the electron temperature and maximum density in the gas-phase of a streamer in an air DBD.

disappointing from the point of view of driving the optimization process with chemical kinetics modeling, but it offers also a clue for an indirect insight of the streamer properties from this strong link between n_e and the composition of radical fluxes outside the streamer. We have also investigated the effects due to the streamer radius Rs. Such a parameter affects mainly the diffusion process. We have varied Rs between 0.05 to 1 mm. The smaller Rs is, the faster diffusion transports radicals and ions outside the streamer. If it happens fast enough it interferes with secondary chemical processes leading to transformation of atomic radicals in O_3, NO_2 and N_2O. A slower diffusion gives time to the system to approach the chemical equilibrium in composition. However equilibrium is approached in times exceeding a few hundreds milliseconds, which is definitely too long respect to any reasonable diffusion time.

3.3 Reactivity of different nitrogen oxides

Plasma remediation is an efficient and promising technology to destroy toxic and greenhouse gases (Manheimer, 1997). These techniques are potentially lower in cost and more efficient than conventional thermal incineration. In these plasmas, the majority of electrical energy is expanded in heating electrons, rather than heating gas, as discussed previously. The understanding of the process and the optimization of the efficiency benefit largely from computational studies of the dynamics of the plasma gas-phase. In particular the air chemical kinetics of high-pressure dielectric barrier discharges. Such systems are considered in the context of volatile organic compound (VOC) and NOx remediation. The air plasma kinetic processes are discussed with the goal of providing insight for optimizing efficiencies. Indeed the most extensively investigated applications of this type are used to treat dilute concentrations of toxic molecules in airstreams. Potential advantages of the high-pressure, nonthermal plasma approach include the highly energy efficient selectivity provided by the plasma chemistry and its capability for minimizing secondary-waste production. Atmospheric pressure operation is preferred for high-throughput waste processing (Shoyama, 2007). Indeed the removal of NO from environment is a relevant problem concerning pollution control (Amoroso, 2008). NO stays in the low atmosphere for several days and enters cycles producing ozone, causing smog. Nitrogen oxides are mainly produced as by-product in combustion processes in free air. For instance in diesel engine exhaust NO can reach 200-500 ppm and NO_2 50 ppm (Srinivasan, 2007). So we applied our simulations to air contaminated by similar level of nitrogen oxides. In Figures 3.3.1 and 3.3.2 we display the results of a simulation, with the same standard parameters but starting with 500 ppm of NO, that is a density of 1.3×10^{16} cm^{-3}. No diffusion of neutrals is considered here, to let the system reach the chemical equilibrium, which however happens only at late times, both considering discharge repetition times (several kHz generally) and diffusion times for the considered streamer radius (a few ms). After the end of the discharge at 2 ns, NO is completely removed, oxidated initially by O atoms and then, when atomic radicals disappear, consumed in reactions with ozone and NO_2. In the final state it is substituted mainly by ozone (about 1000 ppm).

A substantial amount of NO_2 (192 ppm) and N_2O (11 ppm) is produced too, while other oxides are not formed with an appreciable concentration. The transition from oxygen atoms to ozone happens after about 10 μs, while NO disappears only after 10 ms. More details are discussed in literature (Barni, 2010). Starting from NO_2 as initial contaminant produces a different kinetic pattern. Oxidation and substitution with ozone in the final state is achieved

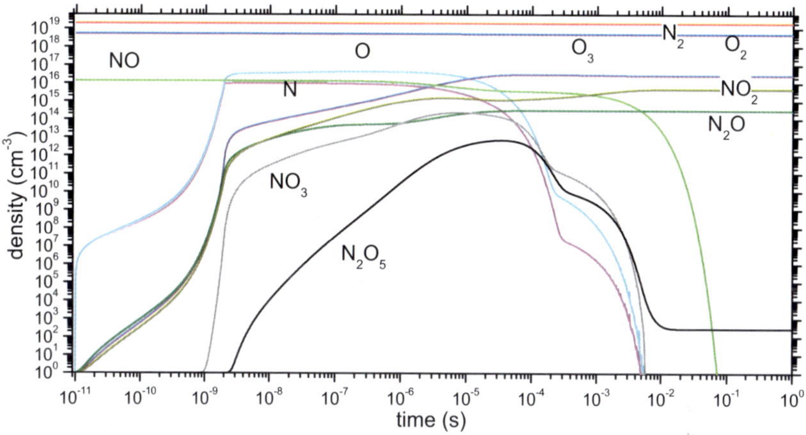

Fig. 3.3.1. Time evolution of the neutral species density in the gas-phase of a streamer. NO is removed to mainly ozone, the transition happening within a few tens of microseconds.

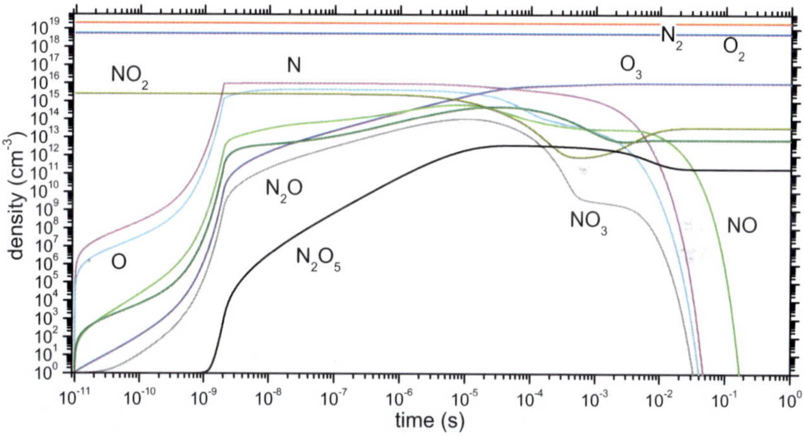

Fig. 3.3.2. Time evolution of the neutral species density in the gas-phase of a streamer. NO_2 is removed to mainly ozone, the transition happening within a few tens of microseconds.

too, but the initial nitrogen oxide is not completely removed and about 2% is not disposed. A similar trend is reported for N_2O which is however better oxidised.

The effect of the repetition of streamer discharges during subsequent cycles of a.c. voltage was studied and displayed in Figure 3.3.4 at 10 kHz. A small number of discharges is needed to remove NO under a few %. To reach an equilibrium in the gas-phase, here producing a constant flux of ozone, consuming mainly atmospheric oxygen, requires a larger number of cycles, in the order of thousands, yet in times less than seconds. In this case substantial amounts of radicals in the form of atomic nitrogen and oxygen are present and could be delivered to materials exposed to the plasma phase, for instance to achieve oxidation of biological matter for sterilization purposes (Moreau, 2008).

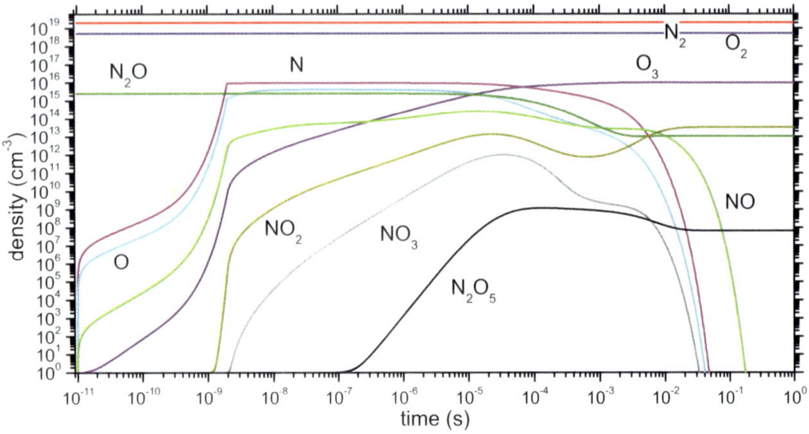

Fig. 3.3.3. Time evolution of the neutral species density in the gas-phase of a streamer. N_2O is removed to mainly ozone, the transition happening within a few tens of microseconds.

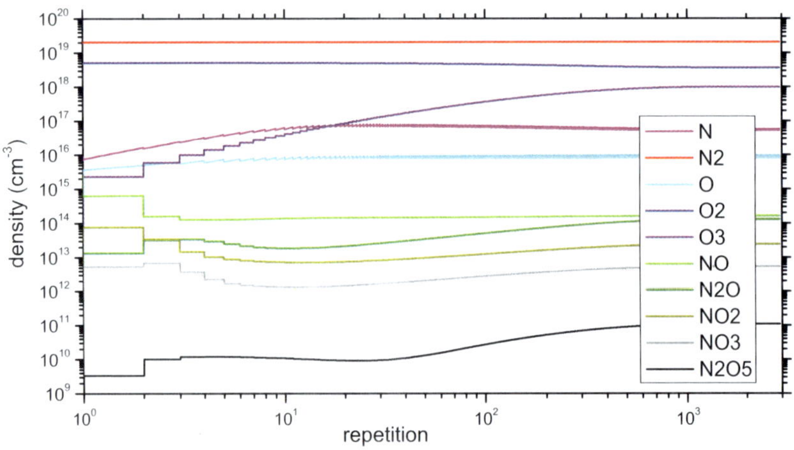

Fig. 3.3.4. Evolution of the neutral species density in the gas-phase of a streamer under subsequent repetitions at a frequency of . N_2O is removed to mainly ozone, the transition happening within a few tens of microseconds.

3.4 Effect of gas temperature

Reaction rates for ion as well as neutral species depends on their temperature, which could depart from the set, that is 300 K. Many neutral gas reactions are quite affected by the gas temperature, so it is interesting to use the theoretical framework we have developed to study what is the impact of a hotter gas phase. In any case, since thermal energy is much smaller than the molecular bond energy, the initial step in the decomposition is presumed to involve again mostly electron-impact dissociation. An idea of the impact the gas temperature has on the chemical kinetics is reported in figure. Taking into account the air temperature within the device to be simulated, the software has been changed adding the temperature dependence in several reactions involving neutral species, rates have been collected through different public databases as coefficients for the Arrhenius equation. The main results was that at low temperature it has been observed a cut down in nitrogen monoxide concentrations, which has been replaced by ozone as principal product. At high temperature nitrogen monoxide remains unperturbed through the discharge while ozone disappears. Thus gas phase temperature, and then the control of a strictly cold plasma condition is crucial for efficient NOx remediation.

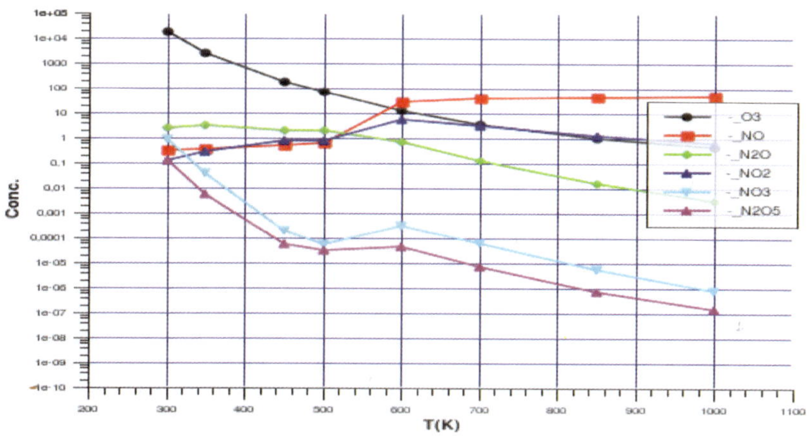

Fig. 3.4.1. Final composition of the neutral species density in the gas-phase of a streamer. NO is removed to ozone only at low temperatures, the transition happening at about 600 K.

4. Chemical kinetics in air steady plasmas

Then we consider application of the modeling to a steady plasma conditions, like the one in a corona discharge. In order to study direct chemical kinetics effect we have chosen an ideal setup, under a well-mixed reactor approximation, and with an uniform plasma background.

Apart from geometry (here 3 mm corona electrode is discussed), we have parametrised our results in terms of two physical values, the effective electron density and temperature. As discussed previously, the former affects mostly the velocity of the chemical kinetics evolution, whereas the latter affects the relative weight of the different electron impact. In order to study the influence of the different parameters we have performed several simulations changing their values in a broad range. The overall temporal evolution appears to be similar to the one reported in figure, even if some particulars are affected. The corona discharge produce mainly NO reaching a steady state after a few hundreds of microseconds. There is a transition from the initial phases of the discharge, where N and NO are the major neutrals. All neutral molecules are accumulating in the gas-phase until 10 microseconds. Then nitrogen atoms start to decline, followed a little after by ozone. The final composition is then reached, with about 90% of NO as final product. In next figure the maximum density of a few neutral species is displayed as a function of the peak electron temperature and density. We made simulations varying Te from 0.5 to 2 eV with a step of 0.25 eV. We found that above 1 eV the density of nitrogen oxides produced in the gas-phase becomes independent from the temperature. Ozone and atomic radicals are minority showing a broad minimum around 1 eV. We have also performed several simulations changing the peak electron density ne from 10^8 cm^{-3} to 10^{12} cm^{-3}. Again, the temporal dynamics appear to be similar, with the same behavior of nitrogen oxides, ozone and atomic radicals and ions.

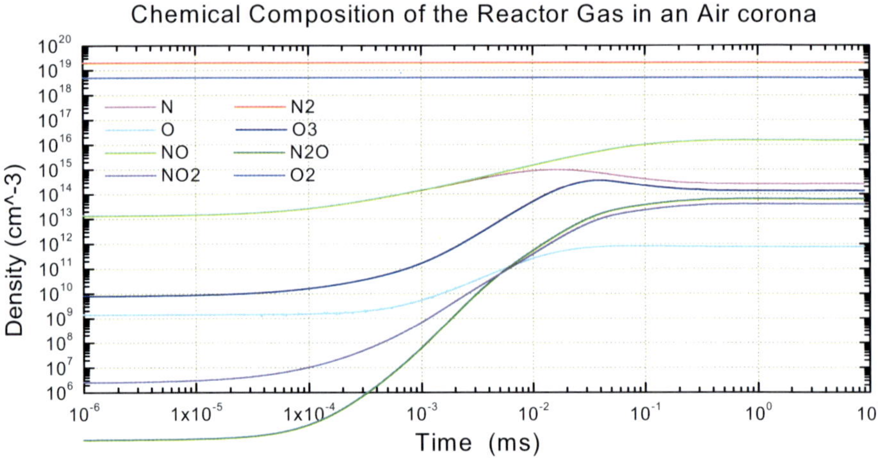

Fig. 4.1. Time evolution of the neutral species density in the gas-phase of an air corona. The neutral gas-phase reaches an equilibrium in about one second, the transition happening between 1 and 100 ms.

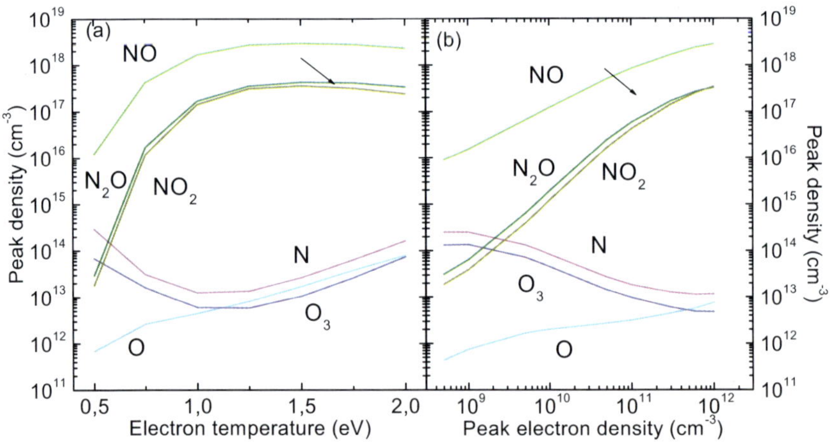

Fig. 4.2. Dependence of the peak density reached by different neutral species on the electron temperature and density in the gas-phase of an air corona.

All the nitrogen oxides densities appear to increase increasing the electron density. The increase is approximately linear on the log-log scale of the figure, showing a trend to saturation at the higher end of the range. The effect is much more pronounced the heavier nitrogen oxides, thus increasing their concentration in the late gas phase. Ozone and nitrogen atoms decrease, becoming comparable to atomic oxygen.

5. Conclusions

A chemical kinetics modeling of atmospheric pressure air discharges in the streamer regime of DBDs as well as in corona steady state plasmas has been presented. The model was used to evaluate the prospect of nitrogen oxides removal from the gas phase. The results obtained show that the chemical system could remove NO and to some extent also other nitrogen oxides up to a certain maximum initial concentration. Under realistic conditions for NO this could be as high as 800 ppm. The system produces mainly ozone through secondary reactions in the gas-phase. This theoretical study shows that important and significant aspects determined by the chemical kinetics effects could be investigated through simulations. Then they could prove worthy in order to study the applications of plasmas at high pressure in streamer regime (for example DBDs) and their capabilities as gas processing units.

6. Acknowledgment

The authors are deeply grateful to their collaborators and students that over several years have partecipated in their research studies, in the laboratory activities and in discussion about plasma science during working hours and not, contributing to the success of the PlasmaPrometeo Center of Excellence. We could enlist M.Piselli, S.Zanini, P.Esena, I.Nardi, E.Grimoldi, F.Fumagalli, I.Biganzoli just to mention a few involved in the topics of this chapter.

7. References

Amoroso, A.; Beine, H.J.; Esposito, G.; Perrino, C.; Catrambone, M. & Allegrini, I. (2008). *Water Air and Soil Pollution*, Vol. 188, pp. 81

Barni, R. & Riccardi, C. (2010). Perspective of NOx removal from numerical simulation of non-thermal atmospheric pressure plasma chemical kinetics, *High Temperature Material Processes*, Vol. 14, pp. 205-210

Barni, R.; Esena, P. & Riccardi, C. (2005). Chemical kinetics simulation for atmospheric pressure air plasmas in a streamer regime, *Journal of Applied. Physics*, Vol. 97, pp. 073301.1-7

Barni, R.; Esena, P. & Riccardi, C. (2005). Chemical kinetics simulations of an atmospheric pressure plasma device, *Surface & Coatings Technology*, Vol. 200/1-4, pp. 924-927

Benson, S.W. (1982). *Thermochemical Kinetics*, Wiley, New York US

Braun, D.; Gibalov, V.I. & Pietsch, G.J. (1991). *Journal of Physics D*, Vol. 24, pp. 564

Chantry, P.J. (1987). *Journal of Applied. Physics*, Vol. 62, pp. 1141

Esena, P.; Riccardi, C.; Zanini, S.; Poletti, G. & Orsini, F. (2005). *Surf. & Coatings Techn*, Vol. 1/4, pp. 664

Guerra, V. & Louriero, J. (1997). *Plasma Sources Science & Technology*, Vol. 6, pp. 373

Kogelschatz, U. (2003). *Plasma Chemistry and Plasma Processing*, Vol.23, pp.1

Kossyi, I.A.; Kostinsky, A.Y.; Matveyev, A.A. & Silakov, V.P. (1992). Kinetic scheme of the non-equilibrium discharges in nitrogen-oxygen mixtures, *Plasma Sources Science & Technology*, Vol. 1, pp. 207-220

Kulikovsky, A.A. (1997). *Journal of Physics D*, Vol.30, pp.441

Kulikovsky, A.A. (1998). *Physical Review E*, Vol.57, pp.7066

Lichtenberg, A.J. ; Lieberman, M.A. ; Kouznetsov, I.G. & Chung, T.H. (2000). *Plasma Sources Science & Technology*, Vol. 9, pp. 45

Malik, D.A. ; Orlov, K.E. ; Miroshnikov, I.V. & Smirnov, A.S. (2008). Spatial and temporal evolution of a dielectric barrier discharge, *Journal of Applied Physics*, Vol. 103, pp. 033303

Manheimer, W.; Sugiyama, L.E. & Stix, T.H. (1997). *Plasma Science and the Environment*, American Institute of Physics, Woodbury, NY US

Mariotti, D & Sankaran, R.M. (2010). Microplasmas for nanomaterials synthesis, *Journal of Physics D*, Vol.43, pp.323001.1-21

Moreau, M. ; Orange, N. & Feuilloley, M.G. (2008). Non-thermal plasma technologies: new tools for biodecontamination, *Biotechnology Advances*, Vol. 26, pp. 610

Raizer, Y.P. (1991). *Gas Discharge Physics*, Springer-Verlag, Heidelberg Germany

Raffaele-Addamo, A.; Riccardi, C.; Selli, E.; Barni, R.; Piselli, M.; Poletti, G.; Orsini, F.; Marcandalli, B.; Massafra, M.R. & Meda, L. (2003). *Surf. & Coatings Techn*, Vol. 174-5, pp. 886

Riccardi, C.; Barni, R.; De Colle, F. & Fontanesi, M.(2000). *IEEE Trans. on Plasma Science*, Vol. 28, pp. 278

Riccardi, C.; Barni, R. & Fontanesi, M. (2001). *Journal of Applied. Physics*, Vol. 90, pp. 3735

Shoyama, T. & Yoshioka, Y. (2007). Theoretical study of methods for improving the energy efficiency of NOx removal from diesel exhaust gases by silent discharge, *Electrical Engineering in Japan*, Vol. 161, pp. 1-9

Siliprandi, R.A.; Roman, H.E.; Barni, R. & Riccardi, C. (2008). Characterization of the streamer regime in dielectric barrier discharges, *Journal of Applied Physics*, Vol. 104, pp. 063309.1-9

Srinivasan, A.D. & Rajanikanth, B.S. (2007). *IEEE Transactions on Industrial Applications*, Vol. 43, pp. 1507

11

Plasma-Chemical Kinetics of Film Deposition in Argon-Methane and Argon-Acetylene Mixtures Under Atmospheric Pressure Conditions

Ramasamy Pothiraja, Nikita Bibinov and Peter Awakowicz
Institute for Electrical Engineering and Plasma Technology,
Ruhr-University Bochum,
Germany

1. Introduction

Understanding chemical kinetics of precursor dissociation and other follow-up plasma chemical reactions at atmospheric pressure plasma conditions is very important area of research for the development of plasma based film coating processes. It is very useful especially for coating on complex geometries like tubes, bottles, etc. Coating thin films on inner surface of tubes improves their functionality in many ways without changing the bulk properties. It improves the value of commercial tubes by improving their surface properties such as hydrophilicity, corrosion or permeation resistance and biocompatibility as in the following cases, 1. Depositing the fluorinated carbon on PVC tubes enhances the biocompatibility for the blood circulating tubes (Babukutty et al., 1999; Prat et al., 2000), 2. Silica coating on PTFE tube increases the wettability of the tube about 3 times (Yoshiki et al., 2006), 3. Carbon or titanium nitride film as protective coating on inner surface of a metallic tube improves its lifetime (Fujiyama, 2000; Hytry et al., 1994; Wang et al., 2008), 4. Deposition of silica on inner surface of PET tubes or bottles reduces the permeation of gases (Deilmann et al., 2008, 2009), 5. Titania coating on inner surface of glass tube improves its surface properties to be suitable for microfluidic devices (Yoshiki & Mitsui, 2008; Yoshiki & Saito, 2008), 6. Coating of nickel/alumina film on inner surface of silica tube and plasma treatment of resultant film increases the catalytic activity of this film for carbon nanofiber synthesis (Agiral et al., 2009). There are many ways film can be coated on various objects. Among those, "cold" plasma based film coating methods have many advantages compared to the conventional thermal film coating methods and spray coating methods. In plasma coating methods, electron will have high temperature (a few eV); however, atomic and molecular species will have low temperature (<0.1 eV). Because of this, precursors can be dissociated at relatively low gas temperature through electron impact. Hence, the plasma technology can be used for film coating on thermo-labile plastic materials. The advantage of using atmospheric pressure plasma source for film deposition is that it does not require vacuum system and hence it is economically favourable method of film coating. Especially for thin film deposition on inner surfaces of tubes, atmospheric pressure plasma is more suitable than low pressure plasma. In this regard, several research groups have developed this process and coated various films like SiO_2 and TiO_2 on inner surface of various metal, quartz, PET and PTFE tubes (Agiral et al., 2009; Babukutty et al., 1999; Deilmann et al., 2008,

2009; Foest et al., 2007; Fujiyama, 2000; Hytry et al., 1993, 1994; Prat et al., 2000; Wang et al., 2008; Yoshiki et al., 2006; Yoshiki & Mitsui, 2008; Yoshiki & Saito, 2008). Mostly microwave or RF driven ICP, CCP and jet based microplasma or magnetron plasma sources were used for their studies. Generally, in several methods used for coating films on inner surface of tubes, precursors are decomposed in the confined electrode region where the plasma is active, chemically active species are transported inside a tube and film coating is carried out by gas flow. In this case, because of polymerization and recombination reactions during the transport process, the nature of chemically active species (constituent of polymer film) is different at different places along the axis of the tube. This phenomenon could reduce the film uniformity along the axis of the tube. Our strategy for film coating on inner surface of tubes is to generate long plasma filaments inside the tube in a gas containing a precursor as an admixture (Pothiraja et al., 2010). The plasma filament, which will be thinner than the diameter of the tube to be coated, will be active for long distance in the region of film coating. This plasma filament can ionize and/or dissociate precursor molecules. Using this method, chemically active species can be generated everywhere along the axis of the tube within close vicinity of inner surface of the tube. In this way, differences in the nature of depositing chemically active species at different places along the axis of the tube can be reduced and films with better uniformity can be deposited. In addition to this, film deposition is supported by ion fluxes, which results the formation of high quality film.

In this regard, pulsed filamentary plasma source has been constructed, and long plasma filaments (longer than 100 mm) are generated inside the tube in the presence of methane or acetylene as a precursor. Using this, carbon based film is coated on inner surface of tubes and deposited film has been characterized using various surface analysis techniques. Understanding film properties on the basis of chemical kinetics of precursor dissociation, other gas phase and inter-phase reactions is very important. Hence chemical kinetics of these reactions is simulated. Since plasma parameters (electron density, electron velocity distribution function (EVDF)) play very important role in these reactions, they have been determined using emission spectroscopy, current-voltage measurement, microphotography and numerical simulation. In this chapter, we describe 1. Reaction schemes considered in our model for the determination of plasma parameters, 2. Influence of plasma parameters on chemical kinetics of precursor dissociation and other gas phase reactions involved in the film growth processes, and 3. Effect of plasma chemical reaction kinetics and nature of precursor on film properties and film growth rates.

2. Experiments and model

Configuration of plasma source used for film coating on inner surface of tubes is discussed below. Following this, methodology used for the determination of plasma parameters, rate constants and high probable plasma chemical reactions are discussed.

2.1 Experimental setup

Our plasma source consists of a cylindrical tungsten driven electrode with a diameter of 1.6 mm. One end of this electrode is sharpened (spike) to a cone angle of 30°, while the other end of the electrode is connected to a high voltage generator (Redline Technologies G2000). The output voltage and the pulse frequency of this generator can be controlled and varied from 0-20 kV and from 4-500 kHz, respectively. Each high voltage pulse exhibits a sequential profile with damped oscillations. A tube made of quartz with the inner diameter of 6 mm, is used in order to test the feasibility of film deposition as well as to characterize the plasma ignited in this setup. Tungsten driven electrode is placed coaxially inside this tube (figure 1). A copper tube (length, 10 mm) is used as a movable grounded electrode, which is placed coaxially on the outer surface of the quartz tube. For all the experiments reported in this chapter, the grounded electrode is fixed at 140 mm away from the spike of the driven electrode.

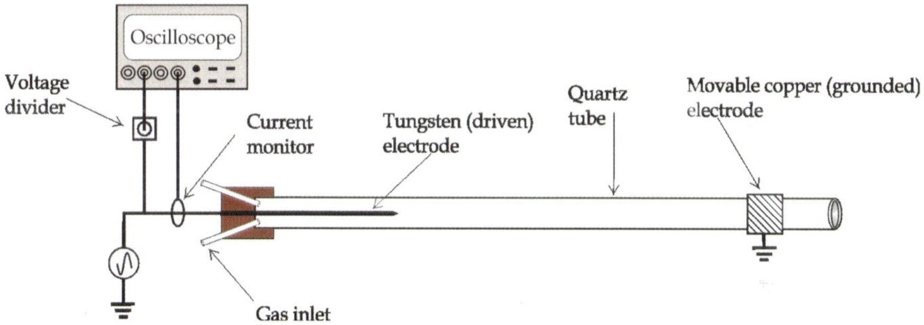

Fig. 1. Schematic view of experimental setup

We have used methane as well as acetylene as precursors. In both cases, we performed two sets of experiments. First set of experiments were carried out in argon and precursor mixture (Ar, 2400 sccm; CH_4, 3 sccm or C_2H_2, 2 sccm) to deposit carbon based film on inner surface of a quartz tube. Films deposited at this condition are characterized using various surface analysis techniques. Second set of experiments were carried out with argon, precursor and nitrogen gas mixture (Ar, 2400 sccm; CH_4 (or C_2H_2), 1 sccm; N_2, 2.5 sccm) for plasma characterization. Emissions of nitrogen molecules and nitrogen molecular ions are used for the determination of plasma parameters. Plasma parameters determined at this condition are considered to be the same as the plasma parameters during the film deposition process in the first set of experiments. The effect of absence of nitrogen on plasma parameters is balanced by increasing the precursor quantity. This fact (balancing of plasma parameters) is confirmed from the similar simulated EVDFs for both sets of experiments (with/without nitrogen). It is also confirmed by measuring argon emission spectra at various places along the axis of the tube in both cases. Argon emission intensities are very close to each other in both cases, and also have the similar trend along the axis of the tube.

Relatively and absolutely calibrated echelle spectrometer (ESA 3000) is used to obtain the emission spectra in a spectral range of 200 to 800 nm (Bibinov et al., 2007). Spectral resolution of the echelle spectrometer amounts to $\Delta\lambda$ = 0.015 nm at λ = 200 nm and $\Delta\lambda$ = 0.060 nm at λ = 800 nm. A Pearson current monitor (model, 6585; output, 1 V = 1 A) is used for plasma current measurement, which is mounted around a cable connecting the generator and the tungsten electrode. The output of the current monitor is connected to an oscilloscope (LeCroy *Wave Runner* 204MXi-A). Discharge duration is determined from the current profile. The actual voltage applied for plasma generation is measured by connecting the output of the generator to the oscilloscope through a capacitive voltage divider with the dividing factor of 2000. The pulse frequency of applied voltage is fixed as 22 kHz for all the experiments. For the plasma volume determination, a high speed sensitive CCD camera (PCO sensicam qe) is used. The spatial resolution of CCD camera amounts to 2 μm for an objective used with this camera.

2.2 Model

For diagnostics purposes, nitrogen is admixed with argon and precursor mixture. Plasma parameters are determined from the emission of neutral nitrogen molecules and molecular nitrogen ions. Our model used to obtain the information about gas temperature, plasma parameters and rate constants, from these emissions, are discussed below.

2.2.1 Plasma gas temperature

Gas temperature in active plasma volume is one of the important parameters, because of its influence on gas density in plasma as well as on the rate constants of chemical reactions. The rotational temperature of diatomic molecules is considered as the gas temperature, since the rotational and the translational degrees of freedom have equal temperatures because of very fast rotational relaxation at atmospheric pressure. For the determination of gas temperature, the rotational intensity distribution in the emission of neutral nitrogen molecule $N_2(C^3\Pi_u, v'=0 \rightarrow B^3\Pi_g, v''=0)$ (abbreviated as N_2(C–B, 0–0)) is used. The emission spectrum is measured perpendicular to the axis of the filament. Since the spectral resolution of our echelle spectrometer is not high enough to determine the intensities of the separate rotational lines in the emission spectrum of neutral nitrogen molecules, the rotational temperature is determined by a fitting procedure. For this purpose, we calculate the intensity distribution in the emission of N_2(C–B, 0–0) (λ = 337.1 nm) for different values of rotational temperature and spectral resolution used in the experiments, applying the program code developed for this purpose (Bibinov et al., 2001). By comparing the measured emission spectrum with the calculated spectra for various rotational temperatures, we determine the actual rotational temperature of nitrogen molecule with an inaccuracy of ±30 K.

When high concentration of the precursor is used, there is an overlap in the emission of N_2(C–B, 0–0) with the emission of NH radical at some places along the axis of the tube (filament). Hence, in this case, the rotational intensity distribution in the emission of CN radical, $CN(B^2\Sigma^+, v'=0 \rightarrow X^2\Sigma^+, v''=0)$ (CN(B–X, 0–0)) is used for the determination of gas temperature. In this case also, the rotational temperature is determined by the fitting procedure. In this regard, we simulate the intensity distribution in the emission of CN(B–X, 0–0) (λ = 388.3 nm) for different values of rotational temperature using the program LIFBASE (Luque & Crosley, 1999). The rotational temperature of CN radical is determined with an inaccuracy of ±30 K.

Under our experimental condition, molecular emissions N_2(C-B) and CN(B-X) are excited by electron impact as well as by collisions with argon metastable atoms (Nguyen & Sadeghi, 1983; Belikov et al., 1988). This effect can influence the rotational spectrum of nitrogen, and has been considered in the model. The angular momentum of heavy nucleus of diatomic molecules changes slightly by electron impact excitation. Therefore rotational distribution in molecular state excited by electron impact is equal to that in ground state, that means corresponds to the gas temperature. By excitation due to argon metastables, the rotational distributions in the excited states N_2(C) and CN(B) can be very different from rotational distributions at gas temperature. It can be approximately described by equilibrium distribution with temperature of about 2000K (Nguyen & Sadeghi, 1983; Belikov et al., 1988). Rotational distribution in measured emission spectrum is formed by initially excited distribution and competition of spontaneous emission, rotational relaxation and quenching process by collisions with surrounding argon atoms. To study the influence of this factor on the reliability of measured gas temperature, we simulate the emission spectrum of N_2(C-B) for our experimental conditions with assumption that all "second positive system" in nitrogen emission spectrum is excited by collisions with argon metastables. To simulate the rotational relaxation, we use the rate constants determined in theoretical and experimental studies of rotational relaxation of nitrogen molecules in ground state by collisions with surrounding argon atoms (Belikov et al., 1988). The measured rotational distribution in N_2(C) excited during collisions with argon metastables (Nguyen & Sadeghi, 1983), and rate constant for quenching of N_2(C-B) emission in argon (Polak-Dingels & Djeu, 1983) are used for this simulation. After simulation of N_2(C-B) emission spectrum, we determine the rotational temperature using Boltzmann plot and estimate the deviation of determined value from the gas temperature assumed for our simulation. For our experimental conditions, this difference amounts to about 1% (e.g. 8 K at gas temperature of 800 K), which is much lower than the inaccuracy of ± 30 K of our fitting procedure.

The CN molecules are produced in $Ar/N_2/C_2H_2$ or $Ar/N_2/CH_4$ mixture through a multi-step reaction. The exact mechanism of formation and the rotational distribution of CN(B) state is not known in the literature. Therefore the rotational relaxation could not be simulated. However, because of the equal rotational temperatures of emission of N_2(C-B) and CN(B-X) determined at the same experimental conditions (see figure 2) and very fast relaxation of CN(B) in argon observed at low pressure conditions (Duewer et al., 1972), we conclude that CN(B)-molecule reach equilibrium rotational distribution before emitting of the photons. Hence, the influence of high rotational distribution after CN formation as well as excitation by collisions with argon metastables on the gas temperature determination by using CN molecular emission is also negligible.

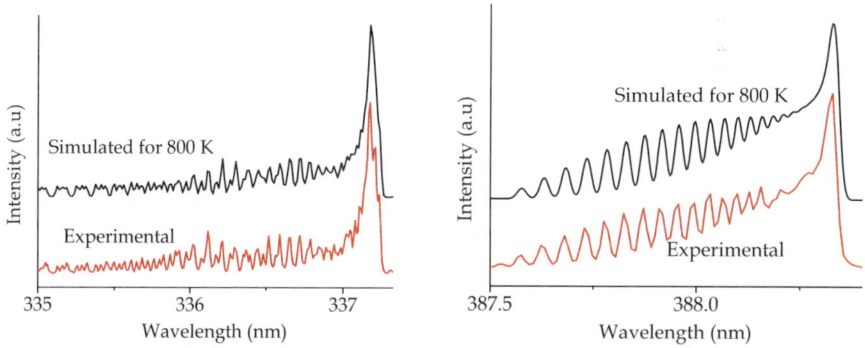

Fig. 2. Comparison of gas temperature determined by using the emission of N_2(C–B, 0–0) (left) and the emission of CN(B–X, 0–0) (right) from the same emission spectrum measured during the discharge. Simulated spectra are shifted for clarity.

2.2.2 Electron velocity distribution functions and rate constants

Electrons are the origin of most of the chemical reactions happening at atmospheric pressure plasma based processes; hence, their energy distribution plays an important role in plasma chemical reactions. The electron velocity distribution function (EVDF) in our system is determined on the basis of the emission of nitrogen molecule (equations 1-13). For this purpose, absolute emission intensities of $N_2(C^3\Pi_u, v'=0 \rightarrow B^3\Pi_g, v''=0)$ (abbreviated as $I_{N_2(C\text{-}B)}$) and $N_2^+(B^2\Sigma_u^+, v'=0 \rightarrow X^2\Sigma_g^+, v''=0)$ ($I_{N_2^+(B-X)}$) are used. Since the threshold energy for the excitation of $N_2(X)$ to $N_2^+(B)$ by electron impact is different from the same for $N_2(X)$ to $N_2(C)$, the relative intensity of $I_{N_2^+(B-X)}$ with respect to the intensity of $I_{N_2(C-B)}$ is depending on the EVDF. On this basis, EVDF is determined using measured $I_{N_2^+(B-X)}$ / $I_{N_2(C-B)}$. For this purpose, we considered the following plasma chemical reactions (equations 1-9) for the determination of intensity of nitrogen emission (equations 10, 11).

$$N_2 + e \xrightarrow{k_{N_2^+(B)}} N_2^+ (B) + 2e \tag{1}$$

$$N_2 + e \xrightarrow{k_{N_2(C)}} N_2 (C) + e \tag{2}$$

$$N_2 + Ar_{met} \xrightarrow{k_{N_2(C)}^{Ar_{met}}} N_2 (C) + Ar \tag{3}$$

$$\longrightarrow N_2 (B) + Ar \tag{4}$$

$$Ar + e \xrightarrow{k_{Ar_{met}}} Ar_{met} + e \tag{5}$$

$$Ar_{met} + e \xrightarrow{k_{qAr_{met}}^{e}} \text{Products} \tag{6}$$

$$Ar_{met} + 2Ar \xrightarrow{k_{qAr_{met}}^{2Ar}} \text{Products} \tag{7}$$

$$Ar_{met} + N_2 \xrightarrow{k_{qAr_{met}}^{N_2}} \text{Products} \tag{8}$$

$$Ar_{met} + Prec \xrightarrow{k_{qAr_{met}}^{Prec}} \text{Products} \tag{9}$$

$$I_{N_2(C-B)} = (k_{N_2(C)} + K_{N_2(C)}^{Ar_{met}}) \cdot n_e \cdot [N_2] \cdot Q_{N_2(C)} \cdot g_f \cdot V_p \cdot t_f \tag{10}$$

$$\frac{I_{N_2^+(B-X)}}{I_{N_2(C-B)}} = \frac{Q_{N_2^+(B)}}{Q_{N_2(C)}} \cdot \frac{k_{N_2^+(B)}}{k_{N_2(C)} + K_{N_2(C)}^{Ar_{met}}} \tag{11}$$

where,

$$Q = \frac{A}{A + k_{qN_2}^{Ar} \cdot [Ar]} \tag{12}$$

$$K_{N_2(C)}^{Ar_{met}} = \frac{[Ar] \cdot k_{N_2(C)}^{Ar_{met}} \cdot k_{Ar_{met}} \cdot (B1) \cdot (B2)}{n_e \cdot k_{qAr_{met}}^{e} + [Ar]^2 \cdot k_{qAr_{met}}^{2Ar} + [N_2] \cdot k_{qAr_{met}}^{N_2} + [Prec] \cdot k_{qAr_{met}}^{Prec}} \tag{13}$$

$k_{N_2^+(B)}$ and $k_{N_2(C)}$ - electron impact excitation rate constants of nitrogen molecular emission, N_2^+(B-X) and N_2(C-B) respectively;
$k_{N_2(C)}^{Ar_{met}}$ - rate constant for the formation of N_2(C) by collision of N_2(X) with argon metastable (2.80x10^{-11} cm^3·s^{-1}) (Polak-Dingels & Djeu, 1983);
$k_{Ar_{met}}$ - electron impact excitation rate constant for argon metastable formation;
$k_{qN_2}^{Ar}$ - rate constant for the quenching of the corresponding excited states of nitrogen during collision with argon (for N_2(C) 8.00x10^{-13} cm^3·s^{-1} (Polak-Dingels & Djeu, 1983); for N_2^+(B) 2.00x10^{-10} cm^3·s^{-1} (Tellinghuisen et al., 1972));
$k_{qAr_{met}}^{e}$ (2.00x10^{-7} cm^3·s^{-1} (Ivanov & Makasyuk, 1990)), $k_{qAr_{met}}^{2Ar}$ (1.20x10^{-32} cm^6·s^{-1} (Kolts & Setser, 1978)), $k_{qAr_{met}}^{N_2}$ (3.50x10^{-11} cm^3·s^{-1} (Kolts et al., 1977)) and $k_{qAr_{met}}^{Prec}$ (5.50x10^{-10} cm^3·s^{-1} and 5.60x10^{-10} cm^3·s^{-1} (Velazco et al., 1978)) - rate constants for quenching of argon metastable during collision with electron, argon, nitrogen and precursors (methane and acetylene), respectively;
A - Einstein coefficient for spontaneous emission (2.38x10^7 s^{-1} for N_2(C-B) (Pancheshnyi et al., 2000); 1.52x10^7 s^{-1} for N_2^+(B-X) (Dilecce et al., 2010));
B1 - branching factor for (3) (value = 0.787) (Zhiglinski, 1994);
B2 - branching factor for N_2(C-B, 0-0) transition by emission from N_2(C,0) (value = 0.5) (Laux & Kruger, 1992);
n_e - electron density (cm^{-3});
$[Ar]$ - density of argon (cm^{-3});
$[N_2]$ - density of nitrogen (cm^{-3});
$[Prec]$ - density of methane or acetylene (cm^{-3});
V_p – observed volume of plasma (cm^3);
g_f - geometrical factor relating the part of photons reaching the entrance hole of the optical fiber in the spectrometer;
t_f - value of fraction of time, in which plasma is active.

The equations (10-13) are derived on the basis that the population of N_2^+(B) from the ground state ion N_2^+(X) is negligible compared to the one from N_2(X). This is because the concentration of N_2^+(X) is negligible compared to the concentration of N_2(X) in the cases we studied. For the generation of N_2(C), only direct electron impact excitation from the ground state of nitrogen molecule N_2(X) and the excitation during collision with argon metastable are considered (Kolts et al., 1977; Sadeghi et al., 1981, 1989; Touzeau & Pagnon, 1978). Other possible mechanism of generation of N_2(C) by 'pooling' reactions of two metastables N_2(A) (Herron, 1999) is negligible because of relatively low density of metastables N_2(A). Quenching of N_2(C) and N_2^+(B) by argon is considered (Polak-Dingels & Djeu, 1983; Tellinghuisen et al., 1972; Touzeau & Pagnon, 1978). However, quenching of N_2(C) and N_2^+(B) by nitrogen and precursor is neglected because of low concentration of these admixtures (Legrand et al., 2001).

For the calculation of rate constants $k_{N_2^+(B)}$ and $k_{N_2(C)}$ for a particular EVDF under our experimental conditions, the following methodology is used.

The EVDF is simulated for our experimental conditions (gas composition, gas temperature, pressure, etc.) by numerical solution of the Boltzmann equation and varied electric field applying the program code "EEDF" developed by Napartovich et al (Stefanovic et al., 2001). In this simulation, "local" approximation is applied, which is valid for atmospheric pressure. This EVDF is normalized to fulfill the equation (14):

$$4\pi\sqrt{2}\int_0^\infty f_v(E)\cdot\sqrt{E}\mathrm{d}E = 1 \tag{14}$$

By using this normalized EVDF and the known collisional cross section σ_{exc} (cm^2) for electron impact excitation of nitrogen emission (Itikawa, 2006), we calculate the rate constants k ($cm^3 \cdot s^{-1}$) for electron impact excitation of N_2(C-B, 0-0) and N_2^+(B-X, 0-0) emissions by using the equation (15):

$$k = 4\pi\sqrt{2}\int_0^\infty f_v(E)\cdot\sqrt{\frac{2C}{m_e}}\cdot E\cdot\sigma_{exc}(E)\mathrm{d}E, \tag{15}$$

where m_e is the mass of electron (g), E is the kinetic energy of electrons (eV) and $C = 1.602 \times 10^{-12}$ erg·eV^{-1}.

From these calculated rate constants and the quenching factors (Q in equation 12), values of ratio of intensities of nitrogen emissions (using equation 11) are calculated for various EVDFs. By comparing the calculated values of ratio of emission intensities with measured one, the actual EVDF and its corresponding reduced electric field are determined.

2.2.3 Electron density

Electron density (n_e in cm^{-3}) is determined by using the equation (16), from the measured absolute intensity of N_2(C-B, 0-0) emission ($I_{N_2(C\text{-}B)}$, phot·s^{-1}), the electron impact excitation rate constant for N_2(C-B, 0-0) emission ($k_{N_2(C)}$), contribution of argon metastable for the formation of N_2(C) ($K_{N_2(C)}^{Ar_{met}}$), density of nitrogen ([N_2]), contribution of the quenching of N_2(C) by Ar ($Q_{N_2(C)}$), the geometrical factor for the fraction of photons produced in plasma volume reaching the optical fiber (g_f), the plasma volume (V_p in cm^3), and value of fraction of time in which plasma is active (t_f).

$$n_e = \frac{I_{N_2(C-B)}}{(k_{N_2(C)} + K_{N_2(C)}^{Ar_{met}})\cdot[N_2]\cdot Q_{N_2(C)}\cdot g_f\cdot V_p\cdot t_f} \tag{16}$$

All measurements with our emission spectrometer are space and time averaged. However, plasma parameters during the discharge are spatially and temporally non-uniform (Veldhuizen et al., 2009). In order to find out the influence of this non-uniformity of the plasma parameters on the reliability of measurements obtained using our spectrometer, we have simulated the total emission spectrum of two plasma regions of equal volume observed simultaneously by our spectrometer. Very different plasma conditions are assumed for these two regions. The composition of gas mixture corresponding to the methane system is used for the simulations. By using the total emission spectrum of nitrogen simulated for these two regions with different plasma parameters, the average plasma parameters are calculated for our optical emission spectroscopic (OES) diagnostics.

By using these averaged plasma parameters, the rate of methane dissociation is calculated. This value is compared with the value of the rate of methane dissociation calculated for these two regions.

For this purpose, the reduced electric field of 300 Td is assumed for the first region while 3000 Td for the second region. Electron density values are assumed as 4.62 $\times 10^{11}$ and 5.00 $\times 10^{11}$ (in cm^{-3}) for the first and the second regions, respectively. In these plasma conditions, the intensity of N_2(C-B, 0-0), which is used for electron density determination, is equal in both regions. On this basis, we have calculated total intensities of emission of nitrogen for the combination of these two regions, in the way our spectrometer would have observed. From these calculated values of intensities, the averaged values of electric field and electron density are calculated as 1800 Td and 3.91 $\times 10^{11}$ cm^{-3}, respectively. The ultimate aim for determination of the plasma parameters is to obtain the dissociation rate of precursor molecule. Hence, by using these averaged values of electron density and the reduced electric field, the rate of methane dissociation is calculated for this combined region. In a similar way, the dissociation rate of methane is calculated for these two regions separately on the basis of the emission spectra simulated for a spatially resolved measurement. The sum of these two values obtained for the spatially resolved measurement, is compared with the value of methane dissociation rate for the combined region calculated using the averaged plasma parameters for the spatially averaged measurement. In this case, there is less than 4% deviation in the rate of methane dissociation in using averaged plasma parameters.

We did similar calculation by assuming very different electron density values for these two regions, as 7.96 $\times 10^{13}$ cm^{-3} and 5.00 $\times 10^{11}$ cm^{-3} for the first (E/N, 300 Td) and the second (E/N, 3000 Td) regions, respectively. For these values of electron density and the electric field, the intensity of N_2^+(B-X, 0-0) for these two regions is equal. In this case, there is 8% deviation in the value of rate of methane dissociation by using spatially averaged plasma parameters.

The low time resolution in OES diagnostics causes an error in electron density determination because of the error in the time factor. The inverse of the same time factor is used for determination of the rate of hydrocarbon dissociation from electron density. Hence, the error in the time factor during electron density determination will be canceled during determination of the rate of methane dissociation. Hence, despite the possible deviation of the averaged plasma parameters determined using our OES diagnostics, from the real spatial and temporal distribution of plasma parameters (EVDF and electron density), the dissociation rate of hydrocarbon molecules obtained using the averaged plasma parameters is reliable.

2.2.4 Temporal and spatial distribution of gas temperature as well as fluxes of chemically active species

In order to determine the temporal and spatial distribution of gas temperature as well as fluxes of chemically active species from the plasma filament towards the surface of the tube, we numerically solve the equations for thermal conductivity (17) and diffusion (18) for a cylindrical symmetry (Bibinov et al., 2007; Rajasekaran et al., 2009):

$$\frac{\partial T}{\partial t} = \nabla \cdot (\alpha(T) \nabla T) \tag{17}$$

$$\frac{\partial [M]}{\partial t} = \nabla \cdot (D(T) \nabla [M]) \tag{18}$$

where,

$$\alpha(T) = \frac{\lambda_{conduction}}{\rho \cdot C_p},$$

$\alpha(T)$ - thermal diffusivity,
$\lambda_{conduction}$- thermal conductivity,
ρ - density,
C_p - specific heat capacity,
D - diffusion coefficient.

3. Results and discussion

3.1 Plasma ignition and film deposition

The pulsed filamentary discharge is ignited (Pothiraja et al., 2010, 2011) in the mixture of argon and methane or acetylene precursor (figure 3). This discharge is similar to a positive streamer discharge in argon (Veldhuizen et al., 2002). This long filament of plasma generated along the axis of the tube during this discharge has a diameter of about 200 μm.

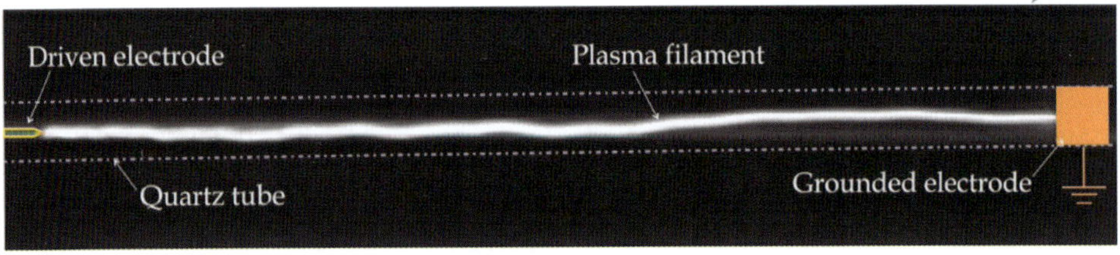

Fig. 3. Plasma filament ignited inside the tube in argon with precursor admixture.

The duration of the positive discharge is 160 ns (figure 4). During plasma operation, the profile and the position of filaments in the tube change with the frequency of several Hz. Because of this fact (profile and position of filaments are stationary for about 100 ms) and the pulse frequency is 22 kHz, about 2000 filaments in series have the same profile and position.

Emission spectra measured using echelle spectrometer for the discharge ignited in Ar/C_2H_2 as well as in Ar/CH_4 mixtures at different regions along the axis of tube indicates similar pattern. Measured spectra show characteristic emissions for the active species like C, C_2, CH, etc.; which indicates the dissociation of precursors, and participation of hydrocarbon radicals in film deposition (figure 5).

Films deposited at this condition are characterized using various surface analysis techniques. FTIR-ATR, XRD, SEM, LSM, Raman spectral and XPS analyses give the conclusion that when methane is used as a precursor, deposited film is amorphous

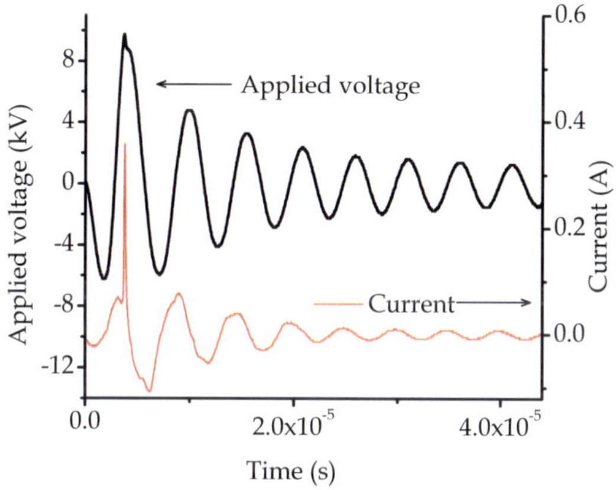

Fig. 4. Current-voltage profile during the positive filamentary discharge inside the tube

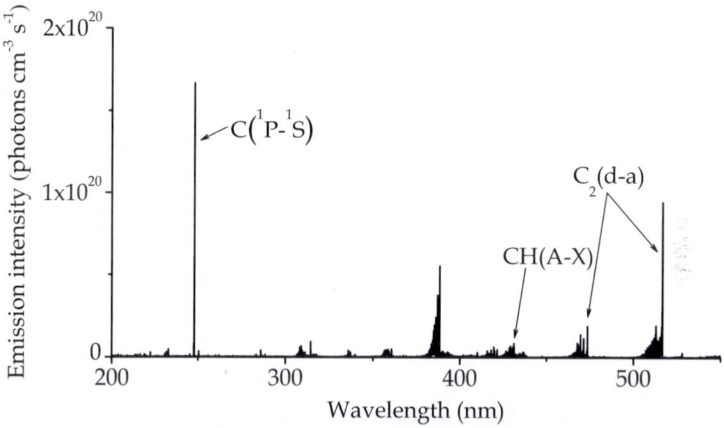

Fig. 5. Emission spectrum measured using echelle spectrometer for the discharge ignited in Ar/CH_4 mixture at the middle region in between the electrodes. Discharge in Ar/C_2H_2 mixture also shows similar emission spectrum

composed of non-hydrogenated sp^2 carbon and hydrogenated sp^3 carbon with traces of O and N (see figure 6, 7) (Murugavel & Pothiraja, 2003; Murugavel et al., 2007). UV-Vis absorption spectra of the film deposited on inner surface of the tube also confirm the presence of doubly bonded sp^2 carbon, which are shortly conjugated. When acetylene is used as a precursor, deposited film contains sp^1 carbon in addition to sp^2 and sp^3 hybridized carbon. Presence of sp^1 carbon in the film reduces the hardness of film, because of its linear structure which cannot form two dimensional or three dimensional structural networks. However, when acetylene is used as precursor, thickness of the film deposited on inner surface of the tubes, between the electrodes is more uniform than the same when methane is used as a precursor (figure 8).

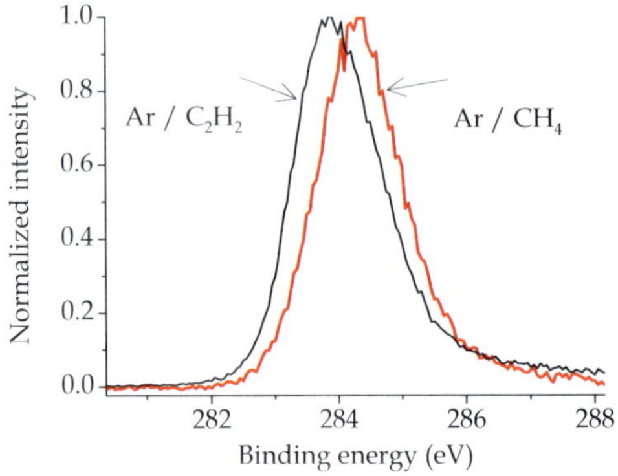

Fig. 6. XPS of carbon of the films deposited in filamentary discharges in Ar/C_2H_2 and Ar/CH_4 mixtures at middle region in between electrodes.

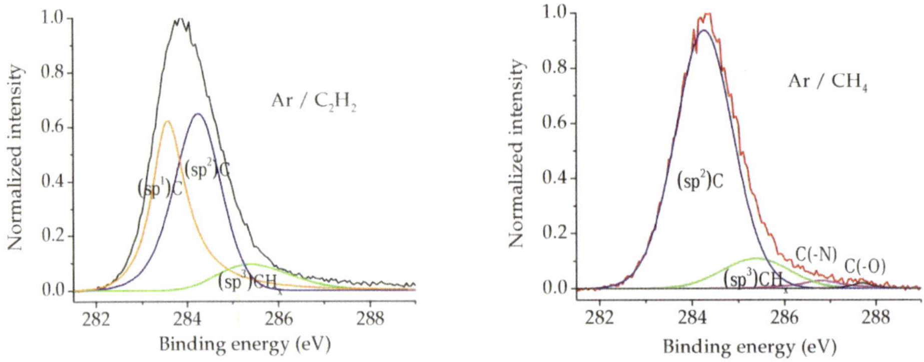

Fig. 7. XPS of carbon of the films deposited in filamentary discharge in Ar/C_2H_2 (left) and Ar/CH_4 (right) mixtures.

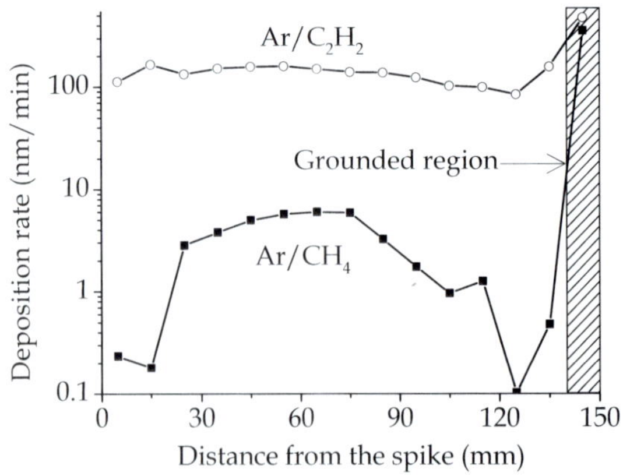

Fig. 8. Deposition rate of carbon based film inside of quartz tube by filamentary discharge in Ar/C_2H_2 and Ar/CH_4 mixtures.

Cross sectional images of the film deposited on quartz tube are obtained using LSM and SEM. From these images, film thickness is determined at 65 mm away from the spike (Pothiraja et al., 2009a, 2009b). By keeping this as reference, film thickness at various places along the axis of the tube is determined by measuring optical thickness of the film at these places on the basis of Beer-Lambert law in UV spectral range. The figure 8 shows growth rate at various places along the axis of the tube for the films deposited in Ar/C_2H_2 and Ar/CH_4 mixtures. For these experiments, similar quantities of methane as well as acetylene are used as precursor. As the figure 8 indicates, film growth rate in the grounded region is similar in both cases, and it is higher compared to the growth rate between the electrodes. When acetylene is used as a precursor, film growth rate between electrodes is about 30 times higher than the case where methane is used as precursor. It clearly indicates that plasma chemical reactions responsible for film growth process between the electrodes are different in these two cases. However, both precursor systems show similar film growth rates in the grounded region, and it is much higher than the film growth rate between the electrodes. This difference is very dominant methane system.

In order to understand these differences in the nature of the film, growth rate and thickness profile, we characterize plasma conditions (gas temperature in plasma filament, electron density, EVDF, etc.) in both cases. Using determined plasma parameters, we calculate production rates of atoms and excited molecules, simulated fluxes of excited chemical species to the inner surface of the tube, and simulated the chemical kinetics. We correlate the differences in the chemical kinetics on the differences in the film properties. OES, microphotography, current-voltage measurements and numerical simulations are used for the characterization of plasma conditions. Since the chemical kinetics depends on plasma conditions, plasma conditions and their differences between methane as well as acetylene cases are discussed first. Following this, differences in chemical kinetics will be discussed.

3.2 Gas temperature and tube temperature

The gas temperature determined in the plasma filament with both precursors at various places along the axis of the tube is shown in figure 9.

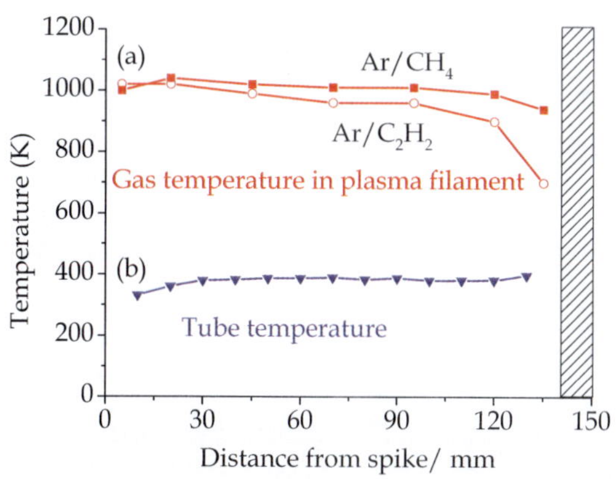

Fig. 9. Gas temperature in the plasma filament obtained using CN (B-X, 0-0) and N_2(C-B, 0-0) emissions (a), and tube temperature (b) along the axis of the tube during the pulsed filamentary discharge (Ar, 99.85%; N_2, 0.11%; CH_4 or C_2H_4, 0.04%; total gas flow rate, 2400 sccm)

The gas temperature in the plasma filament is about 1000 K. Although it is high (figure 9), duration of the discharge pulses is short: 160 ns (pulse frequency, 22 kHz). Therefore, the actual (stationary) temperature of tube will be much lower than the gas temperature in the plasma filament. The actual temperature of the tube during the discharge is measured using a thermocouple. It shows that tube temperature is less (about 330 K) close to the spike and it reaches about 400 K close to the grounded electrode (figure 9). Gas flow could be one of the reasons for this trend in tube temperature, since the gas mixture at room temperature is entering the spike region and relatively hot (or warm) gas mixture is entering the region close to the grounded electrode. With these data, equation for thermal conductivity is numerically solved to simulate the gas temperature in afterglow phase with temporal and spatial resolution. The results of this simulation presented in figure 10 show that the steady state conditions in the tube will be reached after 500 pulses. It is to be noted that, as mentioned before, about 2000 filaments in series have the same profile and position.

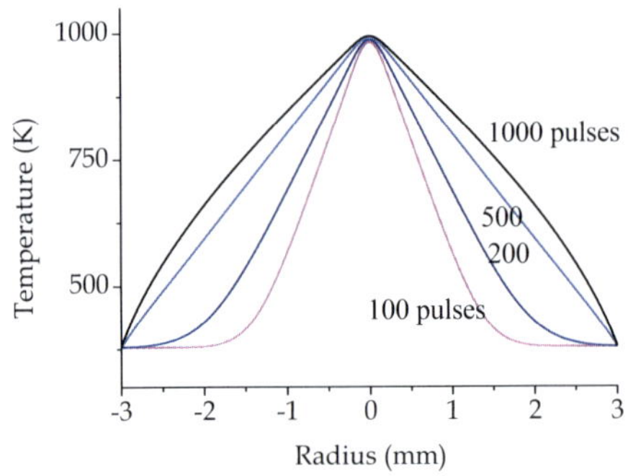

Fig. 10. Spatial distribution (in the radial direction) of the gas temperature from the plasma filament towards the surface of the tube. The filament diameter, 200 µm, is used for the simulations on the basis of micro-photographic images of the filaments

3.3 Plasma parameters

The reduced electric fields determined at different places along the axis of the tube during the discharge are shown in figure 11. It reveals that the reduced electric field has the same trend along the axis of tube, when methane is replaced with acetylene. However it reduces the magnitude of field to about 500 Td (figure 11). Reason for this trend in E/N along the axis of the tube is not clear now.

This change in E/N as methane is replaced with acetylene strongly influences the EVDF, as shown in figure 12. As a result of this, kinetics of electron impact plasma chemical reactions is not the same at different precursors as well as at different region along the axis of tubes.

As expected, difference in the reduced electric field also influences the electron density, when methane is replaced with acetylene. The electron density is almost constant in most part of the region in between the electrodes (figure 13). It is about 1.7×10^{12} cm^{-3} to 2.8×10^{12} cm^{-3}, when methane is used as precursor. However, when methane is replaced with acetylene, it is increased to about 8×10^{12} cm^{-3} to 3.8×10^{13} cm^{-3}. This increase in electron density could be due to the additional mechanism of acetylene ionization during Penning ionization with argon metastables. These electron densities are about two orders of magnitude lower than the related streamer discharge known in the literature (Aleksandrov et al., 1999, 2001). This is because; we have determined the electron densities by assuming that plasma is active continuously between electrodes for all current pulse duration. In reality, the positive streamer head of length about a few mm with the diameter of about 200 μm is moving from one electrode to other electrode with the velocity of about 10^7 cm·s^{-1}. When this factor is considered, the electron densities determined through our method is well in agreement with the value reported in the literature for similar kind of plasma streamer. However, as discussed previously, this less temporally and spatially resolved plasma parameters will not affect considerably the determined overall plasma chemical kinetics parameters.

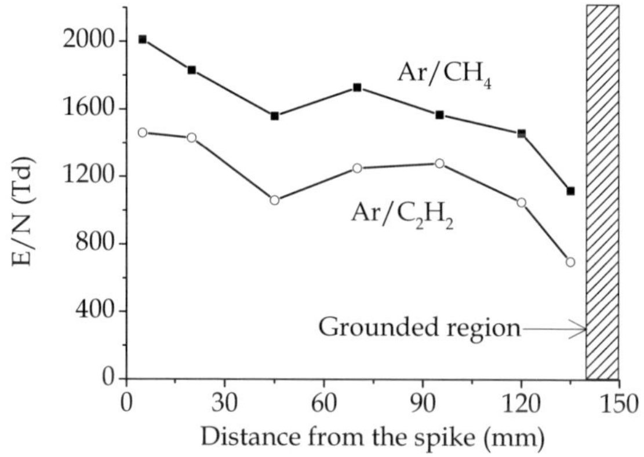

Fig. 11. Variation of the reduced electric field along the axis of the tube during the pulsed filamentary discharge

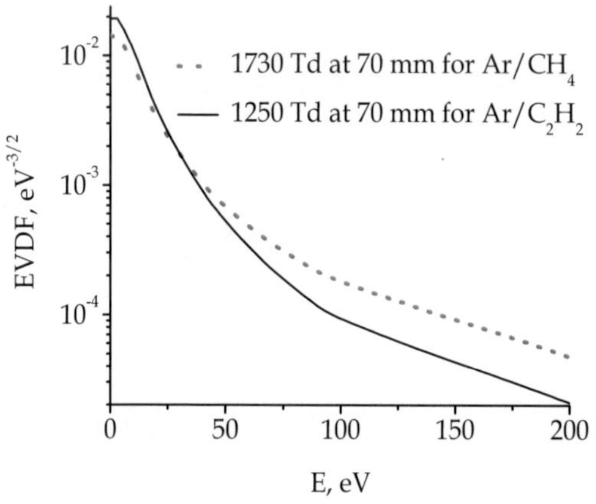

Fig. 12. The change in EVDF as methane admixture is replaced with acetylene in argon filamentary discharge.

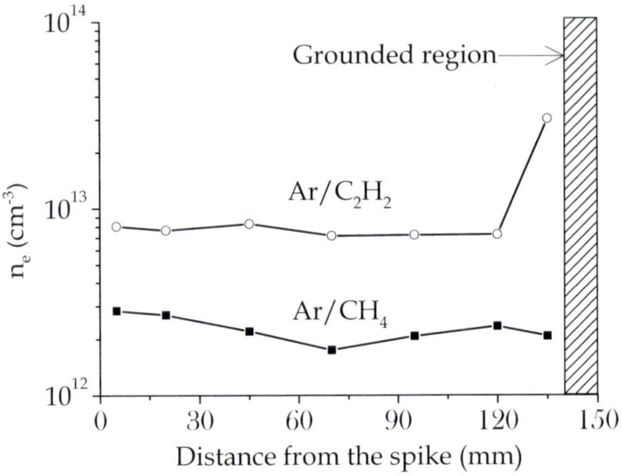

Fig. 13. Electron densities determined applying optical emission spectroscopy along the axis of tube for methane and acetylene plasma system.

3.4 Chemical kinetics

As mentioned previously, electron density and electron velocity distribution function play very important role in plasma (electron impact) chemical reactions. Therefore, the change in electron density and EVDF up on changing the precursor also changes the rate of electron impact excitation processes. The rate constants for electron impact acetylene and methane dissociation, argon ionization and argon metastables formation are determined (figure 14) using the equation (15), from the known values of cross-section for the corresponding process (Ballou et al., 1973; Belic et al., 2010; Garcıa & Manero, 1998; Khakoo et al., 2004) and the determined EVDF. Electron impact dissociation rate constant of precursor molecule is higher than the electron impact ionization rate constant of argon atom (figure 14). Despite this fact, because of the higher concentration of argon than precursor in the supplied gas mixture, electron impact argon ionization rate is much higher than the electron impact dissociation rate of precursor. Since the charge exchange reactions of argon ions with hydrocarbon molecules have big cross sections (Shul et al., 1987), mainly these reactions are

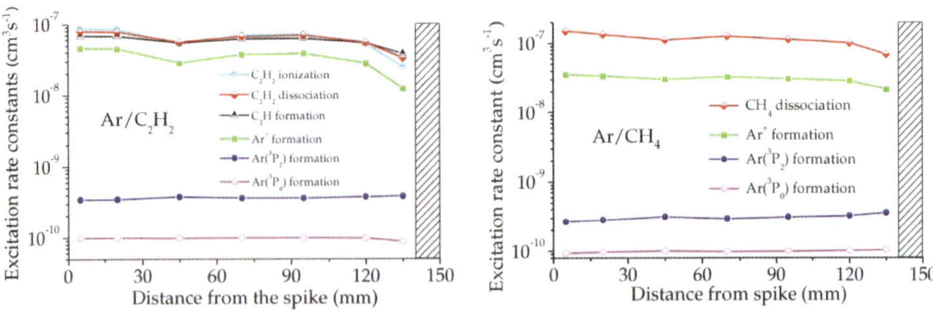

Fig. 14. Variation in the rate constants for electron impact acetylene dissociation, methane dissociation, argon ionization and argon metastables formation along the axis of the tube.

involved in the ionization and dissociative ionization of hydrocarbon species. Hence, argon ions play dominant role in the acetylene and methane ionization, dissociation and consequent film deposition processes. This is in contrast to the low pressure plasma chemical kinetics, where electron impact plays dominant role in acetylene and methane ionization, dissociation and consequent film deposition processes (Behringer, 1991; Moller, 1993; Pastol & Catherine, 1990).

Since the exact densities of various chemically active species and their diffusion coefficients are not known, methane diffusion in argon is simulated in order to have some hints about the diffusion of various chemically active species. Simulated results for methane diffusion in the figure 15 show that it takes about 10 to 20 ms for a chemically active species generated in the filament, which is approximately placed at the middle of the tube, to reach the tube surface. During this transport process, it may undergo several chemical reactions. Gas velocity is 1.4 m·s^{-1} for the gas flow rate of 2.4 slm. Hence, in the duration of 10 to 20 ms, neutral radicals will be moved to a distance of 1.5 to 3 cm along the axis of the tube.

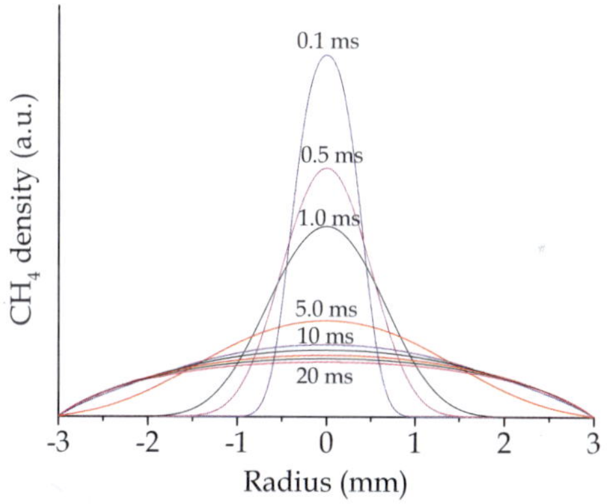

Fig. 15. Spatial distribution of chemically active species generated in the filament towards the surface of tube. Since several chemically active species are generated in the filament, CH_4 diffusion in Ar is simulated.

The next step is to find out differences in the plasma chemical reactions and their chemical kinetics between methane and acetylene cases. Since the same quantity of argon is used in both cases, a main difference on the basis of atomic composition of precursors is the following. In the case of methane, carbon and hydrogen ratio is 1:4, but it is 1:1 for acetylene. The difference in the quantity of hydrogen with respect to carbon is important for chemical kinetics. Because of small size of hydrogen atom, it has high mobility compared to all other elements in the plasma system. Second reason is that atomic hydrogen (hydrogen radical) is the most reactive part of neutral element in our plasma system. Hence a small change in the quantity of hydrogen especially with respect to carbon will have strong influence on the chemical kinetics of carbon based film growth process. The second important difference among the precursors is their reactivity. From chemical structure and bonding point of view, acetylene is more reactive than methane. This will have considerable influence on the film coating process. Acetylene is the monomer of polymer, polyacetylene. It is more prone to undergo polymerization even without plasma in the presence of catalyst. Hence under plasma conditions, it can undergo polymerization reaction leading to high film growth rate. Other difference, which may affect the hardness of deposited film, is the hybridization of carbon in the precursor. Methane has sp^3 hybridized carbon, but acetylene has sp^1 hybridized carbon. It is well known that presence of sp^1 hybridized carbon will reduce the film hardness because of its linear structure, compared to a film composed of sp^2 and sp^3 carbon based materials. Also it is reported in the literature that methane is better precursor for hard film coating compared to acetylene (Fedosenko et al., 2001). By considering all above stated facts (nature of the precursor, plasma conditions and film properties), the most probable reactions among others are calculated using the equation (19), from the known values of densities of argon, methane and electron, as well as rate constants of various processes determined from the plasma parameters and known in the literature (Alman et al., 2000; Baulch et al., 1994; Denysenko et al., 2004; Pitts et al., 1982; Shiu & Biondi, 1978; Sieck & Lias, 1976; Tsang & Hampson, 1986),

$$P = ([M] \cdot k)^{-1} \tag{19}$$

where, P is the probability, $[M]$ is the density of reactant species (cm^{-3}), and k is the rate constant ($cm^3 \cdot s^{-1}$). The possible important chemical reactions for our experimental conditions are shown in the following scheme (figure 16 and 17). The high probable

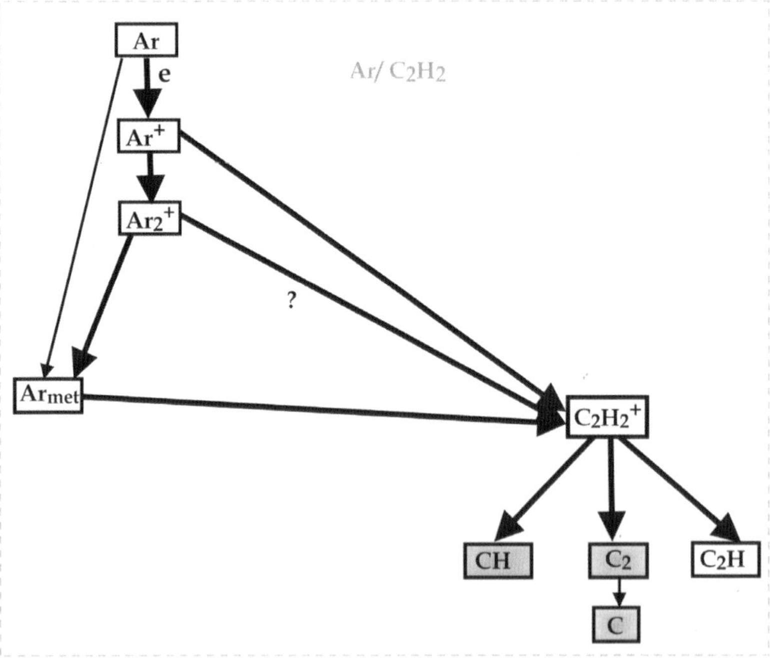

Fig. 16. Chemical reactions involved in the film growth process in filamentary discharge in Ar/C_2H_2 mixture. Thick arrow indicates high probable reaction.

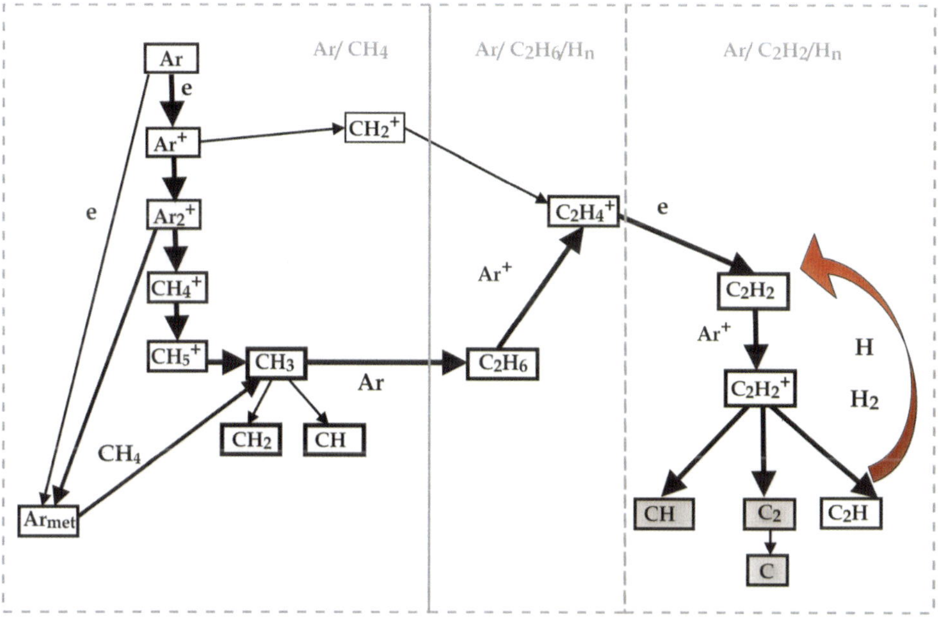

Fig. 17. Chemical reactions involved in the film growth process in filamentary discharge in Ar/CH_4 mixture. Thick arrow indicates high probable reaction. Species shown in gray boxes are observed through their characteristic emission.

reactions among others are shown in thick arrows in the scheme. Analyses of many possible reaction under our plasma conditions indicates that argon ion formation is more probable reaction than argon metastable formation reaction in both methane as well as acetylene cases. This is because of high reduced electric field in both plasma conditions. At atmospheric pressure conditions, Ar^+ ion produces molecular ion, Ar_2^+ through a three particles collision reaction. This is in contrast to the low pressure plasma, where the probability for three particles collision reactions is very low (Pastol & Catherine, 1990; Behringer, 1991; Moller, 1993; Bauer et al., 2005; Awakowicz et al., 2001; Horn et al., 1994). These argon ions undergo charge exchange reaction with precursors. In the case of acetylene, it produces $C_2H_2^+$. The charge exchange reaction of Ar^+ with C_2H_2 is known in the literature. Even though, similar charge exchange reaction of Ar_2^+ with C_2H_2 is not known, to our knowledge; under atmospheric pressure condition, it should have similar high probability.

In the case of methane, the charge exchange reactions produce CH_x^+. These ions through multistep reactions lead to the formation of C_2H_2. This process is very efficient, and it is known in the literature that methane can efficiently be converted in to acetylene in the spark discharge under atmospheric pressure plasma conditions (Leutner & Stokes, 1961; Yao et al., 2002). It indicates that even though it is started with methane, most of the methane will be converted in to acetylene under our plasma conditions. The acetylene produced in the methane system has high probability to undergo charge exchange reactions with argon ions to produce $C_2H_2^+$, as in the case of acetylene system. This indicates that whether it is methane precursor or acetylene precursor, both lead to the formation of mainly $C_2H_2^+$.

In both systems, $C_2H_2^+$ produces reactive species, CH, C_2, C, C_2H, etc., for film deposition process. The presence of reactive species, CH, C_2 and C are observed experimentally (figure 5) through their characteristic emissions in the emission spectra measured for both cases. The reactive species C_2H has very high probability to undergo addition reaction with hydrogen to produce C_2H_2 (Farhat et al., 1993; Kovacs et al., 2010). In other words, presence of hydrogen in the plasma system regenerates acetylene, and hinders the film growth process. The hydrogen quantity with respect to carbon in methane system is four times higher than the same for acetylene. This indicates that film growth hindering reaction due to the presence of hydrogen in methane system is much higher than the same for acetylene system. Hence film growth rate in methane system is very less compared to the same for acetylene system. This fact is verified by externally adding hydrogen into the acetylene system. When three molar ratio of hydrogen molecule with respect to acetylene is added into acetylene system, the film growth rate is drastically reduced compared to the acetylene system without externally added hydrogen.

In the case of methane, at steady state conditions, precursor is fully ionized and dissociated in the tube at the distance of approximately 20 mm from the spike. However, the film deposition rate has sharp maxima under the grounded area, which is at 140 mm away from the spike. The film deposited in the area between the spike and the grounded electrode has different thickness at different places, but with similar properties and components. This film is dense and amorphous; has smooth surface and low content of hydrogen. We suppose that this film is deposited during ion fluxes (Bauer et al, 2005) on the wall after ambipolar diffusion and drift. In the frame of this assumption, we can explain different observed facts such as i) higher deposition rate in the region under grounded electrode because of higher drift velocity in comparison to the velocity of ambipolar diffusion, and ii) low deposition rate near the grounded area because of high axial component of electric field in this region. The hydrocarbon film deposited in the region beyond the grounded area is differed strongly from the film deposited before and under the grounded area. This film is soft, rough and low dense. This film may be deposited by flux of neutral hydrocarbon species which are produced by collisions of hydrocarbon ions with the surface of the tube under the grounded area. The kinetic energy of these ions is high enough for their partial dissociation. The neutral hydrocarbon species formed in this process flow with gas along the tube and deposit on the wall after diffusion. The mechanism of ions transport from the spike area to the grounded area is under investigation.

4. Conclusion

Chemical kinetics of methane and acetylene dissociation and other gas phase reactions are studied for film coating applications under atmospheric pressure plasma conditions. In order to determine the plasma parameters, OES, V-I measurement, micro-photography and numerical simulations are used. From the determined EVDF and n_e, electron impact plasma chemical reaction rates are determined. On the basis of rate of different possible reaction, most probable reactions among others are calculated. From this information and atomic composition of precursors, film deposition rate and film properties are explained as follows, 1. Precursor molecules are ionized and dissociated mainly through charge exchange reaction of argon ions with precursor molecules. 2. Because of low quantity of hydrogen in acetylene, C_2H species dominates in the film deposition process, which facilitates the incorporation of sp^1 carbon in the film. 3. Presence of high quantity of hydrogen in methane facilitates the regeneration of acetylene from the reactive species C_2H; thus reducing film growth rate in methane plasma system in the region between electrodes. 4. Hydrocarbon ion fluxes plays dominant role in methane system, which is responsible for high growth rate in the grounded region. From this study, it can be concluded that atomic composition between carbon and hydrogen in the precursor plays very important role in carbon based film deposition process. Presence of atomic hydrogen in the plasma system improves the film hardness, but in the expense of film growth rate.

5. Acknowledgment

This work is supported by the 'Deutsche Forschungsgemeinschaft' (DFG) within the frame of the research group 'FOR1123 - Physics of Microplasmas'.

6. References

Ağıral, A.; Lefferts, L. & Gardeniers, J. G. E. (2009). Catalyst activation by microplasma for carbon nanofiber synthesis in a microreactor. *IEEE Trans. Plasma Sci.*, Vol.37, pp.985-992

Aleksandrov, N. L.; Bazelyan, E. M.; Gorunov, A. Y. & Kochetov, I. V. (1999). A non-thermal mechanism of spark breakdown in Ar. *J. Phys D: Appl. Phys.*, Vol.32, pp. 2636-2644

Aleksandrov, N. L.; Bazelyan, E. M. & Novitskii, G. A. (2001). The effect of small O_2 addition on the properties of a long positive streamer in Ar. *J. Phys D: Appl. Phys.*, Vol. 34, pp. 1374-1378

Alman, D. A.; Ruzic, D. N. & Brooks, J. N. (2000). A hydrocarbon reaction model for low temperature hydrogen plasmas and an application to the Joint European Torus. *Phys. Plasmas*, Vol. 7, pp. 1421-1432

Awakowicz, P.; Schwefel, R.; Scheubert, P. & Benstetter, G. (2001). Deposition of a-C:H films with an ECWR-reactor at 27 MHz: plasma diagnostics and film properties. *Surf. Coat. Technol.*, Vol. 142-144, pp. 342-347

Babukutty, Y.; Prat, R.; Endo, K.; Kogoma, M.; Okazaki, S. & Kodama, M. (1999). Poly(vinyl chloride) surface modification using tetrafluoroethylene in atmospheric pressure glow discharge. *Langmuir*, Vol. 15, pp. 7055-7062

Ballou, J. K.; Lin, C. C. & Fajen, F. E. (1973). Electron-impact excitation of the argon atom. *Phys. Rev.* A, Vol. 8, pp. 1797-1807

Bauer, M.; Schwarz-Selinger, T.; Jacob, W. & von Keudell, A. (2005). Growth precursors for *a*-C:H film deposition in pulsed inductively coupled methane plasma. *J. Appl. Phys.*, Vol. 98, p. 073302 (11pp)

Baulch, D. L.; Cobos, C. J.; Cox, R. A.; Frank, P.; Hayman, G.; Just, T.; Kerr, J. A.; Murrells, T.; Pilling, M. J.; Troe, J.; Walker, R. W. & Warnatz, J. (1994). Evaluated kinetic data for combustion modeling. Supplement I. *J. Phys. Chem. Ref. Data,* Vol. 23, pp. 847-848

Behringer, K. (1991). Diagnostics and modelling of ECRH microwave discharges. *Plasma Phys. Contr. Fusion,* Vol. 33, pp. 997-1028

Belic, D. S.; Lecointre, J. & Defrance, P. (2010). Electron impact multiple ionization of argon ions. *J. Phys. B: At. Mol. Opt. Phys.,* Vol. 43, p. 185203 (10pp)

Belikov, A. E.; Burshtein, A. I.; Dolgushev, S. V.; Storozhev, A. V.; Strekalov, M. L.; Sukhinin, G. I. & Sharafutdinov, R. G. (1989). Rate constants and rotational relaxation times for N_2 in argon. *Chem. Phys.,* Vol. 139, pp. 239-259

Bibinov, N. K.; Fateev, A. A. & Wiesemann, K. (2001). On the influence of metastable reactions on rotational temperatures in dielectric barrier discharges in He-N_2 mixtures. *J. Phys. D: Appl. Phys.,* Vol. 34, pp. 1819-1826

Bibinov, N.; Halfmann, H.; Awakowicz, P. & Wiesemann, K. (2007). Relative and absolute intensity calibrations of a modern broadband echelle spectrometer. *Meas. Sci. Technol.,* Vol. 18, pp. 1327-1337

Deilmann, M.; Theiß, S. & Awakowicz, P. (2008). Pulsed microwave plasma polymerization of silicon oxide films: Application of efficient permeation barriers on polyethylene terephthalate. *Surf. Coat. Technol.,* Vol. 202, pp. 1911-1917

Deilmann, M.; Halfmann, H.; Steves, S.; Bibinov, N. & Awakowicz, P. (2009). Silicon oxide permeation barrier coating and plasma sterilization of PET bottles and foils. *Plasma Process. Polym.,* Vol. 6, pp. S695-S699

Denysenko, I. B.; Xu, S.; Long, J. D.; Rutkevych, P. P.; Azarenkov, N. A. & Ostrikov, K. (2004). Inductively coupled $Ar/CH_4/H_2$ plasmas for low-temperature deposition of ordered carbon nanostructures. *J. Appl. Phys.,* Vol. 95, pp. 2713-2724

Dilecce, G.; Ambrico, P. F. & Benedictis, S. D. (2010). On the collision quenching of $N_2^+(B^2\Sigma_u^+$, v=0) by N_2 and O_2 and its influence on the measurement of *E/N* by intensity ratio of nitrogen spectral bands. *J. Phys. D: Appl. Phys.,* Vol. 43, p. 195201 (7pp)

Duewer, W. H.; Coxon, J. A. & Setser, D. W. (1972). Collisional transition probabilities for rotational levels of CN($B^2\Sigma^+$). *J. Chem. Phys.,* Vol. 56, pp. 4355-4362

Farhat, S. K.; Morter, C. L. & Glass, G. P. (1993). Temperature dependence of the rate of reaction of C_2H with H_2. *J. Phys. Chem.,* Vol. 97, pp. 12789-12792

Fedosenko, G.; Schwabedissen, A.; Korzec, D. & Engemann, J. (2001). Diamond-like carbon film deposition by a 13.56 MHz hollow cathode RF-RF system using different precursor gases. *Surf. Coat. Technol.,* Vol. 142-144, pp. 693-697

Foest, R.; Kindel, E.; Lange, H.; Ohl, A.; Stieber, M. & Weltmann, K. -D. (2007). RF capillary jet – a tool for localized surface treatment. *Contrib. Plasma Phys.,* Vol. 47, pp. 119-128

Fujiyama, H. (2000). Inner coating of long-narrow tube by plasma sputtering. *Surf. Coat. Technol.,* Vol. 131, pp. 278-283

García, G. & Manero, F. (1998). Electron scattering by CH_4 molecules at intermediate energies (400–5000 eV). *Phys. Rev.* A, Vol. 57, pp. 1069-1073

Herron, J. T. (1999). Evaluated chemical kinetics data for reactions of N(^2D), N(^2P), and $N_2(A^3\Sigma_u^+)$ in the gas phase. *J. Phys. Chem. Ref. Data*, Vol. 28, pp. 1453-1483

Horn, A.; Schenk, A.; Biener, J.; Winter, B.; Lutterloh, C.; Wittmann, M. & Küppers, J. (1994). H atom impact induced chemical erosion reaction at C:H film surfaces. *Chem. Phys. Lett.*, Vol. 231, pp. 193-198

Hytry, R.; Möller, W.; Wilhelm, R. & von Keudell, A. (1993). Moving-coil waveguide discharge for inner coating of metal tubes. *J. Vac. Sci. Technol.* A, Vol.11, pp. 2508-2517

Hytry, R.; Möller, W. & Wilhelm, R. (1994). Running waveguide discharge for inner coating of metal tubes. *Appl. Phys. Lett.*, Vol. 64, pp. 3401-3403

Itikawa, Y. (2006). Cross section for electron collisions with nitrogen molecules. *J. Phys. Chem. Ref. Data*, Vol. 35, pp. 31-53

Ivanov, V. A. & Makasyuk, I. V. (1990). Destruction of Ar4s($^3P_2$) metastable atoms by slow electrons. *Opt. Spectrosc. (USSR)*, Vol. 69, pp. 308-310

Khakoo, M. A.; Vandeventer, P.; Childers, J. G.; Kanik, I.; Fontes, C. J.; Bartschat, K.; Zeman, V.; Madison, D. H.; Saxena, S.; Srivastava, R. & Stauffer, A. D. (2004). Electron impact excitation of the argon 3p^{5}4s configuration: differential cross-sections and cross-section ratios. *J. Phys. B: At. Mol. Opt. Phys.*, Vol. 37, pp. 247-281

Kolts, J. H.; Brashears, H. C. & Setser, D. W. (1977). Redetermination of $N_2(C)$ and $N_2(B)$ branching ratio from the Ar($^3P_{0,2}$) + N_2 reaction. *J. Chem. Phys.*, Vol. 67, pp. 2931-2933

Kolts, J. H. & Setser, D. W. (1978). Decay rates of Ar(4s,^{3}P$_2$), Ar(4s′,^{3}P$_0$), Kr(5s,^{3}P$_2$), and Xe(6s,^{3}P$_2$) atoms in argon. *J. Chem. Phys.*, Vol. 68, pp. 4848-4859

Kovacs, T.; Blitz, M. A. & Seakins, P. W. (2010). H-atom yields from the photolysis of acetylene and from the reaction of C_2H with H_2, C_2H_2, and C_2H_4. *J. Phys. Chem. A*, Vol. 114, pp. 4735-4741

Laux, C. O. & Kruger, C. H. (1992). Arrays of radiative transition probabilities for the N_2 first and second positive, no beta and gamma, N_2^+ first negative, and O_2 Schumann-Runge band systems. *J. Quant. Spectrosc. Radiant. Transfer*, Vol. 48, pp. 9-24

Legrand, J. C.; Diamy, A. M.; Hrach, R. & Hrachová, V. (2001). *Advances in Plasma Physics Research*, Vol. 1, ed Boriotti, S. & Dennis, D. (New York: Nova) pp. 10-19

Leutner, H. W. & Stokes, C. S. (1961). Producing acetylene in a plasma jet. *Industrial and Engineering Chemistry*, Vol. 53, pp. 341-342

Luque, J. & Crosley, D. R. (1999). "*LIFBASE: Database and spectral simulation (version 1.5)*", *SRI International Report MP 99-009*

Möller, W. (1993). Advances in plasma physics research. *Appl. Phys.* A, Vol. 56, pp. 527-546

Murugavel, R. & Pothiraja, R. (2003). Synthesis, spectral characterization and crystal structures of organophosphonic diamides: pyramidal nitrogen centers and hydrogen bonding in [PhP(O)(NH^{t}Bu)$_2$], [PhP(O)(NHDipp)$_2$](Dipp = 2,6-^{i}Pr$_2$C$_6$H$_3$) and [^{t}BuP(O)(NH^{i}Pr)$_2$]. *New J. Chem.*, Vol. 27, pp. 968-974

Murugavel, R.; Pothiraja, R.; Gogoi, N.; Clérac, R.; Lecren, L.; Butcher, R. J. & Nethaji, M. (2007). Synthesis, magnetic behaviour, and X-ray structures of dinuclear copper complexes with multiple bridges. Efficient and selective catalysts for polymerization of 2,6-dimethylphenol. *Dalton Trans.*, pp. 2405-2410

Nguyen, T. D. & Sadeghi, N. (1983). Rotational and vibrational distributions of $N_2(C\ ^3\Pi_u)$ excited by state-selected $Ar(^3P_2)$ and $Ar(^3P_0)$ metastable atoms. *Chem. Phys.*, Vol. 79, pp. 41-55

Pancheshnyi, S. V.; Starikovskaia, S. M. & Starikovskii, A. Y. (2000). Collisional deactivation of $N_2(C^3\Pi_u, v= 0,1,2,3)$ states by N_2, O_2, H_2 and H_2O molecules. *Chem. Phys.*, Vol. 262, pp. 349-357

Pastol, A. & Catherine, Y. (1990). Optical emission spectroscopy for diagnostic and monitoring of CH_4 plasmas used for a-C:H deposition. *J. Phys. D: Appl. Phys.*, Vol. 23, pp. 799-805

Pitts, W. M.; Pasternack, L. & McDonald, J. R. (1982). Temperature dependence of the $C_2(X^1\Sigma_g^+)$ reaction with H_2 and CH_4 and $C_2(X^1\Sigma_g^+$ and a $^3\Pi_u$ equilibrated states) with O_2. *Chem. Phys.*, Vol. 68, pp. 417-422

Polak-Dingels, P. & Djeu, N. (1983). Determination of $N_2(B^3\Pi_g)$ and $N_2(C^3\Pi_u)$ vibrational temperatures in *e*-beam pumped $Ar\text{-}N_2$ and $He\text{-}Ar\text{-}N_2$ mixtures. *J. Appl. Phys.*, Vol. 54, pp. 6818-6821

Pothiraja, R.; Milanov, A. P.; Barreca, D.; Gasparotto, A.; Becker, H. W.; Winter, M.; Fischer, R. A. & Devi, A. (2009). Hafnium carbamates and ureates: new class of precursors for low-temperature growth of HfO_2 thin films. *Chem. Commun.*, pp. 1978-1980

Pothiraja, R.; Milanov, A.; Parala, H.; Winter, M.; Fischer, R. A. & Devi, A. (2009). Monomeric malonate precursors for the MOCVD of HfO_2 and ZrO_2 thin films. *Dalton Trans.*, pp. 654-663

Pothiraja, R.; Bibinov, N. & Awakowicz, P. (2010). Pulsed corona plasma source characterization for film deposition on the inner surface of tubes. *J. Phys. D: Appl. Phys.*, Vol. 43, p. 495201 (10pp)

Pothiraja, R.; Bibinov, N. & Awakowicz, P. (2011). Amorphous carbon film deposition on the inner surface of tubes using atmospheric pressure pulsed filamentary plasma source. *J. Phys. D: Appl. Phys.*, Vol. 44, p. 355206 (10pp)

Prat, R.; Koh, Y. J.; Babukutty, Y.; Kogoma, M.; Okazaki, S. & Kodama, M. (2000). Polymer deposition using atmospheric pressure plasma glow (APG) discharge. *Polymer*, Vol. 41, pp. 7355-7360

Rajasekaran, P.; Mertmann, P.; Bibinov, N.; Wandke, D.; Viöl, W. & Awakowicz, P. (2009). DBD plasma source operated in single-filamentary mode for therapeutic use in dermatology. *J. Phys. D: Appl. Phys.*, Vol. 42, p. 225201 (10pp)

Sadeghi, N. & Setser, D. W. (1981). Primary $N_2(B)$ vibrational distributions from excitation-transfer reactions between $Kr(^3P_2)$ or $Xe(^3P_2)$ atoms and N_2. *Chem. Phys. Lett.*, Vol. 82, pp. 44-50

Sadeghi, N.; Cheaib, M. & Setser, D. W. (1989). Comparison of the $Ar(^3P_2)$ and $Ar(^3P_0)$ reactions with chlorine and fluorine containing molecules: Propensity for ion–core conservation. *J. Chem. Phys.*, Vol. 90, pp. 219-231

Shul, R. J.; Passarella, R.; Yang, X. L.; Keesee, R. G. & Castleman, J. A. W. (1987). Studies of the energy dependence of reactions of Ar^+ and Ar_2^+ with CH_4 and CS_2. *J. Chem. Phys.*, Vol. 87, pp. 1630-1636

Shiu, Y. J. & Biondi, M. A. (1978). Dissociative recombination in argon: Dependence of the total rate coefficient and excited-state production on electron temperature. *Phys. Rev.* A, Vol. 17, pp. 868-872

Sieck, L. W. & Lias, S. G. (1976). Rate coefficients for ion-molecule reactions I. Ions containing C and H. *J. Phys. Chem. Ref. Data*, Vol. 5, pp. 1123-1146

Stefanović, I.; Bibinov, N. K.; Deryugin, A. A.; Vinogradov, I. P.; Napartovich, A. P. & Wiesemann, K. (2001). Kinetics of ozone and nitric oxides in dielectric barrier discharges in O_2/NO_x and $N_2/O_2/NO_x$ mixtures. *Plasma Sources Sci. Technol.*, Vol. 10, pp. 406-416

Tellinghuisen, J. B.; Winkler, C. A.; Freeman, C. G.; McEwan, M. J. & Phillips, L. F. (1972). Quenching rates of N_2^+, N_2O^+, and CO_2^+ emission bands excited by 58.4 nm irradiation of N_2, N_2O, and CO_2. *J. Chem. Soc., Faraday Trans. 2*, Vol. 68, pp. 833-838

Touzeau, M. & Pagnon, D. (1978). Vibrational excitation of $N_2(C)$ and $N_2(B)$ by metastable argon atoms and the determination of the branching ratio. *Chem. Phys. Lett.*, Vol. 53, pp. 355-360

Tsang, W. & Hampson, R. F. (1986). Chemical kinetic data base for combustion chemistry. Part I. Methane and related compounds. *J. Phys. Chem. Ref. Data*, Vol. 15, pp. 1087-1279

Velazco, J. E.; Kolts, J. H. & Setser, D. W. (1978). Rate constants and quenching mechanisms for the metastable states of argon, krypton, and xenon. *J. Chem Phys.*, Vol. 69, pp. 4357-4373

Veldhuizen, E. M. v.; Rutgers, W. R. & Ebert, U. (2002). *Int. Symp. HAKONE VIII*, Pühajärve, Estonia, pp. 33-37

Veldhuizen, E. M. v.; Nijdam, S.; Luque, A.; Brau, F. & Ebert, U. (2009). 3D properties of pulsed corona streamers. *Eur. Phys. J. Appl. Phys.*, Vol. 47, p. 22811 (5pp)

Wang, L.; Huang, L.; Wang, Y.; Xie, Z. & Wang, X. (2008). Duplex diamond-like carbon film fabricated on 2Cr13 martensite stainless steel using inner surface ion implantation and deposition. *Surf. Coat. Technol.*, Vol. 202, pp. 3391-3395

Yao, S. L.; Suzuki, E.; Meng, N. & Nakayama, A. (2002). A high-efficiency reactor for the pulsed plasma conversion of methane. *Plasma Chemistry and Plasma Processing*, Vol. 22, pp. 225-237

Yoshiki, H.; Abe, K. & Mitsui, T. (2006). SiO_2 thin film deposition on the inner surface of a poly(tetra-fluoroethylene) narrow tube by atmospheric pressure glow microplasma. *Thin Solid Films*, Vol. 515, pp. 1394-1399

Yoshiki, H. & Mitsui, T. (2008).TiO_2 thin film coating on a capillary inner surface using atmospheric-pressure microplasma. *Surf. Coat. Technol.*, Vol. 202, pp. 5266-5270

Yoshiki, H. & Saito, T. (2008). Preparation of TiO_2 thin films on the inner surface of a quartz tube using atmospheric-pressure microplasma. *J. Vac. Sci. Technol.* A, Vol. 26, 338-343

Zhiglinski A G 1994 *Handbook of Rate Constants of Process of Atoms, Electrons and Photons* (St. Petersburg: St. Petersburg university press) (in Russian)

Part 4

Recent Developments

12

Nanoscale Liquid is Second Liquid

Boris A. Mosienko
Siberian Research Institute of Geology, Geophysics and Mineral Resources, Novosibirsk, Russia

1. Introduction

In the beginning of the 20th century liquid was considered nonstructural (i.e. similar to a very dense gas). But as it is proved by experiment in 1933, liquid has complicated *intermolecular structure* [1]. This was the first important broadening of our notions of liquid. From that time on, the liquid structure is studying in many scientific laboratories of the world [2-5]. The second broadening had been developing for a long time in some stages; it is concerned with phase transitions of first kind, in particular, with melting. It turned out that the melting of crystal on its surface begins at the temperature essentially more low than it was considered before. This phenomenon for the first time was noticed and studied by M. Faraday (1850), but the results of his investigations did not gain recognition in that time. The existence of this phenomenon was definitely proved experimentally in 1985 only [6]; it was named *premelting*. Premelting of ice enables to interpret plenty of natural phenomena (the flow of glaciers, ice slippery, heaving of frozen ground and so on). Investigations on these subjects are carried out now on a large scale in many countries [7-10].

Author of this article has made an attempt to extend further our notions of liquid [11, 12]. It is considered now that sublimation is a direct transition from solid (crystalline) state of matter into gas. The author has propounded and substantiated the principle of least time for first-order phase transitions [11, 13]; it is shown by means of this principle that sublimation goes in two steps through a certain intermediate state in the form of surface film. It is concluded that this film consists of nonstructural liquidlike substance which is a certain antipode of liquid; this liquidlike state of matter is named *second liquid* [12].

In this work, the mentioned subject is continued and developed. From theoretical reasons, it is assumed that second liquid can exist not only in the lower part of phase plane (on the sublimation curve) but also in its upper part, in all existence area of ordinary liquid. The point comes to the sizes of liquid objects: if only one dimension of a liquid object does not exceed a certain critical size h_c, this object has to consist of second (not ordinary) liquid. This conclusion ought to be of an important applied significance.

It seems that, logically, notion of second liquid is simple and clear [12]; however, it is uncustomary, and therefore difficult for comprehension. For this reason, and also for a coherence of exposition, we shall dwell upon the second liquid notion in the concise form (section 2). In more detail it is considered in [12].

The new data are set forth in sections 3-5.

2. Preliminary information

2.1 Second liquid

It is believed at present that the phase transitions G→L, L→S, and G→S happen owing to forces of intermolecular interactions, which are called Van der Waals forces. These forces are due to the quantum mechanism (proposed by F. London in 1929).

As known, intermolecular potentials have only one minimum. Since Van der Waals forces are assumed to be the only mechanism of intermolecular interaction, it is reasonable to expect that gaseous molecules should always condense immediately into the solid state (which happens, according to the existing notions, if the process goes along the line 2-2 in Fig. 1). A question arises: Why does liquid exist?

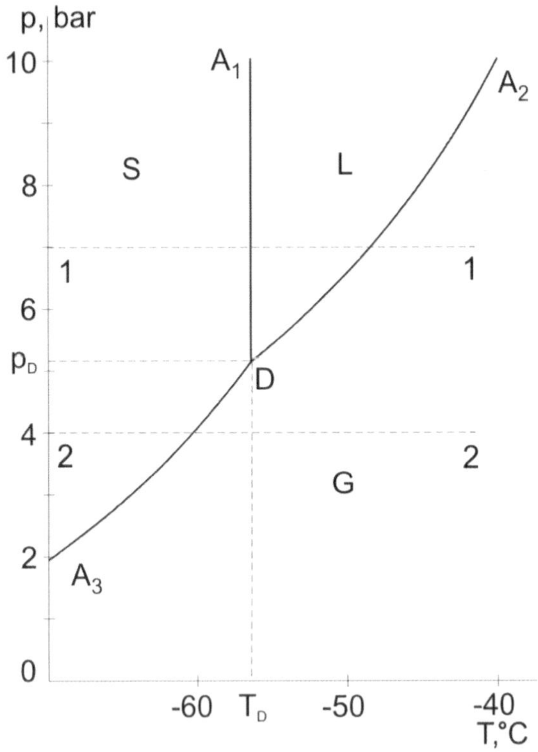

Fig. 1. Typical phase diagram (of carbon dioxide) in coordinates T (temperature) and p (pressure). D is the triple point; DA_1, DA_2 and DA_3 are the curves of melting, boiling and sublimation, respectively; S, L and G are the areas of existence of solid (crystal), liquid and gaseous states of matter.

This question is not as naive as it seems at first sight. Indeed, based on the current notions, molecules of gas, in the upper part of the diagram (if the process goes along the line 1-1), descend to the same potential well in two stages: during the G→L and L→S transitions. Of course, it is hardly the case. Therefore, we assume that, probably, *two different independent mechanisms of intermolecular interaction exist, which are realized by the phase transitions G→L and L→S*. Let us denote them by symbols M_1 and M_2, respectively.

Since the mechanisms of intermolecular interaction are independent, they apparently have different physical nature and cannot be combined into a single mechanism at the triple point of phase diagram. So the curves of melting and vaporization do not merge but intersect at the triple point.

It is quite easy to understand that the mechanisms of phase transition {G→S}, in the upper and lower parts of the phase plane, are realized in different successions. Depending on which mechanism is the first to "switch on" by the transition G→S, the intermediate state can be either an ordinary liquid L_1=L (as it happens in the upper part of the phase plane) or another modification of liquid which may naturally be called a second liquid L_2. As the states L_1 and L_2 are generated by different physical mechanisms, the second liquid must substantially differ from ordinary liquid by its characteristics.

2.1.1 Second liquid of helium

As known, at a temperature of 4.2 K under normal pressure, gaseous helium turns into a liquid (helium 1), but at 2.2 K helium 1 transforms into another modification of liquid which is called helium 2. Helium 1 is an ordinary liquid which differs from other liquids by nothing but low temperature. Helium 2, on the contrary, has unusual properties, the most interesting of which is superfluidity. By its anomalous properties helium 2 radically differs not only from helium 1 but also from all other liquids in nature. However, what is stranger is the very existence of two quite different liquids of helium. The existence of helium 2, the second liquid of helium, is an exception to the rule, which displays itself as a unique physical and logical anomaly.

Given that a second liquid exists, this anomaly is classified as a norm.

The existence of helium 2 is an established fact; meanwhile, the existent idea of sublimation reflects only the level of our present-day knowledge. The facts are admitted to be of greater logical weight than theoretical notions. So, it should be more correct to agree that our notion of sublimation, rather than the existence of second liquid of helium, is a real anomaly.

Now we demonstrate that the phase diagram of helium is a typical diagram of substance with a bulk second liquid.

Formal phase transition curves for different mechanisms of molecular interaction are shown in Fig. 2a. Since these mechanisms are independent, the curves after intersection continue to keep their course and divide the phase plane into four sections. The point D turns out to be not triple but quadruple. The area of existence of second intermediate state, second liquid L_2, together with that of liquid, L_1, appears on the phase plane.

Simple thermodynamic reasoning implies that the quadruple point D cannot actually exist; it will fall apart into two triple points D_S and D_G, connected by a line of the second-order phase transition $L_1 \rightleftarrows L_2$ (Fig. 2b).

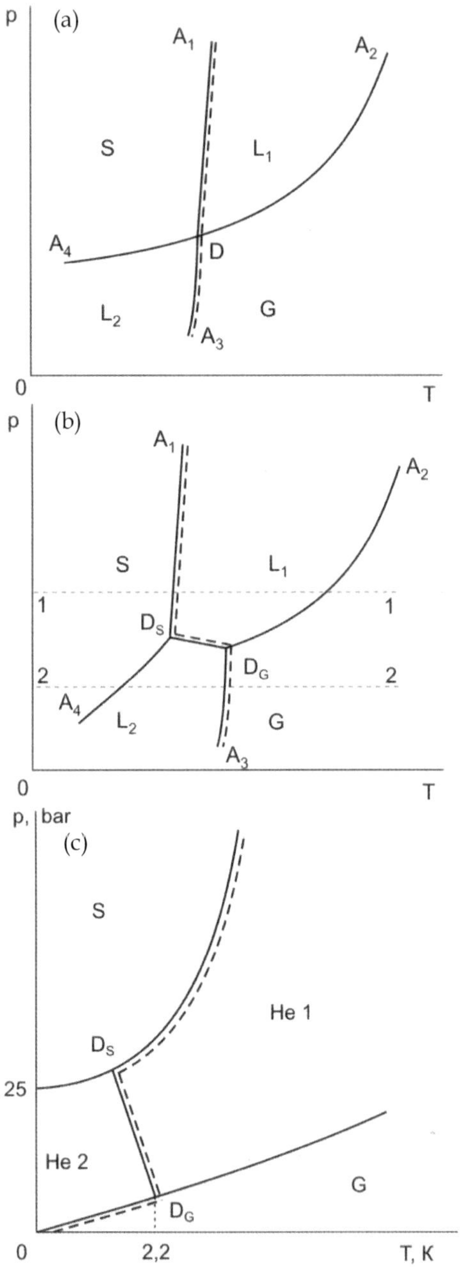

Fig. 2. Scheme explaining the origin of second liquid. **a.** Diagram with the quadruple point D; A_2A_4 and A_1A_3 are the lines of "switching-on" of the mechanisms M_1 and M_2, respectively. **b.** Diagram with a quadruple point fallen apart into the triple points D_S and D_G. **c.** Helium phase diagram (with vertical exaggeration of scale for clearness).

It is reasonable to suppose that near the point D_S potential barriers of the phase transitions $S \rightarrow L_1$ and $S \rightarrow L_2$ are equal; so, there ought to be no sharp bend of the curve $A_1D_sA_4$ at the point D_S. The same is true for the point D_G. Therefore, the phase diagram resembles that of helium (Fig. 2c).

With the area of existence of second liquid tending to zero, we obtain, in the limit, a phase diagram with second liquid in the form of surface film. Obviously, this diagram is similar to that of CO_2 (Fig 1).

2.2 Classical version of superfluidity

The superfluidity phenomenon was discovered by P. L. Kapitsa in 1938 and in just three years it was interpreted in theory proposed by L. D. Landau. This theory (supported by quantum-mechanical premises) has gained recognition, since it has satisfactorily explained the results of experiments with superfluid helium 2.

Meanwhile, atoms and molecules (as opposed to electrons) are commonly known as quite classical objects. That is why we may expect that the superfluidity phenomenon can be explained in the context of classical physics by the behavior of molecules, namely by the molecular-kinetic theory.

Let us assume that the expression "liquid structure" is clear and well-known. We denote the structure property by symbol *Con* (from the word "connection") and accept it as characteristic property of liquid.

Next we consider the mechanism of internal friction (viscosity) of flowing liquid or gas. It consists in the following: the neighboring layers which move with different velocities exchange impulses; these impulses are transferred by particles which diffuse through the boundary between layers. Besides, the intermolecular bonds of structural elements (normally – i.e., perpendicularly – orientated to the sliding surface) deform and tear up; this is the second factor of viscosity inherent to liquid only.

It is easy to comprehend (at least, formally) that if the above factors, which condition the mechanism of liquid viscosity, are eliminated, we would get a certain model of superfluidity. Let us show that such a model is possible.

We know that by the transition $L \rightarrow S$, which is the result of the mechanism M_2, molecules, in a sense, really come to a stop: by crystallization molecules are localized, and diffusion of molecules practically ceases. Of course, it is only the translational motion of molecules which ceases; the thermal movement continues in the form of vibration of molecules relative to strictly defined localized positions which form crystal lattice. Since the transition $G \rightarrow L_2$ is realized through the mechanism M_2 as well (see Fig. 2), such localization should occur in this case too. The localization of molecules, apparently, may be considered the characteristic property of second liquid; let us denote it by symbol *Loc*. Thus, liquid has the property {*Con*, -}, second liquid has the property {-, *Loc*}, and crystal has the property {*Con*, *Loc*}. Hence, the second liquid is a certain antipode of liquid.

Emphasize that the property *Loc* suggests that diffusion (or, to tell more exactly, self-diffusion) of molecules in second liquid is practically absent.

As we see, the second liquid lacks the both factors of viscosity. This allows draw the following heuristic prediction: *second liquid should be very different from ordinary liquid by its higher fluidity.*

Note that out of caution we speak here of comparatively high fluidity of second liquid, not of superfluidity. This precaution might seem unwarranted if temperature and pressure are expressed in relative form: $T^*=T/T_D$ and $p^*=p/p_D$. The combination of inequalities

$$T^*<1 \ \& \ p^*<1 \tag{1}$$

might be considered as the existence condition for second liquid.

The condition (1) is common for all substances. It may be proposed that the property of superfluidity is caused by the low relative temperature T^* (not by the low absolute temperature T, as it is presently assumed). In such definition the assumption of second liquid superfluidity of any substance looks more acceptable.

Note that this point of view could lead to the significant simplification of our understanding of the superfluidity physical nature.

3. This strange second liquid

Second liquid properties in broad outline were considered in preceding section. But these properties appear somewhat abstract. In this section we shall dwell upon them in more detail and consider them in the frame of habitual notions (fluidity, diffusion, evaporation, and viscosity).

3.1 Fluidity

Liquid has the property *Con* (structuration), but second liquid has not it. How it manifest itself?

The existence of structural elements (clusters) in liquid causes supplementary resistance during the movement through a tube (canal, capillary); this resistance increases with a diminution of the tube cross-section. In very thin tubes (nanocapillaries), if their diameters are compared with the sizes of structural elements, ordinary liquid apparently could not flow. Meanwhile, the second liquid fluidity, with a diminution of the tube cross-section, even increases owing to the reduction of turbulence.

3.2 Diffusion and evaporation

Second liquid has the property *Loc* (localization), but ordinary liquid has not it. What this lead to?

It is known, that the molecule diffusion of ordinary liquid is a cause of evaporation. As second liquid lacks of diffusion (see section 2.2), one might believe that the rate of its evaporation is much less than that of liquid. By this property, second liquid radically differs from ordinary liquid. Let us accept (as a postulate) the assumption that second liquid does not evaporate at all by temperature $T<T_{vap}$, where T_{vap} is the boiling heat.

Superfluidity is the wonderful and extraordinary phenomenon, but it does not arouse a doubt because it is corroborated with the direct experiment carried out at first by P. L. Kapitsa. Lack of evaporation from the second liquid surface is a different matter. It presents itself not only wonderful but impossible phenomenon too. Really, it is difficult to imagine a liquid which does not evaporate from the free surface. An unaccustomed thing perfectly can be taken for the impossible one; therefore, a doubt arises: is it like this indeed? That's why we adduce one more argument based on the superfluidity.

It is known, that viscosity of liquid is in a direct dependence upon the diffusion coefficient. If the molecules of helium 2 were capable to diffuse (and, therefore, to evaporate), the viscosity of helium 2 could not be equal to zero; it means that superfluidity could not exist. However, as we know, it does exist.

3.3 The third condition of superfluidity

It is obvious, that the presence of the property *Loc* and the lack of the property *Con* are necessary for superfluidity. But there is one more obvious and important condition for superfluidity: molecules of second liquid must have the central symmetry; ideally, they must be spherical (as it takes place for helium). For this reason, the most perspective for superfluidity in the bulk phase are elements of the eighth group (neon, argon and so on), whose molecules (atoms) have the central symmetry. Nonspherical molecules (for instance, the lineal molecules CO_2: O – C – O) cannot bring superfluidity, as they are a cause of viscosity.

4. Dimension factor

4.1 Theoretical considerations

The notion of liquid as a state of substance with a certain intermolecular structure has almost the century history. This notion has appeared at the definite stage of experimental technology development and continued to get more accurate with its improvements [5]. Emphasize that structural elements of liquid are substantially three-dimensional objects.

Let us carry out an imaginary experiment. Consider the very beginning of melting process (in the ideal case) when on the crystal surface, at first, the film with a thickness h of one molecule appears, then of two molecules, of three molecules and so on. Let us put a question: at which stage (i.e., by which critical thickness h_c of a film) do the structural elements of liquid arise? We consider, for the simplicity, that the structure elements are only isometric clusters which can be approximated by spheres of a certain diameter d_{cl}. It is obvious, that the relation $d_{cl}>d_{mol}$, where d_{mol} is the diameter of molecule, take place even for the very small clusters. The clusters cannot arise till the film thickness is smaller of cluster diameter; they simply could not get in. Moreover, one must take into account that the formation of three-dimensional structure elements of liquid is a statistical process; it is possible only when a certain freedom of the movement of molecules in the all three dimensions takes place. Taking into consideration this condition (*dimension factor*), we come to the following inequality:

$$h_c>>d_{cl},$$

i.e., the critical thickness must be some times as much as the cluster diameter; let it be by an order of magnitude greater. The diameter of simple molecules is equal 0.5 nm. It means that the diameter of the minimal cluster is equal 1 nm. So, the minimal critical thickness of film is equal 10 nm. Let the maximal one be 50 nm.

Thus, the intermolecular structure of the liquid film can form only when the film thickness reaches a certain critical size h_c, which might be estimated on the order of some tens of nanometer; let it be 50 nm. The exact value of it could be stated only by experiments. One might put a question: what liquid is the film made of, when $h<h_c$? As one might see in the case of helium, liquid has only two modifications [12] – L_1 (ordinary structural liquid) and L_2 (second nonstructural liquid). To introduce any third modification for consideration would be superfluous: this would be a violation of the principle of simplicity. Therefore, the answer is definitive: when $h<h_c$, the film consists of second liquid L_2.

So, at first, during melting, the film of nonstructural second liquid is formed on the surface of crystal substance. When the film thickness gets equal h_c, the phase transition of second kind happens, and second liquid transforms into ordinary structural liquid.

It is obvious, that similar transformation happens with drop growing. The growth stages of liquid drops by condensation of vapor are shown in Fig. 3.

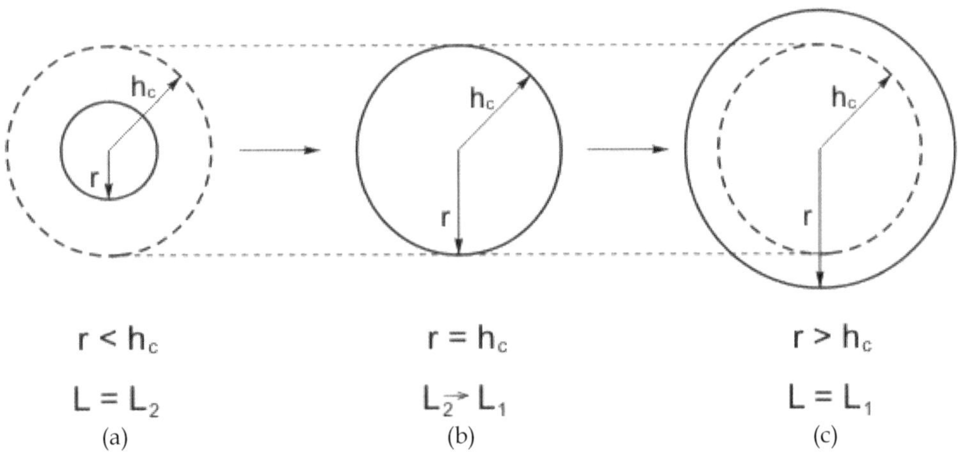

Fig. 3. Growth stages of drops in the upper part of phase diagram. **a.** A very small drop (nanodrop), $r<h_c$; the drop consists of second liquid L_2. **b.** A drop grown up to the critical size, $r=h_c$; the phase transition $L_2 \rightarrow L_1$ takes place. **c.** A drop grown out the critical size (microdrop), $r>h_c$; the drop consists of liquid L_1.

Thus, we have come to a new approach in our conception of liquid. We formulate this conclusion in the general form.

Let us perceive the expression "physical D-space" as an aggregate of n physical bodies (n is any natural number) which have the same dimensionality. Consider, that physical D-space is incomplete-dimensional, if only one dimension does not exceed h_c (we name such dimensions "truncated"). Below we state the following postulates of the new conception of liquid.

1. There are two modifications of three-dimensional physical D-spaces of liquid: structural liquid L_1, in the upper part of the phase plane, and nonstructural second liquid L_2 in the lower one (see Fig. 2c).
2. The incomplete-dimensional physical D-spaces of liquid – two-dimensional (nanofilms), one-dimensional (nanothreads) and zero-dimensional (nanodrops) – exist only in the form of nonstructural second liquid L_2 (Fig. 3a). Or else, in the concise form: *any nanoscale liquid is second liquid.* Note that this formulation might be considered a definition of the notion "dimension factor".

3. When the truncated dimensions of objects of the incomplete-dimensional physical D-space of liquid, in the upper part of phase plane, increase and reach the critical size h_c, the second-order phase transition $L_2 \rightarrow L_1$ happens, i.e. second liquid transforms into ordinary liquid (Fig. 3b).

4.2 On the size correlation of solid and liquid nanoobjects

As known, solid nanomaterials have unusual, unique physical and chemical properties. They contain structural elements, whose geometrical sizes, if only in one dimension, do not exceed the value h_o=100 nm; it is, first of all, nanoparticles (zero-dimentional elements) and nanofilms (two-dimensional elements).

The above-mentioned critical size of liquids (h_c=50 nm) lies in the accepted nanometric range (1 - 100 nm). Note that the cited here sizes (50 nm and 100 nm) are tentative; the value h_c, by somewhat different estimation, perfectly well could be equal 100 nm and even more.

Imagine that we have the concrete and sufficiently exact sizes h_c and h_0 of a certain chemical substance, obtained experimentally. In which relation could be these sizes? Let us assume that they must be equal. This assumption has important heuristic contents which might be used to understand and substantiate the uniquity of properties of nanomaterials. Indeed, if one would take this assumption, *the accepted nanometric range would acquire a profound physical meaning: it is the existence area of corresponding second liquid.*

5. Second water on the Earth

Consider, in which phenomena do nanoobjects of water take part. Let us begin with nanofilms.

5.1 Water nanofilms on the surface of ice

It has been mentioned above, that melting of crystalline substance begins at temperature which is essentially below the melting temperature T_{mel}. This phenomenon (premelting) is studied already for some decades. It is established with experiments, that premelting begins at the temperature about $0{,}9T_{mel}$, and the liquid film thickness on a crystalline surface increases together with the temperature [6]. According to the new approach, the liquidlike film of premelting consists of second liquid. At T=T_{mel} the thickness of the film reaches the value h_c, and the phase transition $L_2 \rightarrow L_1$ happens.

Let us appeal to premelting of water. In this case, we certainly recollect the notorious problem "why is ice slippery". We shall not go into the history of it. The last point in this history was put about 15 years ago [14]: ice is slippery because its surface, from the outset, is covered with a thin film of water (premelting). The ice slippery is getting worse perceptibly with a decreasing of the temperature, when the film thickness approaches to zero. At T<–30^{0}C a certain role for the slippery plays also the friction [14].

We make only one essential alteration in this interpretation: the film on the surface of ice (in the course of premelting) consists of second liquid L_2, not of ordinary liquid L_1. In the light of this alteration becomes clearly, why the ice slippery considerably diminishes in the days of thaw; this phenomenon is well known to the skaters. Indeed, in this case, the phase transition $L_2 \rightarrow L_1$ happens in the surface film, and fluidity of the liquid film falls.

The film of second liquid covers also the surface of snow crystals. So, the slippery of a snowy sleigh-road and ski-track is explained similarly.

5.2 Water nanodrops in atmosphere

Note that in any historical period (for example, 50 or 100 years ago), for the people which are far from science, the situation looks as if all mysteries of atmosphere are studied and explained. In reality, it is far not so.

Let us listen to opinion of the prominent physicist R. Feynman. This is what he said on the mechanisms of electric charging in a thunder-cloud: "Nobody exactly knows how they work. We know only that a lightning happens from the thunderstorm (and know, of course, that a thunder happens from the lightning…)". These words were said a half of century ago [15], but they are of present interest. Moreover, they might be attributed to other mechanisms of the thunderstorm. At present, the thunderous electricity phenomenon contains more secrets than positive solutions.

The problem of thunderstorm can be subdivided into three principal items. 1). How arise and accumulate charged particles (ions)? 2). How happens the spatial separation of the electric charges in a cloud? 3). What is the discharge mechanism of the thunder-cloud? We shall deal with the first item only.

There is only one reliable source of the electric charges in troposphere. It is the cosmic radiation; the radio-activity of mining rocks, which play an important part in the lower troposphere stratum, might be also ascribed to this category. The ions accumulate to some balance concentration when the rate of the ion arising in the volume unit (which can be measured by experiments) becomes equal to the rate of their recombination.

But it turned out that this concentration is insufficient to initiate a thunderous discharge – the lightning. A series of auxiliary ionization mechanisms was proposed [6, 16-20], but they were hypothetical and therefore could not lead to the satisfactory solution of the problem.

Let us proceed to nanodrops. One may put a question: what we see as looking on a cloud or a dense cover of a fog? Raindrops – that's quite another thing; they are macroscopic objects. As to a cloud (or a fog), it contains microscopic drops of 0.2-100 mc in sizes. One cold see them, each separately, with microscope only. But even with the best optical microscope it is impossible to see drops whose sizes are smaller 0.2 mc. As known, we see owing to the reflected light. The very short waves of the visible light have the length about 0.4 mc. If the size of a drop is under 0.2 mc, the light does not reflect from it; it means that nanodrops are invisible for us.

But this trouble is not the only one. According to the existent theory, nanodrops cannot arise and exist in atmosphere in general.

Indeed, the pressure of saturated vapor over a spherical drop of radius r is equal

$$p=p_0+2a/r$$

where p_0 is the pressure of saturated vapor over the plane, α is the coefficient of a surface tension (Laplas formula). Hence, additional pressure $2a/r$ over little drops is more than that over large ones. It means that the vapor saturated over large drop can be unsaturated over little one. Therefore, very little drops (nanodrops), originated by chance, are unstable; they must evaporate immediately. That's why it is considered, that clouds consist only of microdrops condensed on the comparatively large solid particles (aerosols) which are numerous in troposphere. These particles, from the outset, ensure considerable radius of the curvature for drops developing on their surfaces.

However, the said above applies to the neutral nanodrops only. As to the electrical charged ones, experiments show, that in this case we have quite a different situation.

Consider the results of experiments carried out 50 years ago with mass-spectrometers installed into geophysical rockets. These experiments were fulfilled in mesosphere, at the altitudes 50-90 km. It was found unexpected ubiquity of hydrated ions $H^+(H_2O)_n$ and $OH^-(H_2O)_n$ where n=1, 2, 3, … [21, 22]. Besides, in the process of investigation, the more and more heavy hydrated ions were discovered. Otherwise, it was observed an initial stage of the growth of water nanodrops. Note that the centers of nucleation are hydrogen and hydroxyl ions. As ions are present in troposphere, a similar process of the origin of nanodrops must happen in this case too.

It is important to note the following. The mentioned observations in mesosphere had shown that at night the concentration of little ions reduced drastically; and it was naturally, since the most ions in mesosphere arise by photons of the harsh (short-wave) ultra-violet radiation coming from the sun. But the concentration of heavy hydrated ions at night remained like that by day. It means, that the charged nanodrops have a high stability in respect to vaporization and recombination. This was unexpected and incomprehensible.

Subsequently, similar phenomenon was discovered in troposphere [23-25]. The distinction was the following: in troposphere, the most centers of nucleation were represented by the charged fragments of molecules of industrial contamination (nitric oxides, ammonia, sulphuric acid and so on). It was obvious that ions play an important role in the production of new aerosol particles (first of all, water nano- and microdrops) in atmosphere. But the problem of stability of the charged water nanodrops is not solved up to now.

Some ideas for solution of this problem were proposed [26-28], but they did not get the proper experimental corroboration. We give the quotation to elucidate the situation which is formed.

"The role of ions in the production of aerosols is among the least understood, but potentially is an important, process in the Earth's atmosphere. Atmospheric and experimental observations have shown that the nucleation of aerosol particles can occur under conditions that cannot be explained by classical nucleation theory" [29].

Let us show, that the new approach to liquid enables to understand and explain the ion-induced nucleation. The point is that nanodrops consist not of ordinary water but of second one. It is shown in section 3 that second liquid practically does not evaporate. Precisely this strange property of second liquid is the key to the problem in question. So, we come to the following.

1. As second liquid does not evaporate, liquid nanodrops are stable to vaporization. Naturally, this takes place for temperatures $T<T_{vap}$ only.
2. An electric charge, which is a centre of nucleation, cannot come out on the surface of water nanodrop because of the lack of diffusion. This means that it cannot recombine

with a little ion of the opposite sign: it is isolated by the coat of some layers (ligands) of molecules H_2O. Therefore, the charged nanodrops are stable to recombination. Of course, the recombination, after all, happens (at least, after the transition $L_2 \rightarrow L_1$, i.e., when the critical size h_c is overcome).

So, "ions are active in continuously generating a reservoir of small thermodynamically stable clusters that can then rapidly grow in the presence of considerable vapors. These results demonstrate that ions probably play an important role in the production of new aerosol particles in the Earth's atmosphere" [29].

The aforesaid does not mean that the problem of arising and accumulation of electric charges in the thunder-cloud is completely solved. However, it is clear, that nanodrops of second water enable to advance in the proper direction.

5.3 Nanocapillarity

In this section, other fields connected with second liquid will be considered in the concise form.

As known, the thin tubes (from one to some tens of microns in diameter), along which liquid moves, are called capillaries. For example, most thin blood-vessels of animals or human beings are capillaries. In more broad meaning, capillaries are the thin cavities with the various shapes of cross-sections (for example, the soil pores). We shall consider capillarity just in such broad meaning.

The capillary liquids in our earthly conditions are, first of all, water and water solutions of diverse chemical compositions. Another instance of natural capillary liquid is oil which fills the pores of sedimentary rocks at different depths from the earth surface.

The value 1 mc is usually taken as the lower limit of capillary sizes. It is no mere chance; this value is near to the lower size of bodies which can be seen in optical microscope. So, capillarity in the existent understanding is microcapillarity. But we are interested in nanocapillarity.

Nanocapillary water causes a serious problem by the production of dry (i.e., completely deprived of water) thin powder which is used in technology processes. Usual drying is not effective in this case: some amount of water (in the form of the smallest capillaries between solid particles), by unknown cause, can not be removed. This remaining moisture can be driven off just by roasting.

According to the new approach, this remaining moisture in nanocapillaries (when the width of cavity $h<h_c$) consists of second liquid. As was mentioned, second liquid is practically deprived of diffusion, i.e., it practically does not evaporate by $T<T_{vap}$. It can be removed only by $T>T_{vap}$.

(Note that expression "width of cavity" hardly yields to the strict definition. Nevertheless, let us try to give it. The width h of cavity (capillary) in the given place is the maximal diameter d_{max} of spherical volume which can be inscribe to the cavity (i.e., $h=d_{max}$). Mathematician most likely would consider such definition incorrect; but for physicists and chemists, I hope, it will be quite acceptable.)

5.3.1 Second liquid in biology

Here we confine ourselves to the very general considerations only.

As is known, intercellular and intracellular cavities of living organisms (including organisms of human beings) have nanometrical sizes [30]. The continuous and intensive movement of water solutions takes place in these cavities. In the last decades, researchers have come to a conclusion that water in intracellular space of living organisms has the special, quite unusual and enigmatic properties. This water was called structurated, quasicrystalline and even living water (see, for example, the works by K. Trincher and also B. V. Deriagin).

According to the new approach, the nanocapillary liquid of living organisms is nonstructural second liquid. As second liquid essentially differs from ordinary liquid (in particular, by high fluidity), at least a part of the existing puzzles of inter- and intracellular water has to get natural explanation. Emphasize that we do not exclude also the influence of other factors.

Note, that we are calling second liquid "nonstructural" only in respect to ordinary liquid which has the property *Con*. In reality, each liquid has a definite structure (*Con* or *Loc*); each liquid, in its way, displays a quality which inherent in solid (crystal). Otherwise, the both liquids are quasicrystalline, but prefix "quasi" should be understood differently, depending on that which liquid is meant.

6. Conclusion

Thus, the liquid objects, which have if only one dimension of nanoscale size, consist of second liquid. This conclusion is obtained from theoretical considerations and is of great applied significance. It is shown that the second liquid conception could throw light upon the following problems: 1) the cause of uniquity of solid nanomaterial properties; 2) the ion-induced nucleation in atmosphere; 3) some unusual properties of liquid water in nanocavities (particularly, in the cells of living organisms). Apparently, this list might be continued.

It is possible, that the reader had perceived that the third modification of incomplete-dimensional physical D-space of liquid – nanothreads – was not considered here. The point is that nanothreads, unlike nanofilms and nanodrops, can exist only in very nonequilibrium conditions. Therefore, nanothreads must be found in nature more rarely than nanodrops. It might be supposed that nanothreads, together with nanodrops, play the determinative role in the phenomenon of thunderstorm. But this is a different theme, it requires a special consideration.

7. References

[1] J.D. Bernal and R.H. Fowler, J. Chem, Phys. 1, 515 (1933).
[2] J.I. Frenkel, *Kinetic theory of liquid,* Oxford: Oxford University Press (1946).
[3] D. Turnbull, J. Chem. Phys. 20, 411 (1952).
[4] J.A. Barker, *Lattice theories of liquid state,* Oxford: Pergamon Press (1963).
[5] H. Reichert, O. Klein, H. Dosh, M. Denk, V. Honkimäki, T. Lippmann, and G. Reiter, Nature (London) 408, 839 (2000).
[6] J.G. Dash, H. Fu, and J.S. Wettlaufer, Rep. Prog. Phys. 58, 115 (1995) and references therein.

[7] S. Engemann, H. Reichert, H. Dosh, J. Bilgram, V. Honkimäki, and A. Snigirev, Phys. Rev. Lett. 92, 205701 (2004).
[8] N. Materer, U. Starke, A. Barbieri, M.A. Van Hove, G.A. Somorjai, G.J. Kroes, and C. Minot, J. Phys. Chem. 99, 6267 (1995).
[9] X. Wey, P.B. Miranda, C. Zhang, and Y.R. Shen, Phys. Rev. B 66, 085401 (2002).
[10] H. Bluhm, D.F. Ogletree, C.S. Fadley, Z. Hussain, and M.G. Salmeron, J. Phys. Condens. Matter. 14, L227 (2002).
[11] B.A. Mosienko, Z. Phys. Chem. 222, 1533 (2008).
[12] B.A. Mosienko, Z. Phys. Chem. 223, 905 (2009).
[13] B.A. Mosienko, Z. Phys. Chem. 224, 1347 (2010).
[14] R. Rosenberg, Phys. Today 58, issue 12, 50 (2005).
[15] R. Feynman, R. Leiton, and M. Sands, *The Feynman lectures on physics*, Vol. 2, Chap. 5, London: Addison-Westley Pub. Co. (1964).
[16] C.T.R. Wilson, J. Franklin Inst. 208, 1 (1929).
[17] R.G. Fleagle and J.A. Businger, *An introduction to atmospheric physics*, New York: Academic (1980).
[18] T. Takahashi, J. Phys. Chem. 87, 4122 (1983).
[19] G.J. Turner and C.D. Stow, Phil. Mag. 49, L25 (1984).
[20] Y. Dong and J. Hallett, J. Geophys. Res. 97, 20361 (1992).
[21] G. Brasseur and S. Solomon, *Aeronomy of the middle atmosphere,* Dordrecht: D. Reidel Pub. Co. (2005).
[22] A.D. Danilov, *Common aeronomy,* Leningrad: Hydrometeoizdat (1978).
[23] D. Smith and P. Spanel, Mass Spectr. Rev. 14, 255 (1995).
[24] S.H. Lee, J.M. Reeves, J.C. Wilson, D.E. Hunton, A.A. Viggiano, T.M. Miller, J.O. Ballenthin, and L.R. Lait, Science 301, 1886 (2003).
[25] K. Nagato, C.S. Kim, M. Adachi, and K. Okuyama, J. Aerosol Sci. 36, 1036 (2005).
[26] F. Arnold, Nature 284, 610 (1980).
[27] F. Raes, A. Janssens, and R. Dingenen, J. Aerosol Sci. 17, 466 (1986).
[28] R.P. Turco, J.X. Zhao, and F. Yu, Geophys. Res. Lett. 25, 635 (1998).
[29] H. Svensmark, J.O.P. Pedersen, N.D. Marsh, M.G. Enghoff, and U.I. Uggerhoj, The Royal Society, Online ISSN, 1471 (2006).
[30] A.R. Rees and M.J.E. Sternberg, *From cells to atoms,* Chap. 1, 3, Oxford, London and so on: Blackwell Scientific Pub. (1984).

13

Recent Developments on the Mechanism and Kinetics of Esterification Reaction Promoted by Various Catalysts

Zuoxiang Zeng, Li Cui, Weilan Xue, Jing Chen and Yu Che
Institute of Chemical Engineering, East China University of Science and Technology, P.R.China

1. Introduction

Esters have played a significant role in daily living and chemical industry, such as plasticizers, fragrance, adhesive and lubricants (Joseph et al., 2005; Mbaraka & Shanks, 2006; Krause et al., 2009; Martínez et al., 2011). The vast majority of esters can be prepared using esterification reaction in the chemical engineering industry. Esterification has acquired further improvement from the engineering side; this mainly depends on the research of esterification kinetics. On the other hand, the need to control chemical reactions at the molecular level, which depends critically on the catalytic mechanism, is rapidly increasing (Salciccioli et al., 2011).

In the recent years, various esterification mechanisms were proposed for homogeneous and heterogeneous systems. Base on the mechanism, numerous kinetic models have been developed to represent the kinetic behaviors of esterification, such as simple orders or the power-law model, the pseudo-homogeneous model, the L-H model, the E-R model, etc.

Herein, we review the mechanisms of esterification catalyzed by inorganic acid, Lewis acid, metallic compounds, solid acids, ion-exchange resin, respectively. Meanwhile, the kinetics for each esterification is also conducted in detail. The study on the mechanism of various catalysts is not only useful in the present applications but it is required to enhance the scope of their applications. Therefore, it is desired to research and develop more efficient catalysts for high yield ester production, under mild reaction conditions. The esterification kinetics is important for simulation and design of a reactor.

A literature survey more than 90 relevant references has been done in this chapter. The studies on esterification are mainly focused on the following aspects: (1) establishing the adequate reaction mechanism according to the research papers, and (2) evaluating the available esterification kinetics.

2. Esterification mechanism and kinetic model

2.1 Inorganic acids

Inorganic acids, such as H_2SO_4, HCl and HI, are still being widely applied in the chemical industry (Liu et al., 2006; Schmitt et al., 2008). Under this condition, they are used as homogenous catalysts for cheap price, high activity and efficiency (greater density of acid sites per gram) (Sanz et al., 2002), stable performance. There is no doubt that mineral acid-catalyzed esterifications have been the subjects of extensive studies because of their long history (Liu et al., 2006; Vahteristo et al., 2008). For instance, it can be mentioned that Berthelot and Saint-Gilles studied the equilibrium of acetic acid with ethanol in 1862(Huiping & Xiaohua, 2006).

Many researchers have conducted a number of experiments to study the mechanism and kinetics of esterifications promoted by mineral acids (Cardoso et al., 2008). Summarizing recent research and development, esterification is an additive-eliminate course in the presence of mineral acid catalyst, generally complying with the following four typical and mature mechanisms.

2.1.1 Bimolecular reaction

In 1895, Emil Fischer discovered that esters are formed simply by heating a carboxylic acid in alcohol solution containing a small amount of strong acid catalyst (Zhang et al., 1995; Rönnback et al., 1997; Otera & Nishikido, 2009). The following mechanism, which includes five elementary reactions, was proposed:

1. Ketonic oxygen is easy to capture hydrogen ion to form protonated carbonyl substrate.
2. The substrate makes carbon atom of carboxyl possess higher electropositive, which is conducive to the attack of nucleophile (RCOH) to generate a tetrahedral intermediate.
3. Transfer of a proton from one oxygen atom to another yields a second tetrahedral intermediate and converts the OH group into a good leaving group.
4. The acyl-oxygen bond disconnects and one water molecule lost.
5. Loss of a proton gives the ester product.

The chemical reaction can be expressed as Figure 1.

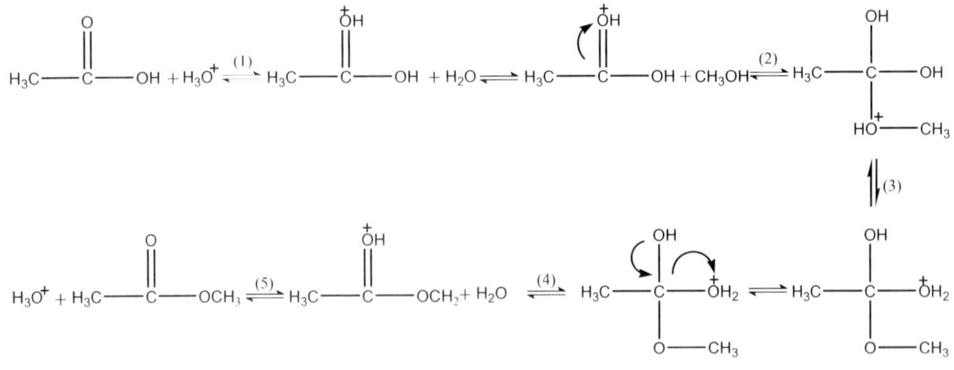

Fig. 1. Mechanism of bimolecular reaction

Streitwieser explained how the proton transfers specifically in 1985(Streitwieser et al., 1985; Liu et al., 2006; Fei & Zhao, 2009). The above chemical step (3) can be written as Figure 2:

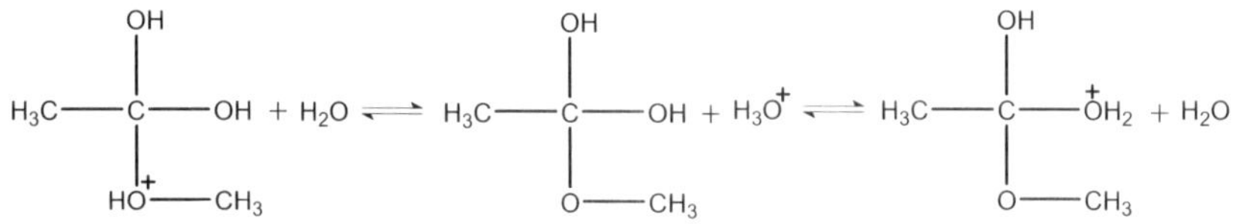

Fig. 2. The proton transfers step

In addition, Streitweiser considered that step (2) is the rate-determining stage. The total reaction is:

$$CH_3COOH + CH_3OH \rightleftharpoons CH_3COOCH_3 + H_2O \tag{1}$$

The result of the reaction is that the rupture of carboxylic acid acyl-oxygen bond occurs, and the hydroxy of acid is replaced by alkoxy, which is a nucleophilic substitution process of carboxylic acids.

Esterifications of primary alcohols, secondary alcohols with carboxylic acids comply with this mechanism usually. According to this mechanism, the intermediate with a tetrahedral structure is more crowd than reactants, which makes the structure of carboxylic acid and alcohol have a significant effect on the easy of esterification.

The activity of different structures of the alcohol and carboxylic acid in esterification obeys the following order: Alcohol: CH_3OH > RCH_2OH > R_2CHOH; Acid: CH_3COOH > RCH_2COOH > $R_2CHCOOH$ > R_3CCOOH (Solomons, 1986; March, 1992; TianQuan 1992; Fei & Zhao, 2009).It shows that straight-chain structure is easier than branched- chain structure to esterification, and the more the branched-chain is, the lower the rate will be.

Based on the above mechanism proposed by Streitweiser, Rönnback, et al. developed a esterification kinetic model of carboxylic acid with methanol in the presence of hydrogen iodide though isothermal batch experiments at 30-60℃. The catalyst concentration varied from 0.05 to 10.0 wt%. Because the proton-donation step (1) as well as the subsequent steps (3)-(5) is assumed to be rapid, the simplified mechanism shown in Figure 3:

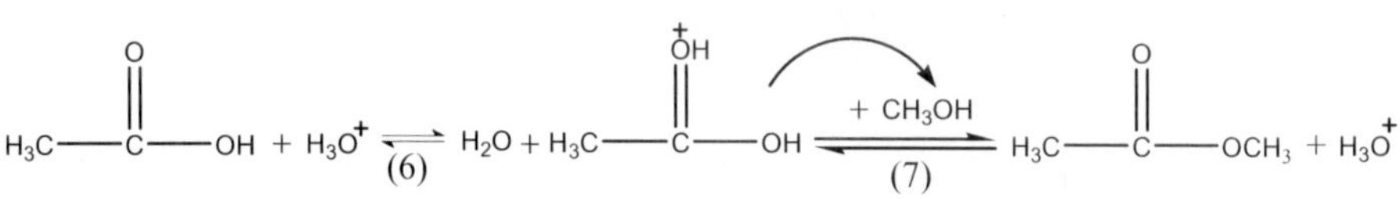

Fig. 3. The simplified mechanism

The reaction rate can therefore be expressed as:

$$r = r_2 = k_2 c_A c_{CH_3OH} - k_{-2} c_E c_{H_3O^+} \tag{2}$$

where r is the total rate, r_2 is the rate of step(2), A is $CH_3C(OH)_2^+$ and E is CH_3COOCH_3.

The concentration of the intermediate A is obtained after applying the quasi-equilibrium hypothesis on the rapid step(6):

$$K_6 = K_1 = c_A \cdot c_{H_2O} / c_{CH_3COOH} \cdot c_{H_3O^+} \tag{3}$$

The rate equation is rewritten as follows,

$$r = r_2 = K_1 k_2 \left(\frac{c_{H_3O^+}}{c_{H_2O}} \right) \left[c_{CH_3COOH} \cdot c_{CH_3OH} - \frac{c_E \cdot c_{H_2O}}{K_1 (k_2/k_{-2})} \right] \tag{4}$$

The product K_1 (k_2/k_{-2}) equals the equilibrium constant of the overall reaction K_{E2}. In addition, the product K_1k_2 is denoted by a lumped constant k_2'. Thus, we obtain for r_2,

$$r = r_2 = k_2' \left(\frac{c_{H_3O^+}}{c_{H_2O}} \right) \left(c_{CH_3COOH} \cdot c_{CH_3OH} - \frac{c_E \cdot c_{H_2O}}{K_{E2}} \right) \tag{5}$$

The kinetic and equilibrium parameters included in Equation (5) are estimated from experimental data with regression analysis. Simulation of the model with the estimated parameters revealed that Equation (5) can predict the experimental trends in the acid-catalyzed esterification correctly.

2.1.2 Single-molecule reaction

The tertiary alcohol is prone to generate carbocation under acidic condition. Therefore, the mechanism of tert- esterification is different from that of the primary and secondary alcohol, it follows the single-molecule reaction process(shown in Figure 4):The tertiary alcohol combines with protons to generate protonated alcohol(1); The protonated alcohol is got rid of a molecule water to produce tert-carbocation(2), which is very stable; Then the electrophilic attacking is taken place between the tert-carbocation and oxygen atom of carboxylate, the protonated ester(3) is yielded; The loss of a proton from the protonated ester gives the product(4) (Bart et al., 1994).

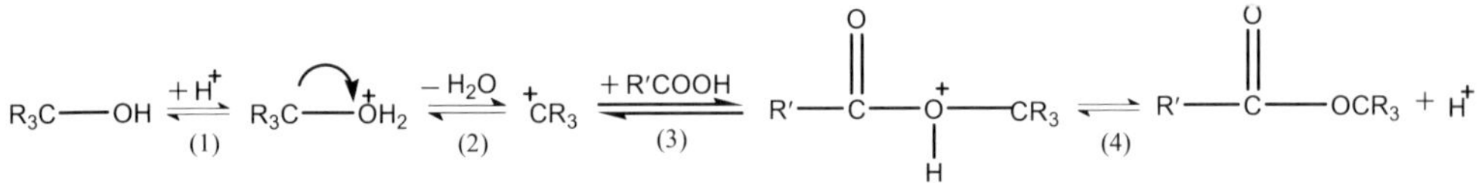

Fig. 4. Mechanism of tert-esterification

2.1.3 Large-steric reaction

Aromatic acid has serious steric hindrance. If there are both ortho-methyls, just as 2.4.6-trimethyl benzoic acid, the alcohol molecule is so difficult to access to carboxyl that the esterification cannot occur. However, if 2.4.6- trimethyl benzoic acid is dissolved in the 100% sulfuric-acid solution, acylilum ion will be formed as shown in Figure 5. Then the added alcohol with the acylilum ion produced ester. The reaction will conduct smoothly (Streitwieser et al., 1985).

This kind of esterification could occur for the reason that carbon atom of the acylilum ion is sp^2 hybridized and coplanar with the benzene ring, Then alcohol molecule can be virtually unhindered to attack the acylilum ion from above or below of the molecular plane. Esterifications conducts with this mechanism are merely few.

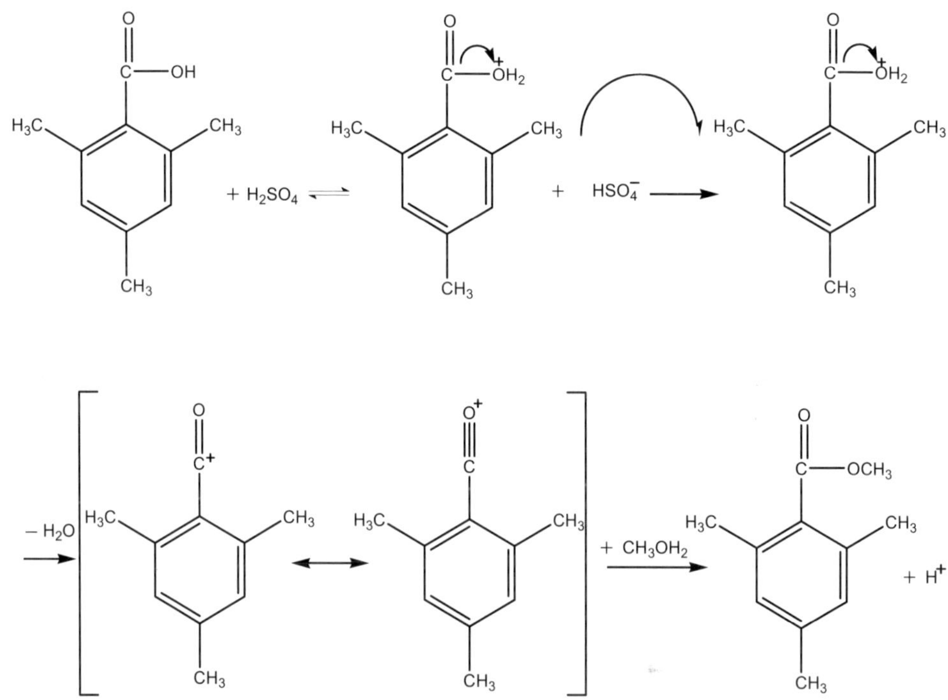

Fig. 5. Mechanism of large-steric reaction

2.1.4 Sulfuric acid

Dhanuka showed that the mechanism of sulfuric acid-catalyzed esterification is the model of alkyl sulfuric intermediate. It's a two-step reaction. R´-O-SO_3H firstly is generated via sulfuric acid with alcohol, which is treated as a catalyst in the second step (Lide, 1994):

$$R'OH + H_2SO_4 \rightleftharpoons R'OSO_3 + H_2O \tag{6}$$

$$RCOOH + R'OH \xrightleftharpoons{R'OSO_3} RCOOR' + H_2O \tag{7}$$

The alkylation reaction of sulfuric acid with alcohol is irreversible (Aranda et al., 2008).Therefore the reaction rate can be expressed as:

$$r = k(C_A C_B - C_W C_E / K) \tag{8}$$

where k is rate constant and K is equilibrium constant; C_A, C_B, C_W, C_E is the concentration of carboxylic acid, alcohol, water and ester, respectively.

In 2009, Fei, *et al.* studied on the esterification behaviors of neo-polyhydric alcohols with fatty acids catalyzed by sulfuric acid. It was found that the esterification follows the above mechanism.

2.2 Lewis acids

Lewis acid is a compound or ionic species that can accept an electron pair from a donor compound to form a Lewis adduct, such as $ZnCl_2$, Mg $(ClO_4)_2$, $Sn[N(SO_2\text{-n-}C_8F_{17})_2]_4$. It is potentially useful on the production of esters as a catalyst, the reason is that it can be easily separated from the reaction media (Sanchez et al., 1992; Cardoso et al., 2009); moreover, comparing with Bronsted acid, template effects are to be expected as Lewis acid sterically bulkier than a proton. In 1964, Anantakrishnan, et al. investigated the esterification reaction of Ac_2O with 50% MeOH, EtOH, PrOH, and iso-PrOH, in 50% Me_2CO or Dioxane as solvent, using Lewis acid ($ZnCl_2$) as catalyst.

Along with the scientific and technological progress and social development, more and more researchers have concerned about this issue, including the kinds of catalysts, the mechanism and kinetics of reaction. Thus, the contents containing the reaction mechanism and esterification kinetics have been significantly reviewed according to the type of catalysts as follows.

2.2.1 Metal chloride

Ethyl oleate was synthesized by the esterification of and ethanol catalyzed by $SnCl_2 \cdot 2H_2O$ (Cardoso et al., 2008). Under the circumstance of excess ethanol, the effects of the concentration of the catalyst and oleic acid, and temperature on the reaction rate were investigated. A related esterification mechanism was presented and described as follows: in presence of Sn^{2+}($SnCl_2 \cdot 2H_2O$) catalyst, the carbonyl of the fatty acid is polarized to activate of substrate, which makes the nucleophilic attack to the molecules by ethanol become more favorable. Cardoso et al. investigated the effect of different carbonic chain of alcohol (methyl alcohol, ethyl alcohol, n-propyl alcohol, n-butyl alcohol) on the conversion of oleic acid into respective ester. The results showed that the conversion rate was down with the increase of carbon chain of alcohol, which indicated that high bulk hindrance occurs on the hydroxyl of the alcohol, and the efficient attack of them to the polarized carbonyl of oleic acid is reduced. However, it is not clear how the carbonyl is polarized by Sn^{2+}.

Kinetic data of esterification of ethanol and oleic acid catalyzed by $SnCl_2$ ($n_{ethanol} : n_{oleic\ acid} : n_{SnCl2} = 120 : 1 : 0.01$) were measured at the reflux temperature, and kinetic model was obtained as follows,

$$\ln C = -0.00278 \times t - 2.3155 \tag{9}$$

where C is the concentration of oleic acid, t is the reaction time.

The effectiveness of the catalyst $SnCl_2 \cdot 2H_2O$ has been investigated in a broad range of concentrations, and the results are approximately concomitant with a first order dependence in relation to the catalyst concentration. The effect of the temperature on the initial rate of the esterification was determined, showing that an increase in the reaction temperature was caused a corresponding improvement on the reaction rate, especially at a range of 45-75°C. The value of activation energy for the reaction was determined from the data of the initial rate to be 46.69 $kJ \cdot mol^{-1}$.

The kinetics of catalytic esterification of castor oil with lauric acid using $SnCl_2 \cdot 2H_2O$ was studied (Kulkarni & Sawant, 2003). Effects of the catalyst concentration and temperature on the progress of the reaction were investigated. The reaction was assumed to be a first order with respect to each reactant. For the irreversible, bimolecular-type second order reaction,

$$A+B \xrightarrow{Catalyst} Product \tag{10}$$

The consumption rate of A ($-r_A$) is expressed by,

$$-r_A = kC_C C_A C_B \tag{11}$$

where C_A, C_B, C_C is the concentration of lauric acid, hydroxyl group and catalyst (mol/mL), respectively.

The catalyst concentration was constant throughout the reaction; therefore, Equation (11) can be rewritten as

$$-r_A = k'C_A C_B\ ,\ k' = kC_C \tag{12}$$

The integrated form of Equation (12) using fractional conversion is,

$$\ln[(1-X_B)/(1-X_A)] = (C_{B0} - C_{A0})k't \tag{13}$$

where X_A, X_B is fractional conversion of the lauric acid and the -OH group, respectively; C_{A0}, C_{B0} is initial concentration of the lauric acid and hydroxyl group (mol/mL), respectively; and k is the second-order rate constant ($mL^2mol^{-2}min^{-1}$).

The esterification reaction of castor oil and lauric acid was carried out using $SnCl_2 \bullet 2H_2O$ as catalyst (0.25,0.5,1.0 and 2.0 % w/w catalyst loadings) at 185°C and the kinetic data were measured. The results showed that there was a good linearity relationship between ln $[(1-X_B)/(1-X_A)]$ and t. The plot of k' versus C_C was close to a straight line. For the given values of C_{B0}, C_{A0} and C_C, the kinetic model of esterification of castor oil and lauric acid was obtained at 185°C,

$$\ln[(1-X_B)/(1-X_A)] = 1.62 \times 10^6 (C_{B0} - C_{A0})C_C t \tag{14}$$

It was investigated the esterification of octanoic acid and n-octyl alcohol utilizing metallic chlorides (KCl, $CoCl_2$, $MgCl_2$, $ZnCl_2$, $FeCl_3$ etc.) in a stirred tank reactor (Santos, 1996). The results showed that the best efficiency of the formatted ester (n-octyl octanoate) was obtained with ferric chloride, indicating that the higher electronegativity of the metallic ion and the existence of free d orbitals in the transition metals are responsible for the higher yield of ester. Thus, the existence of free d orbitals in Fe^{3+} (its configuration: $3d^3$) gives the possibility of the formation of complexes with OH groups of the reactants, which explains the highest activity found for $FeCl_3 \bullet 6H_2O$ in this way. Generally, in the catalytic systems whose bases were constituted by a transition metal, such as Fe, Co, Mn, Zn, the mechanism of esterification can similarly be ascribed to the above mentioned.

The esterification reaction of octanoic acid and n-octyl alcohol was carried out using $CoCl_2 \bullet 2H_2O$ as catalyst (0, 0.0385, 0.077 mol/l) at 70℃ and the kinetic data were measured. The experimental curves suggest that the kinetics of esterification between octanoic acid and n-octyl alcohol can be described by an irreversible second order power model, considering the catalyst concentration as a constant in the kinetic model proposed. The activation energy is seen to have a value of 53 kcal/mol (Urteaga et al., 1994).

The reaction rate went on a power law model of second order, one for the alcohol and one for the acid,

$$r = kC_{alcohol}C_{acid} \quad (15)$$

where k is kinetic constant (l mol^{-1}min^{-1})

$$r = 9.30 \times 10^{-4} C_{alcohol}C_{acid} \quad (16)$$

Catalyst	**k[l mol^{-1} min^{-1}]**	**R^2**
KCl	0.95×10^{-4}	0.988
$CaCl_2$•$6H_2O$	0.83×10^{-4}	0.980
$NiCl_2$•$6H_2O$	1.86×10^{-4}	0.805
$CoCl_2$•$6H_2O$	1.69×10^{-4}	0.994
$MgCl_2$•$6H_2O$	5.87×10^{-4}	0.986
$MnCl_2$•$6H_2O$	1.20×10^{-4}	0.852
$FeCl_2$•$6H_2O$	1.62×10^{-4}	0.977
$BaCl_2$•$2H_2O$	0.96×10^{-4}	0.955
$SnCl_2$•$2H_2O$	10.00×10^{-4}	0.943
$ZnCl_2$•XH_2O	1.54×10^{-4}	0.876
$AlCl_3$•$6H_2O$	6.91×10^{-4}	0.876
$SnCl_4$	9.50×10^{-4}	0.896
$FeCl_3$•$6H_2O$	9.30×10^{-4}	0.845

Table 1. Kinetic constant for homogeneous reactions

It was also observed that the homogeneous reactions were fitted much better than the pseudo-homogeneous reactions to proposed kinetics model. The reason for it is that an important influence of the physical steps that could have place in the global mechanism of this reaction.

2.2.2 Perchlorate

Perchlorates are of great chemical interest and importance. The high electronegativity, together with the relatively low charge density, results in poor complexing ability of the perchlorate ion. Metal perchlorates can therefore act as powerful Lewis acids, with this character mainly being exploited to activate bidentate compounds (Bartoli et al., 2007). Magnesium perchlorate is one of the most active Lewis acids for esterification. By 2003, Gooβen & Döhring synthesized various esters through a decarboxylative esterification of alkyl and aryl carboxylic acids with dialkyl dicarbonates in the presence of 1 mol% of $Mg(ClO_4)_2$. However, more in-depth investigations on the mechanism of this reaction are underway.

Until 2006, Bartoli, et al. explored the efficiency of Perchlorates (such as $Mg(ClO_4)_2$, $LiClO_4$, $Zn(ClO_4)_2$) as catalyst to activate diethyl dicarbonate for preparing alkyl and aryl ethyl carbonates. The results showed that among the above catalysts, $Mg(ClO_4)_2$ is the most efficient one. The reactions between diethyl dicarbonate and various alcohols including aliphatic alcohols and aryl alcohols were studied, and the results obtained suggest that the reaction rate depends on the acidity of the starting hydroxy compound, and not on its nucleophilicity. Herein, the reaction mechanism was presented to explain the observed reaction characteristics. In fact, the more acidic and less nucleophilic phenols react faster than aliphatic alcohols. Thus, the release of the alcoholic proton should be involved in the rate-determining step. A reasonable mechanistic hypothesis is depicted as follows (Figure 6),

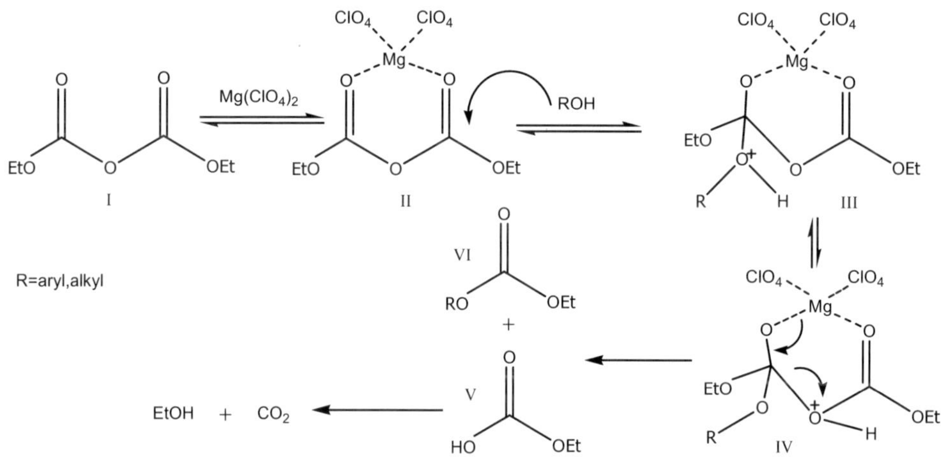

Fig. 6. Mechanism for preparing alkyl and aryl ethyl carbonates catalyzed by $Mg(ClO_4)_2$

Due to the ability of coordinating with 1,3-dicarbonyl compounds, $Mg(ClO_4)_2$ reacts with diethyl dicarbonate to form complex (II), which can undergo the addition of the alcohol to form intermediate (III). An internal proton shift in (III) can produce intermediate (IV), which can irreversibly decompose to the mixed carbonate (VI) and to the carbonic acid monoester (V). Owing to its high instability, (V) immediately produces EtOH and CO_2. The irreversibility of the last two steps drives the overall process towards (III). This explanation accounts for the formation of the mixed carbonate (VI) as the major product of the reaction (Jousseaume et al., 2003).

Nevertheless, this is a speculative hypothesis; more studies are in progress to find experimental evidence to elucidate the reaction mechanism.

2.3 Organometallic compound

Organometallic compounds containing bonds between carbons and metals provide a source of nucleophilic carbon atoms which can react with electrophilic carbon to form a new carbon-carbon bond (Banach et al., 2001; Finelli et al., 2004). Organometallics find practical uses in catalytic processes. For example, Titanium tetrabutoxide, Butylhydroxyoxo-stannane are well-known catalysts for the esterification between diacid and diol in polyester industry (Grzesik et al., 2000; Prabhakarn et al., 2011). The catalytic mechanism and kinetic model of related catalysts are reviewed in the following discussions.

2.3.1 Titanate

Titanium-based catalysts have been known for many years and actually are widely used for the production of poly (butylene terephthalate) (PBT), poly (trimethylene terephthalate)

(PTT), and so on. Recently, the developments of titanium-based catalysts make a marvelous progress (Liu et al., 2006), such as titanium dioxide based catalyst (C-94) mainly focusing on designing to be stable and having good activity and color.

The mechanism of the mono-esterification between terephthalic acid (TPA) and 1,4-butanediol (BDO) catalyzed by $Ti(OBu)_4$ was proposed (Tian et al., 2010). As shown in Figure 7, the reaction involves the formation of an adduct between a carbonyl group and Ti atom.

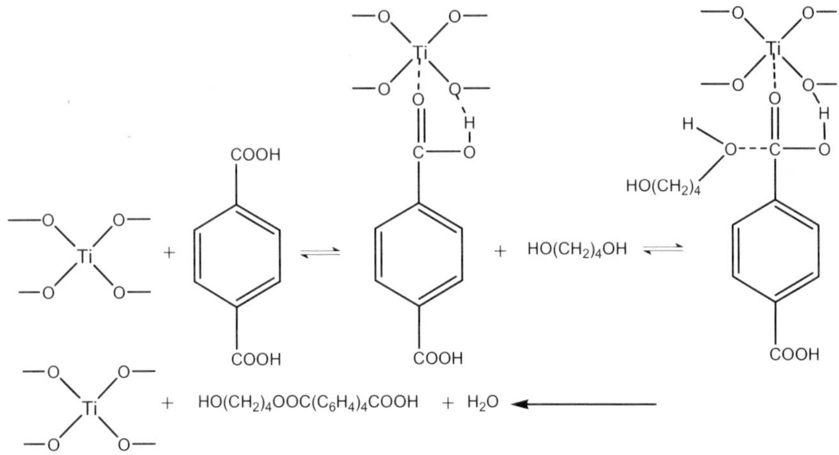

Fig. 7. Mechanism of the mono-esterification between BDO and TPA catalyzed by $Ti(OBu)_4$

Although the reaction system of TPA and BDO is heterogeneous, it can be assumed that the esterification occurs only in the liquid phase. The initial rate method is used to predict the reaction rate. The kinetic model of mono-esterification between TPA and BDO catalyzed by $Ti(OBu)_4$ in the temperature of 463-483K was investigated (Bhutada & Pangarkar, 1986). The reaction rate r can be described as,

$$r = kC_{A}^{n}C_{B}^{m} \tag{17}$$

where C_A, C_B is the concentrations of TPA and BDO, respectively, k is the reaction rate constant, n and m is the reaction order with respect to A and B.

The reaction order can be obtained from experiments in which the initial rates are measured at a series of initial reactant concentrations. The results show that the reaction order for TPA and BDO is nearly a constant of 0.7 and 0.9, respectively. Therefore, the rate equation of the esterification is written as follows,

$$r = k_{Ti}C_{B}^{0.9}C_{A}^{0.7} \tag{18}$$

$$\ln k_{Ti} = 11.73 - 7.67 \times 10^{3} / T(R^{2} = 0.997) \tag{19}$$

where k_{Ti} is the rate constant ($L^{0.6} \cdot mol^{-0.6} \cdot min^{-1}$), R^2 is the correlation coefficient.

The reaction of behenic acid with fatty alcohols (decanol, lauryl alcohol, myristyl alcohol and cetyl alcohol) was studied by Tiwari, et al. (Tiwari & Sawant, 2005) using TBT as catalyst in the temperature range of 165-185℃.The reaction rate for the catalytic reaction is the sum of the rates of both the uncatalyzed (Equation (20)) and the catalyzed reactions (Equation (21)),

$$CH_3(CH_2)_{20}COOH+CH_3(CH_2)_8CH_2OH \rightleftharpoons CH_3(CH_2)_{20}COOCH_2(CH_2)_8CH_3+H_2O \quad (20)$$

$$CH_3(CH_2)_{20}COOH+CH_3(CH_2)_8CH_2OH \xrightarrow{Catalyst} CH_3(CH_2)_{20}COOCH_2(CH_2)_8CH_3+H_2O \quad (21)$$

Excess of the acids is used to get almost complete conversion of the alcohols, and the unreacted acid was easily removed from the ester as a sodium salt. Assuming that it is first order dependence of the reaction rate on each reactant and the catalyst, the overall rate expression in the integrated form becomes,

$$X_A / (1 - X_A) = C_{A0}kt \quad (22)$$

where X_A is fractional conversion of behenic acid; C_{A0} is initial concentration of behenic acid; $k = k_c C_c + k_{uc}$, k_c is catalyzed reaction rate constant, k_{uc} is uncatalyzed reaction rate constant; C_C is catalyst concentration.

The kinetic data show that there is a reasonably good agreement between experimental points and the ones calculated by Equation (22). The values of activation energy obtained for the uncatalyzed (ΔE_{uc}) and catalyzed (ΔE_c) reaction of behenic acid with decanol, lauryl alcohol, myristyl alcohol and cetyl alcohol are shown in Table 2.The model Equation (22) is also appropriate for the reaction of erucic acid with cetyl alcohol and oleyl alcohol using TBT as a catalyst (Tiwari & Sawant, 2005).

Alcohol	ΔE_{uc}(kJ mol^{-1})	ΔE_c (kJ mol^{-1})
decanol	68.1	86.2
lauryl alcohol	69.2	79.6
myristyl alcohol	64.5	78.6
cetyl alcohol	67.3	87.1

Table 2. Activation energy value for uncatalyzed and catalyzed reaction

2.3.2 Butylhydroxyoxo-stannane

Stannum-based catalysts such as butylhydroxyoxo-stannane (BuSnOOH) are commonly used for the synthesis of poly (ethylene terephthalate) (PET) (Patel et al., 2007), poly (butylene terephthalate) (PBT) and so on. Due to the similarity in coordination number and electronegativity between Ti and Sn, as shown in Figure 8, the mechanism of BuSnOOH catalyst is also proposed by TIAN, et al.

The initial rate method will also be used in this reacting system. The kinetic model of mono-esterification reaction between terephthalic acid (TPA) and 1,4-butanediol (BDO) is expressed as follow,

$$r = k_{Sn} C_B^{0.9} C_A^2 \quad (23)$$

$$\ln k_{Sn} = 9.58 - 6.42 \times 10^3 / (R^2 = 0.999) \quad (24)$$

where C_A and C_B is the concentrations of TPA and BDO, respectively; k_{Sn} is the rate constant ($L^{1.9} \cdot mol^{-1.9} \cdot min^{-1}$) .

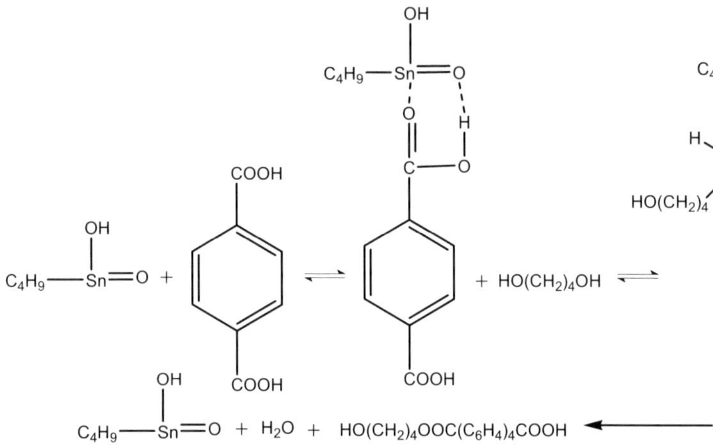

Fig. 8. Mechanism of the mono-esterification between BDO and TPA catalyzed by BuSnOOH

2.3.3 Fluorous metaloxide

In 2004, Otera investigated the transesterification and esterification of various acids and alcohols using 1, 3-disubstituted tetraalkyldistannoxanes as catalyst, and found that the catalytic mechanism different from that proposed for tetraalkyldistannoxanes. In the latter case, the initial step is substitution of the bridging X group to give an alkoxydistannoxane intermediate, $(YR_2SnOSnR_2OR)_2$, which works as an alkoxyl donor. In contrast, for 1, 3-disubstituted tetraalkyldistannoxanes, no substitution takes place at the bridging position by an alkoxy group. As described above, the bridging chlorine in 1, 3-disubstituted tetraalkyldistannoxanes is never substituted by isothiocyanate ion, but experiences strong association.

A related mechanism of the esterification is proposed that both alcohol and acid coordinate on the terminal tin atom (Yoshida et al., 2006), on which the interchange between the hydroxyl groups of carboxylic acids and the alkoxy groups of alcohols takes place. Meanwhile, since water, one of the products, is less fluorophilic, the esterification of carboxylic acids with alcohols should proceed efficiently.

Fluorous distannoxanes exhibit unusually high preference for fluorous solvents over common organic solvents thanks to coverage of the molecular surface with fluoroalkyl groups. While the fluorous biphase technology had been high-lighted mainly in terms of facile separation of products and fluorous catalysts, it has now been revealed that the equilibrium is also controllable under fluorous biphase conditions. Thus, the esterification has been completely driven in the desired direction by use of a 1:1 ratio of starting materials without recourse to any dehydration technique.

2.4 Solid acids

The research for solid acids has become active since the early 1970s. In 1971, Isao, et al. investigated the esterification of ethanol with acetic acid on silica-alumina, and a simple kinetic model based on a Langmuir-Hinshelwood mechanism was proposed. Since then, the esterification catalyzed by solid acids is widely studied and largely reported (Jiang et al., 2008; Jothiramalingam & Wang, 2009; Li et al., 2010). Herein, the esterification mechanisms and kinetic models according to the different types of solid acids are reviewed, such as sulfate-supported metal oxides (SO_4^{2-}/M_xO_y), TPA/SnO_2.

2.4.1 TPA/SnO_2

The esterification of palmitic acid with methanol using 12-Tungstophosphoric acid (TPA)/SnO_2 was investigated (Srilatha et al., 2011). The reaction is shown as follows:

$$\underset{(A)}{C_{15}H_{31}COOH}+\underset{(B)}{CH_3OH} \underset{}{\overset{k}{\rightleftharpoons}} \underset{(C)}{C_{15}H_{31}COOCH_3}+\underset{(D)}{H_2O} \tag{25}$$

As shown in Figure 9, the mechanism of this esterification is proposed,

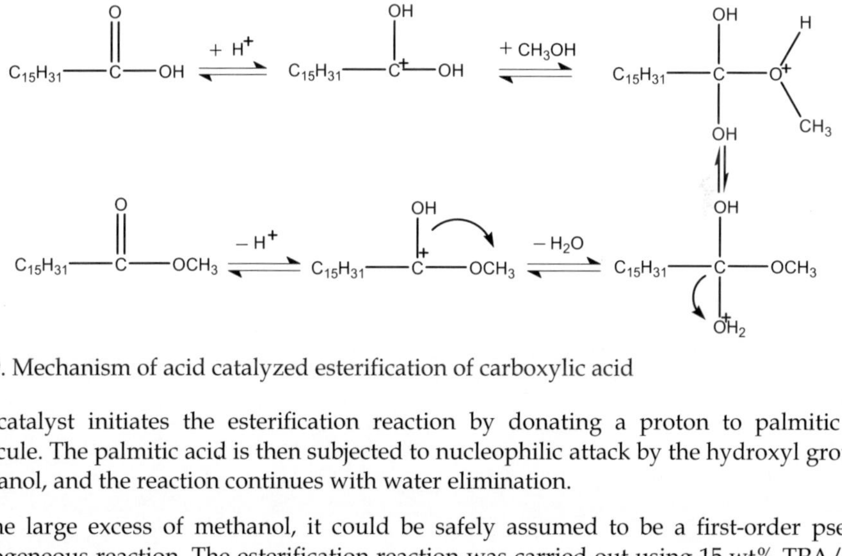

Fig. 9. Mechanism of acid catalyzed esterification of carboxylic acid

The catalyst initiates the esterification reaction by donating a proton to palmitic acid molecule. The palmitic acid is then subjected to nucleophilic attack by the hydroxyl group of methanol, and the reaction continues with water elimination.

As the large excess of methanol, it could be safely assumed to be a first-order pseudo-homogeneous reaction. The esterification reaction was carried out using 15 wt% TPA/SnO_2 as catalyst (w_A: w_{cat}=5:1) in the temperature range of 45-65℃and the kinetic data were measured.

The reaction rate can be described as follows:

$$-ln(1-X_A)=kt \tag{26}$$

where X_A is the conversation of palmitic acid, t is the reaction time, k is the reaction rate constant.

The plots of $-\ln(1-X_A)$ versus t at different temperatures showed that there was a good linearity relationship. Linear fitting to ln$k$ - 1/T curve was carried out and the reaction rate constant can be described as follows:

$$k = \exp(8.66 - 4369 / T) \quad (27)$$

The activation energy was obtained as 36.33 kJ mol^{-1}.

2.4.2 SO_4^{2-} /M_xO_y

The solid superacid (SO_4^{2-} /M_xO_y) is a new type of catalyst used in esterification (Jiang et al., 2004). M_xO_y are usually some transition metal oxides such as ZrO_2 and TiO_2.

In 2010, Rattanaphra, et al. investigated the esterification of myristic acid with methanol catalyzed by sulfated zirconia. The mechanism of esterification is probably following Langmuir-Hinshelwood model (Arata, 2009; Reddy & Patil, 2009). It is possible that methanol and myristic acid are preferentially adsorbed on the Bronsted acid sites of sulfated zirconia during esterification. The hydroxyl group of methanol is protonated by Bronsted acid on the catalyst surface while the protonation of myristic acid on an adjacent site leads to the carbocation. Deprotonation of methanol oxygen produces the nucleophile, which attacks the carbocation to generate a tetrahedral intermediate. As shown in Figure 10, the tetrahedral intermediate eliminates water to form ester.

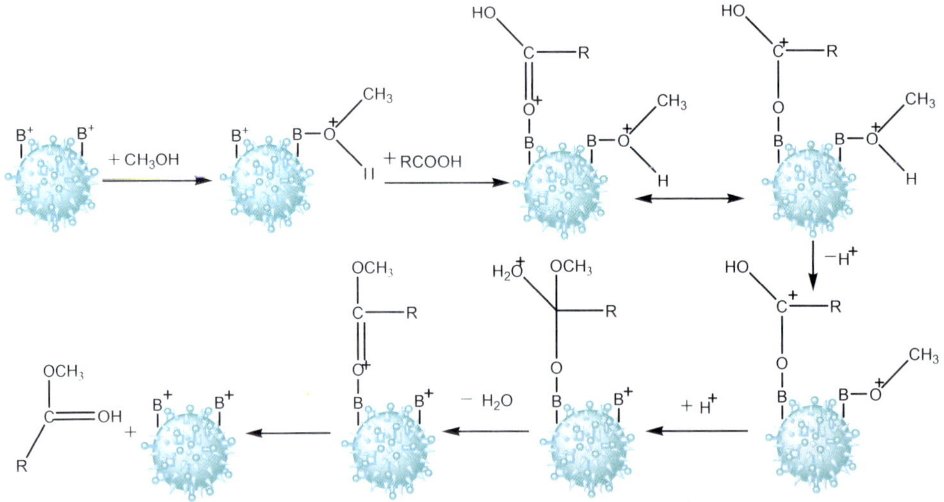

Fig. 10. Mechanism of esterification catalyzed by sulfated zirconia

In 2011, Rattanaphra, et al. also investigated the kinetic model of myristic acid esterification with methanol using sulfated zirconia as catalyst. The reaction is shown as follows:

$$CH_3(CH_2)_{12}COOH + CH_3OH \underset{k_{-1}}{\overset{k_1}{\rightleftharpoons}} CH_3(CH_2)_{12}COOCH_3 + H_2O \quad (28)$$

(A) (B) (E) (W)

The stirring rate is sufficient to overcome the diffusion limitation of reactive species. Therefore, the performance of pseudo-homogeneous model can be considered as satisfactory to correlate the kinetic data for the esterification. The rate equation can be written as follows:

$$-r_A = -\frac{dC_A}{dt} = k_1 C_A C_B - k_{-1} C_E C_W \quad (29)$$

where C_A, C_B, C_E and C_W is the concentration of myristic acid, methanol, myristic acid methyl ester and water respectively, k_1 is the forward rate constant and k_{-1} is the backward rate constant.

The equation can be rearranged to be:

$$\frac{dX_A}{dt} = k_1 C_{A0}[(1 - X_A)(M - X_A) - \frac{1}{K_e} X_A^2] \quad (30)$$

where X_A is the conversion of myristic acid， C_{A0} is the initial concentration of myristic acid, K_e is the equilibrium constant, M is the concentration ratio of methanol to myristic acid (M=C_{B0}/C_{A0}).

$$K_e = \frac{k_1}{k_{-1}} = \frac{X_{Ae}^2}{(1 - X_{Ae})(M - X_{Ae})} \quad (31)$$

The relationship between temperature and the forward rate constant in the temperature range of 393-443K is given as following equations,

$$k_1 = \exp(2.88 - 2707 / T) \quad (32)$$

The linear coefficient is 0.996, and the activation energy is 22.51 kJ /mol.

In 2004, Jiang, et al. studied the esterification of n-pentanol with benzoic acid using Al-pillared clay (PILC) supported SO_4^{2-} /TiO_2 superacid catalyst (Fang et al., 2010), and find that it is known that the generation of super acid sites in the system of SO_4^{2-} /M_xO_y solid superacid is necessarily promoted by the sulfur of the metal oxides, the more acid sites formed, the higher catalytic activity exhibited. Therefore, Al-PILC carrier can effectively enhance the catalytic activity.

In 2010, Zubir, et al. investigated the kinetic behavior of the heterogeneous catalyzed esterification of oleic acid with ethanol using tungstated zirconia as a catalyst in the temperature range of 303.15- 323.15K (Otera, 1993).

$$\underset{(A)}{CH_3(CH_2)_7CH{=}CH(CH_2)_7COOH} + \underset{(B)}{CH_3CH_2OH} \rightleftharpoons \underset{(C)}{CH_3(CH_2)_7CH{=}CH(CH_2)_7COOCH_2CH_3} + \underset{(D)}{H_2O} \quad (33)$$

The kinetics of esterification reaction can be expressed using a pseudo-homogeneous second-order equilibrium model in the absence of any intraparticle diffusional limitation as follows:

$$-r_A = k(C_A C_B - C_C C_D / K_e) \quad (34)$$

where C_A ,C_B, C_C, C_D is the concentration of oleic acid, ethanol, ethyl oleate and water, respectively, k is the kinetic constants for the forward reaction, K_e is the equilibrium constant.

$$K_e = \exp(29.42 - 10536 / T) \tag{35}$$

$$k = \exp(23.43 - 6242 / T). \tag{36}$$

The value of activation energy is 51.9 $kJ \cdot mol^{-1}$. The goodness-of-fit of the experimental data to the proposed model is assessed by comparing the experimental reaction rate with the theoretical prediction, and the experimental data are reproduced with errors not greater than 10%.

2.5 Ion-exchange resin

Ion-exchange resins, especially the cation-exchange resins such as Dowex, Amberlyst series are manufactured mainly by sulfonation of ethylbenzene first, followed by a cross-link with divinylbenzene (Liu & Tan, 2001; Alexandratos, 2008; Tesser et al., 2010). Because of their selective adsorption of reactants, surface acid site features, and swelling nature, these resins not only catalyze the esterification reaction but also affect the equilibrium conversion. They also show excellent performance such as reusable, mechanical separation, continuous operation as a heterogeneous catalyst in esterification (Yang et al., 2007; JagadeeshBabu et al., 2011; Ju et al., 2011; Toor et al., 2011).

By 1965, Bochner, et al. evaluated the performance of Dowex 50WX-8 as a catalyst for the esterification of salicylic acid with methanol. Through analyzing the experimental results, the Langmuir-isotherm applied to this system to describe the reaction rate. Since then, various mechanisms and kinetics of esterification between acids and alcohols catalyzed by cation- exchange resins were proposed. Here is an overview of the reaction mechanisms and kinetic models according to the type of cation-exchange resins.

2.5.1 Dowex

Dowex, a common cation-exchange resin, is widely used as catalysts in esterification (Vahteristo et al., 2009). In 2005, Kulawska, et al. investigated the esterification of maleic anhydride with octyl, decyl or dodecyl alcohol over Dowex 50Wx8-100, and the kinetic data were measured in the temperature range of 403-433 K (C_{0ALC}/C_{0MA} =5:1). Based on the data, a first order reaction was found- first order with respect to acid and zero order with respect to alcohol. The reaction rate can be described as follows,

$$r = -\frac{dc_M}{dt} = kc_M \tag{37}$$

where c_M is the concentration of maleic monoester, t is reaction time.

The values of activation energy are 66.0 (±0.65) kJ/mol, 58.6 (±0.4) kJ/mol, and 66.1(±0.4) kJ/mol for dioctyl, didencyl, and didodecyl maleate formation, respectively. However, the effects of the catalyst (the particle size and the concentration) and the mass transfer resistance on the reaction rate were not taken into account.

The esterification kinetics of acetic acid with iso-butanol catalyzed by Dowex 50 Wx2 was studied (Izci & Bodur, 2007). It is considered to be reversible reactions and can be described by pseudo-homogeneous (PH) model. The general reaction rate expression can be written as follows,

$$-r_A = k_1\left(C_A \times C_B - C_E \times C_W / K\right) \tag{38}$$

where subscripts A, B, E and W is acid, alcohol, ester and water, respectively, k_1 is forward reaction rate constant (L mol^{-1} min^{-1}), K is the equilibrium constant of the reaction.

It is found that this bimolecular type is second order reaction. The values of k_1 for different temperatures are 0.24x10^3 (318K), 1.00x10^3 (333K), 3.07x10^3 (348K). The activation energy was found to be 1.745 kJ$\cdot$mol^{-1} in the presence of Dowex 50 Wx2. However, the PH model does not take into account the resin swelling ratio, adsorption of the components and the non-ideal thermodynamic behavior of reactants and products (Ali &Merchant, 2006; Patel & Saha, 2007; Jeřábek et al., 2010; Erdem & Kara, 2011).

The kinetics of Dowex 50 Wx8-catalyzed esterification was studied between acetic acid and benzyl alcohol (Ali & Merchant, 2009). The swelling ratio of Dowex 50 Wx8 in different solvent was measured, and the results show that it decreases in the order of water, benzyl alcohol, acetic acid, benzyl acetate. Water appears to be preferentially adsorbed by the catalyst from a binary solution of acetic acid and water, and hinders the approach of butanol to the protonated acid. Therefore, the water exerts an adverse effect on the esterification rate.

The initial reaction rates of esterification between acetic acid and benzyl alcohol were measured at various conditions, and the Eley-Rideal (ER) model was used to correlate the data and showed a high degree of fit, indicating that the surface reaction between adsorbed alcohol and acid in the bulk is the rate-limiting step during the initial stage of the reaction. The ER model of this esterification can be described as follow,

$$ri = \frac{\left[M_{cat}k_f K_{alc}\left(a_{acid}a_{alc} - \left(a_{ester}a_{water} / K_a\right)\right)\right]}{\left[1 + K_{alc}a_{alc} + K_{water}a_{water}\right]} \tag{39}$$

$$k_f = 55770 \times \exp(-6661.4 / T) \tag{40}$$

$$\text{In}\left(K_a\right) = \left(-1279 / T\right) + 6.810 \tag{41}$$

where M_{cat} is the mass of the catalyst, g; a_{acid}, a_{alc}, a_{ester}, a_{water} is the activity of acid, alcohol, ester, water in the liquid phase, respectively; k_f is forward reaction rate constant for the esterification, mol g^{-1} s^{-1}. K_a is activity reaction equilibrium constant. K_{acid}, K_{alc}, K_{water} is adsorption equilibrium constant for the alcohol present in the system, respectively.

The activation energy form the above relationship was found to be 55.4kJ/mol.

However, as the reaction proceeds, the acid adsorption term might have to be introduced and in such an event the reaction kinetics would be represented by a dual site mechanistic, such as Langmuir-Hinshelwood (LH) model.

In 2011, Ju, et al. measured the kinetic data for the esterification of butyric acid with n-butanol over Dowex 50Wx8-400, and correlated with various types of kinetic models. Strong resin water affinity was taken into account, and the non-ideality of the system was considered by applying the no-random two liquid (NRTL) model. The comparisons of the conversion of butyric acid with reaction time between experimental data and ones predicted by these kinetic models reveal that the ER model and LH model are the most reasonable fit for describing the mechanism, with the total average error 12.52%. Surface reaction is the rate determining step, and the affinity between resin and water is found to be not strong. Therefore, the most possible esterification reaction mechanisms can be proposed as following lists:

1. Single site mechanism: the adsorbed butyric acid onto the catalysts reacts with non-adsorbed n-butanol in the bulk.
2. Single site mechanism: the adsorbed n-butanol onto the catalyst reacts with non-adsorbed butyric acid in the bulk.
3. Dual site mechanism: both the reactants adsorbed on the catalyst surface and react there.

In 2007, Ali, et al. studied the esterification of 1-propanol with propionic acid catalyzed by Dowex 50Wx8-400. The experiments were carried out over a temperature range of 303.15-333.15K, and the reaction mechanism for the esterification was proposed (Lilja et al., 2002). The reaction is initiated by the transfer of a proton from the catalyst to the carboxylic acid , and the carbonium ion is formed during the reaction. The ion is accessible for a nucleophilic attack by the hydroxyl group from the alcohol. After that, a molecule of water is lost from the ion. Finally, the catalyst is recovered by the transfer of proton from the ion to the catalyst surface. This mechanism is represented by the following scheme (Figure 11):

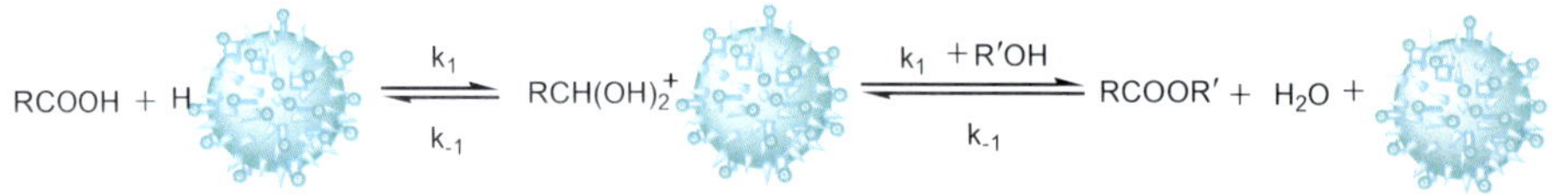

Fig. 11. Mechanism for the esterification catalyzed by Dowex 50Wx8-400

The donation of a proton is commonly assumed to be a fast step, and the nucleophilic substitution is usually assumed to be the rate determined step.

Based on the above reaction mechanism, external and internal diffusion can be negligible, and the E-R model (Equation (39)) is applied. The activity coefficients of components can be predicted using UNIFAC model. Meanwhile, by taking into account the strong water affinity for Dowex 50Wx8-400, a correction term (a) was added to the activity term for water in rate expression. The experimental results for the esterification between 1-propanol and propionic acid were modeled according to the above kinetic model. The total average error between the predicted and experimental mole fractions of acid is 1.65%. The activation energy for the forward reaction was estimated to be 67.3 kJ /mol.

The effect of different alcohols on the conversion of propionic acid was investigated using methanol, ethanol, 1-propanol and 1-butanol. The results reveal that the conversion of propionic acid at the same time intervals decreases with increasing the chain length of the alcohol, indicating that the chain length of alcohol has a retarding effect on the reaction rate. It is ascribing to the steric hindrance. Meanwhile, the LH model is used to correlate the above experimental data, and the total average error between the predicted and experimental mole fractions of acid is 5.71%.

Interestingly, the kinetic study of esterifications between the same acid (acetic acid) and different alcohol (benzyl alcohol, 2-propanol) in the presence of Dowex 50x8 reveal that the ER model and the LH model is the most suitable predictive model, respectively. These observations seem to indicate that the type of acid and alcohol play an important role in determining the number of sites involved in this heterogeneously catalyzed reaction.

2.5.2 Amberlyst

Amberlyst, acidic cation-exchange resin bead, was widely used as excellent heterogeneous acid catalysts for a wide variety of organic reactions owing to its macroreticular and continuous open pore structure (Pöpken et al., 2000; Kolah et al., 2007; Pereira et al., 2008; Tsai et al., 2011).

In 2011, Tsai, et al. investigated the kinetic behavior of heterogeneous esterification of dibasic acids such as glutaric acid with methanol over Amberlyst 35. As shown in Equation (42) and Equation (43), the esterification includes two reversible reactions in series accompanying with an intermediate of monomethyl glutarate (MMG):

$$\underset{(A)}{HOOC(CH_2)_3COOH} + \underset{(B)}{CH_3OH} \underset{k_2}{\overset{k_1}{\rightleftharpoons}} \underset{(C)}{HOOC(CH_2)_3COOCH_3} + \underset{(D)}{H_2O} \quad (42)$$

$$\underset{(C)}{HOOC(CH_2)_3COOCH_3} + \underset{(B)}{CH_3OH} \underset{k_4}{\overset{k_3}{\rightleftharpoons}} \underset{(E)}{CH_3OOC(CH_2)_3COOCH_3} + \underset{(D)}{H_2O} \quad (43)$$

where A, B, C, D, E is glutaric acid, methanol, monomethyl glutarate, water, dimethyl glutarate, respectively, k_1, k_3 is forward reaction rate constants, and k_2, k_4 is backward reaction rate constants, respectively,($cm^6g^{-1}min^{-1}mol^{-1}$).

The large excess of methanol was taken in this study due to the low solubility of glutaric acid in methanol. The kinetic data which had been determined experimentally for the esterification were correlated with quasi-homogeneous (*QH*) model (Schmitt & Hasse, 2006). Comparing with the experimental values, the QH model represents well the conversions of glutaric acid and the mole fractions of each constituent component varying with the contact time. The values of the rate constants were determined by fitting the kinetic data to the reaction rate expressions simultaneously. The temperature dependent k_1, k_2, k_3, k_4 were listed in Table 3,

$$k_i = k_{i0} \exp(-\Delta E / RT) \; (i = 1,2,3,4) \quad (44)$$

It should be noted that the kinetic constants reported above include the swelling effects of Amberlyst 35 beads and just for this two-stage esterification system. However, the non-ideal thermodynamic behavior of reactants and products was not taken into account.

	k_1	k_2	k_3	k_4
k_0	3.346x10⁷±1.01	6.416x10³±1.00	3.487x10⁵±1.01	1.958x10⁹±1.01
$\Delta E/R$	4417.4±1.7	84.5±0.001	2042.2±1.7	5974.6±4.0

Table 3. Each of reaction rate constant for the esterification

In 2008, Schmid, et al. investigated the reaction kinetics of the consecutive, reversible liquid-phase esterification of ethylene glycol with acetic acid to ethylene glycol monoacetate and ethylene glycol diacetate using Amberlyst 36 as catalyst in the temperature range from 333.15K to 363.15K. As shown in Equation (45) and Equation (46), the reaction contains two parts: the formation of the mono-acetylated ethyleneglycol and its hydrolysis as backward reaction; the consecutive esterification of the mono-acetylated ethylene glycol to ethylene glycol diacetate and its hydrosis:

$$\underset{(A)}{CH_3COOH}+\underset{(B)}{(CH_2OH)_2} \underset{k_{-1}}{\overset{k_1}{\rightleftharpoons}} \underset{(C)}{CH_3OOC(CH_2)_2OH}+\underset{(D)}{H_2O} \tag{45}$$

$$\underset{(A)}{CH_3COOH}+\underset{(C)}{CH_3COO(CH_2)_2OH} \underset{k_{-2}}{\overset{k_2}{\rightleftharpoons}} \underset{(E)}{CH_3COO(CH_2)_2OOCCH_3}+\underset{(D)}{H_2O} \tag{46}$$

The acetic acid initiates swelling of the resin, which results in easy accessible acid groups for the reaction and free mobility of all the components. Therefore, a pseudo-homogeneous (PH) kinetic model is applicable. For the reaction, there is,

$$r_{\mathrm{m}} = \frac{1}{m_{cat}}\frac{1}{v_i}\frac{dn_i}{dt} = k_1 a_{\mathrm{A}} a_{\mathrm{B}} - k_{-1} a_{\mathrm{C}} a_{\mathrm{D}} + k_2 a_{\mathrm{C}} a_{\mathrm{A}} - k_{-2} a_{\mathrm{E}} a_{\mathrm{D}} \tag{47}$$

where k_1, k_2, k_{-1}, k_{-2} is the forward and backward rate constants, respectively, (mol g^{-1} s^{-1}), a_i is the activity of each component, and it is calculated using the UNQUAC model, m_{cat} is the mass of catalyst.

The values of k_1, k_2, k_{-1}, k_{-2} is 539.14, 156.43, 114.41, 95.68, respectively, and the mean squared deviation between calculated and experimental mole fractions is 4.53×10^{-2}.

The kinetic behavior of esterification of lactic acid with isopropanol over Amberlyst 15 was investigated (Toor et al., 2011; Kirbaslar et al., 2001), at different temperatures from 323K to 353K. The ER model was used to describe the reaction mechanism that takes place between adsorbed molecules of isopropanol and the molecules of lactic acid in bulk. The adsorption of ester is reported to be negligible. Hence the rate equation can be described as follows,

$$\frac{dX_{\mathrm{A}}}{dt} = k_1 C_{\mathrm{A0}}(w/V)\left[(1-X_{\mathrm{A}})(M-X_{\mathrm{A}}) - \frac{X_{\mathrm{A}}^2}{K_{\mathrm{e}}}\right] \tag{48}$$

where k_1 is Rate constant for esterification reaction, M is molar ratio of isopropanol to lactic acid, K_e is equilibrium rate constant.

The value of activation energy is found to be 221 J/mol, and at each different temperature, the rate constants is 1.058×10^{-5} (323.15 K), 1.235×10^{-5} (333.15 K), 1.588×10^{-5} (343.15 K),

2.117×10^{-5} (353.15 K), respectively. The predicted values of lactic acid fractional conversion are in close agreement with the experimental within the range of experimental error.

The heterogeneous esterification of propionic acid with n-butanol over Amberlyst 35 for the synthesis of n-butyl propionate was investigated (Lee et al., 2002). The esterification is shown as follows,

$$CH_3CH(OH)COOH + CH_3(CH_2)_3OH \underset{k_{-1}}{\overset{k_1}{\rightleftharpoons}} CH_3CH(OH)COO(CH_2)_3CH_3 + H_2O \quad (49)$$

(A) (B) (C) (D)

The kinetics data of the liquid-solid catalytic esterification are correlated with various kinetic models, over wide ranges of temperature and feed composition. The activity coefficients calculated using the NTRL model are utilized to represent the non-ideality behavior of the species in the liquid solutions. Meanwhile, the effects of film diffusion and pore diffusion appear to be negligible at the experimental conditions. The results reveal that the Langmuir-Hinshelwood (LH) model yielded the best representation for the kinetic behavior of the liquid-solid catalytic esterification:

$$-r_A = \frac{2.9782\times10^{10}\exp(-7664/T)\left[a_A a_B - 0.01847\exp(819.06/T)a_C a_D\right]}{\left[1+3.70a_D\right]^2} \quad (50)$$

The activation energy of reaction is about 6.81kJmol^{-1}. This model is capable of representing the kinetic behavior of the liquid-solid catalytic esterification at temperatures from 353.15 to 373.15 K over entire range of the experimental feed compositions.

The kinetics of esterification between acrylic acid and propylene glycol in the presence of Amberlyst 15 was investigated (Altıokka & Ödeş, 2009). Taking into account the general esterification reaction as well as polymerization of acrylic acid and products, the overall reaction mechanism is proposed to be:

$$CH_2CHCOOH + CH_3CHOHCH_2OH \underset{k_2}{\overset{k_1}{\rightleftharpoons}} CH_2CHCOOC_3H_6OH + H_2O \quad (51)$$

(A) (P) (T) (W)

$$2CH_2CHCOOH \overset{k_3}{\rightleftharpoons} CH_2CHCOOOCCHCH_2 + H_2O \quad (52)$$

(A) (T1) (W)

$$2CH_2CHCOOC_3H_6OH \overset{k_4}{\rightleftharpoons} C_{12}H_{18}O_5 + H_2O \quad (53)$$

(T) (T2) (W)

Some of the dimer molecules formed here may transform into polymer. Assuming that each reaction step is elementary, the corresponding rate expression can be written.

$$\begin{aligned}
\frac{dC_A}{dt} &= -k_1 C_A C_P + k_2 C_T C_W - k_3 C_A^2 \\
\frac{dC_P}{dt} &= -k_1 C_A C_P + k_2 C_T C_W \\
\frac{dC_T}{dt} &= k_1 C_A C_P - k_2 C_T C_W - k_4 C_T^2 \\
\frac{dC_W}{dt} &= k_1 C_A C_P - k_2 C_T C_W
\end{aligned} \tag{54}$$

The reaction rate constants k_1, k_2, k_3 and k_4, in Equation (54) are determined, and shown in Table 4, where k_1, k_2 is forward and backward reaction rate constants in Equation(51), and k_3, k_4 is forward reaction rate constants in Equation(52) and Equation(53), respectively,(L min^{-1} mol^{-1}), T is absolute temperature in K.

Together with the experimental data, the concentration-time curves based on the model were obtained under given reaction conditions; there is a reasonably good agreement between calculated curves and experimental points.

	k_1	k_2	k_3	k_4
k_0	4.249x10^{9}	1.015x10^{6}	1.584x10^{27}	1.871x10^{13}
$\Delta E/R$	9667	7797	24710	12340

Table 4. Each of reaction rate constant for the esterification

3. Conclusions

This chapter discussed esterification mechanisms, and evaluated the kinetics objectively and quantitatively, which provided a most effective way to select catalyst and design reactor for different esterification systems. It is discovered that some new catalysts (such as lipases, room temperature ionic liquids) have being used in esterification; nevertheless, there are few research on the case. Herein, it is worthy to be investigated deeply.

4. References

Alexandratos, S. D. (2008) Ion-exchange resins: a retrospective from industrial and engineering chemistry research. *Industrial & Engineering Chemistry Research,* 48, 388-398,ISSN 0888-5885.

Ali, S. H. & S. Q. Merchant (2006) Kinetics of the esterification of acetic acid with 2-propanol: Impact of different acidic cation exchange resins on reaction mechanism. *International Journal of Chemical Kinetics,* 38, 593-612,ISSN 05388066.

Ali, S. H. & S. Q. Merchant (2009) Kinetic study of dowex 50 Wx8-catalyzed esterification and hydrolysis of benzyl acetate. *Industrial & Engineering Chemistry Research,* 48, 2519-2532,ISSN 0888-5885.

Ali, S., A. Tarakmah, S. Merchant & T. Alsahhaf (2007) Synthesis of esters: Development of the rate expression for the Dowex 50 Wx8-400 catalyzed esterification of propionic acid with 1-propanol. *Chemical Engineering Science,* 62, 3197-3217,ISSN 00092509.

Altıokka, M. R. & E. Ödeş (2009) Reaction kinetics of the catalytic esterification of acrylic acid with propylene glycol. *Applied Catalysis A: General,* 362, 115-120,ISSN 0926860X.

Aranda, D. A. G., R. T. P. Santos, N. C. O. Tapanes, A. L. D. Ramos & O. A. C. Antunes (2008) Acid-catalyzed homogeneous esterification reaction for biodiesel production from palm fatty acids. *Catalysis Letters,* 122, 20-25,ISSN 1011-372X.

Arata, K. (2009) Organic syntheses catalyzed by superacidic metal oxides: sulfated zirconia and related compounds. *Green Chemistry,* 11, 1719,ISSN 1463-9262 1463-9270.

Banach, T., C. Berti, M. Colonna, M. Fiorini, E. Marianucci, M. Messori, F. Pilati & M. Toselli (2001) New catalysts for poly (butylene terephthalate) synthesis:: 1. Titanium-lanthanides and titanium-hafnium systems. *Polymer,* 42, 7511-7516,ISSN 0032-3861.

Bart, H. J., J. Reidetschlager, K. Schatka & A. Lehmann (1994) Kinetics of esterification of levulinic acid with n-butanol by homogeneous catalysis. *Industrial & Engineering Chemistry Research,* 33, 21-25,ISSN 0888-5885.

Bartoli, G., M. Bosco, A. Carlone, M. Locatelli, E. Marcantoni, P. Melchiorre, P. Palazzi & L. Sambri (2006) A New, Mild, General and Efficient Route to Aryl Ethyl Carbonates in Solvent-Free Conditions Promoted by Magnesium Perchlorate. *European Journal of Organic Chemistry,* 2006, 4429-4434,ISSN 1434-193X 1099-0690.

Bartoli, G., M. Locatelli, P. Melchiorre & L. Sambri (2007) Taking Up the Cudgels for Perchlorates: Uses and Applications in Organic Reactions under Mild Conditions. *European Journal of Organic Chemistry,* 2007, 2037-2049,ISSN 1434193X 10990690.

Bhutada, S. & V. Pangarkar (1986) Esterification of phthalic anhydride with 2 ethylhexanol. *Journal of Chemical Technology & Biotechnology,* 36, 61-66,ISSN 1097-4660.

Bochner, M., S. Gerber, W. Vieth & A. Rodger (1965) Ion exchange resin-catalyzed esterification of salicylic acid with methanol. *Industrial & Engineering Chemistry Fundamentals,* 4, 314-317,ISSN 0196-4313.

Cardoso, A. L., R. Augusti & M. J. Silva (2008) Investigation on the Esterification of Fatty Acids Catalyzed by the H3PW12O40 heteropolyacid. *Journal of the American Oil Chemists' Society,* 85, 555-560,ISSN 0003-021X 1558-9331.

Cardoso, A. L., S. C. G. Neves & M. J. da Silva (2008) Esterification of Oleic Acid for Biodiesel Production Catalyzed by SnCl2: A Kinetic Investigation. *Energies,* 1, 79-92 ,ISSN 1996-1073.

Cardoso, A. L., S. C. G. Neves & M. J. da Silva (2009) Kinetic study of alcoholysis of the fatty acids catalyzed by tin chloride (II): An alternative catalyst for biodiesel production. *Energy & Fuels,* 23, 1718-1722,ISSN 0887-0624.

Erdem, B. & A. Kara (2011) Sulfonic acid functionalized poly (ethylene glycol dimethacrylate-1- vinyl-1,2,4-triazole) as an efficient catalyst for the synthesis of methyl propionate. *Reactive and Functional Polymers,* 71, 219-224 ,ISSN 13815148.

Fang, J., F.C. Shi, J. Bu, J. J. Ding, S.T. Xu, J. Bao, Y. S. Ma, Z.Q. Jiang, W. P. Zhang, C. Gao & W.X. Huang (2010) One-step synthesis of bifunctional TiO2 catalysts and their photocatalytic activity. *The Journal of Physical Chemistry C,* 114, 7940-7948 ,ISSN 1932-7447.

Fei, J. Q. & W. Zhao (2009) Study on Esterification Behaviors of Neo-Polyhydric Alcohols with Fatty Acids Catalyzed by Sulfuric Acid. *Lubricating Oil,*

Finelli, L., C. Lorenzetti, M. Messori, L. Sisti & M. Vannini (2004) Comparison between titanium tetrabutoxide and a new commercial titanium dioxide based catalyst used for the synthesis of poly (ethylene terephthalate). *Journal of applied polymer science,* 92, 1887-1892 ,ISSN 1097-4628.

Gooßen, L. & A. Döhring (2003) Lewis Acids as Highly Efficient Catalysts for the Decarboxylative Esterification of Carboxylic Acids with Dialkyl Dicarbonates. *Advanced Synthesis & Catalysis,* 345, 943-947,ISSN 1615-4150 1615-4169.

Grzesik, M., J. Skrzypek & T. Gumu a (2000) The effect of the catalyst used on the kinetics of di-2-ethylhexyl maleate synthesis. *Reaction Kinetics and Catalysis Letters,* 71, 13-18,ISSN 0133-1736.

Izci, A. & F. Bodur (2007) Liquid-phase esterification of acetic acid with isobutanol catalyzed by ion-exchange resins. *Reactive and Functional Polymers,* 67, 1458-1464,ISSN 13815148.

JagadeeshBabu, P. E., K. Sandesh & M. B. Saidutta (2011) Kinetics of Esterification of Acetic Acid with Methanol in the Presence of Ion Exchange Resin Catalysts. *Industrial & Engineering Chemistry Research,* 50, 7155-7160,ISSN 0888-5885 1520-5045.

Jeřábek, K., L. Hanková & L. Holub (2010) Working-state morphologies of ion exchange catalysts and their influence on reaction kinetics. *Journal of Molecular Catalysis A: Chemical,* 333, 109-113,ISSN 13811169.

Jiang, T., Q. Zhao, M. Li & H. Yin (2008) Preparation of mesoporous titania solid superacid and its catalytic property. *J Hazard Mater,* 159, 204-9 0304-3894 (Print) ,ISSN 0304-3894 (Linking).

Jiang, Y.-X., X.-M. Chen, Y.-F. Mo & Z.-F. Tong (2004) Preparation and properties of Al-PILC supported SO42−/TiO2 superacid catalyst. *Journal of Molecular Catalysis A: Chemical,* 213, 231-234,ISSN 13811169.

Joseph, T., S. Sahoo & S. B. Halligudi (2005) Brönsted acidic ionic liquids: A green, efficient and reusable catalyst system and reaction medium for Fischer esterification. *Journal of Molecular Catalysis A: Chemical,* 234, 107-110,ISSN 13811169.

Jothiramalingam, R. & M. K. Wang (2009) Review of Recent Developments in Solid Acid, Base, and Enzyme Catalysts (Heterogeneous) for Biodiesel Production via Transesterification. *Industrial & Engineering Chemistry Research,* 48, 6162-6172,ISSN 0888-5885.

Jousseaume, B., C. Laporte, M.-C. Rascle & T. Toupance (2003) Dichlorodistannoxane transesterification catalysts, pure Lewis acids. *Chemical Communications,* 1428 1359-7345,ISSN 1364-548X.

Ju, I. B., H.-W. Lim, W. Jeon, D. J. Suh, M.-J. Park & Y.-W. Suh (2011) Kinetic study of catalytic esterification of butyric acid and n-butanol over Dowex 50Wx8-400. *Chemical Engineering Journal,* 168, 293-302,ISSN 13858947.

Kirbaslar, S. I., Z. B. Baykal & U. Dramur (2001) Esterification of acetic acid with ethanol catalysed by an acidic ion-exchange resin. *TURK. J. ENG. ENVIRON. SCI.,* 25, 569-577 ,ISSN 1300-0160.

Kolah, A. K., N. S. Asthana, D. T. Vu, C. T. Lira & D. J. Miller (2007) Reaction kinetics of the catalytic esterification of citric acid with ethanol. *Industrial & Engineering Chemistry Research,* 46, 3180-3187 ,ISSN 0888-5885.

Krause, P., L. Hilterhaus, G. Fieg, A. Liese & U. Bornscheuer (2009) Chemically and enzymatically catalyzed synthesis of C6-C10alkyl benzoates. *European Journal of Lipid Science and Technology,* 111, 194-201 ,ISSN 14387697 14389312.

Kulawska, M., J. Z. Sad owski & J. Skrzypek (2005) Kinetics of the esterification of maleic anhydride with octyl, decyl or dodecyl alcohol over dowex catalyst. *Reaction Kinetics and Catalysis Letters,* 85, 51-56 ,ISSN 0133-1736.

Kulkarni, M. G. & S. B. Sawant (2003) Kinetics of the catalytic esterification of castor oil with lauric acid using n-butyl benzene as a water entrainer. *Journal of the American Oil Chemists' Society,* 80, 1033-1038 ,ISSN 0003-021X.

Lee, M. J., J. Y. Chiu & H. Lin (2002) Kinetics of catalytic esterification of propionic acid and n-butanol over Amberlyst 35. *Industrial & Engineering Chemistry Research,* 41, 2882-2887,ISSN 0888-5885.

Li, K. T., C. K. Wang, I. Wang & C. M. Wang (2010) Esterification of lactic acid over TiO2-ZrO2 catalysts. *Applied Catalysis A: General,*,ISSN 0926-860X.

Li, T. Q.(1992) *The basis of organic synthesis chemistry(in chinese).* Higher Education Press

Lide, D. R. 1994. *Handbook of chemistry and physics.* CRC, ,ISBN 084930475X.

Lilja, J., D. Y. Murzin, T. Salmi, J. Aumo, P. Maki-Arvela & M. Sundell (2002) Esterification of different acids over heterogeneous and homogeneous catalysts and correlation with the Taft equation. *Journal of Molecular Catalysis A: Chemical,* 182, 555-563 ,ISSN 1381-1169.

Liu, D. Z., S. H. Sun, J. G. Wei & P. Q. Sun (2006) Study on the consecutive reaction kinetics of synthesis of di(2-ethylhexyl) terephthalate under nonisothermal conditions. *International Journal of Chemical Kinetics,* 38, 577-584,ISSN 0538-8066 1097-4601.

Liu, W. T. & C. S. Tan (2001) Liquid-phase esterification of propionic acid with n-butanol. *Industrial & Engineering Chemistry Research,* 40, 3281-3286,ISSN 0888-5885.

Liu, Y. , E. Lotero & J. Goodwinjr (2006) Effect of carbon chain length on esterification of carboxylic acids with methanol using acid catalysis. *Journal of Catalysis,* 243, 221-228,ISSN 00219517.

Liu, Y., E. Lotero & J. G. Goodwin (2006) Effect of water on sulfuric acid catalyzed esterification. *Journal of Molecular Catalysis A: Chemical,* 245, 132-140,ISSN 13811169.

Liu, Y., E. Lotero & J. Goodwinjr (2006) A comparison of the esterification of acetic acid with methanol using heterogeneous versus homogeneous acid catalysis. *Journal of Catalysis,* 242, 278-286,ISSN 00219517.

March, J. 1992. *Advanced organic chemistry.* Wiley New York

Martínez, M., R. n. Oliveros & J. Aracil (2011) Synthesis of Biosurfactants: Enzymatic Esterification of Diglycerol and Oleic Acid. 1. Kinetic Modeling. *Industrial & Engineering Chemistry Research,* 50, 6609-6614 ,ISSN 0888-5885 1520-5045.

Mbaraka, I. K. & B. H. Shanks (2006) Conversion of oils and fats using advanced mesoporous heterogeneous catalysts. *Journal of the American Oil Chemists' Society,* 83, 79-91,ISSN 0003-021X.

Mochida, I., Y. Anju, A. Kato & T. Seiyama (1971) Elimination reactions on solid acid catalysts: II. Esterification of ethanol with acetic acid. *Journal of Catalysis,* 21, 263-269,ISSN 0021-9517.

Otera, J. & J. Nishikido. 2009. *Esterification: methods, reactions, and applications.* Vch Pub, ,ISBN 3527322892.

Otera, J. (1993) Transesterification. *Chemical reviews,* 93, 1449-1470 0009-2665.

(2004) Toward ideal (trans) esterification by use of fluorous distannoxane catalysts. *Accounts of chemical research,* 37, 288-296 , 0001-4842.

Patel, D. & B. Saha (2007) Heterogeneous kinetics and residue curve map (RCM) determination for synthesis of n-hexyl acetate using ion-exchange resins as catalysts. *Industrial & Engineering Chemistry Research,* 46, 3157-3169,ISSN 0888-5885.

Patel, H., G. Feix & R. Schomäcker (2007) Modeling of Semibatch Esterification Process for Poly(ethylene terephthalate) Synthesis. *Macromolecular Reaction Engineering,* 1, 502-512,ISSN 1862832X 18628338.

Pereira, C. S. M., S. P. Pinho, V. M. T. M. Silva & A. E. Rodrigues (2008) Thermodynamic equilibrium and reaction kinetics for the esterification of lactic acid with ethanol catalyzed by acid ion-exchange resin. *Industrial & Engineering Chemistry Research,* 47, 1453-1463,ISSN 0888-5885.

Pöpken, T., L. Götze & J. Gmehling (2000) Reaction kinetics and chemical equilibrium of homogeneously and heterogeneously catalyzed acetic acid esterification with methanol and methyl acetate hydrolysis. *Industrial & Engineering Chemistry Research,* 39, 2601-2611,ISSN 0888-5885.

Prabhakarn, A., J. A. Fereiro & C. Subrahmanyam (2011) Esterification of Methacrylic acid with Ethylene glycol over Heteropolyacid supported on ZSM-5. *Journal of the Korean Chemical Society,* 55, 14-18 ,ISSN 1017-2548.

Rattanaphra, D., A. Harvey & P. Srinophakun (2010) Simultaneous Conversion of Triglyceride/Free Fatty Acid Mixtures into Biodiesel Using Sulfated Zirconia. *Topics in Catalysis,* 53, 773-782,ISSN 1022-5528 1572-9028.

Rattanaphra, D., A. P. Harvey, A. Thanapimmetha & P. Srinophakun (2011) Kinetic of myristic acid esterification with methanol in the presence of triglycerides over sulfated zirconia. *Renewable Energy,* 36, 2679-2686,ISSN 09601481.

Reddy, B. M. & M. K. Patil (2009) Organic syntheses and transformations catalyzed by sulfated zirconia. *Chemical reviews,* 109, 2185-2208,ISSN 0009-2665.

Ronnback, R., T. Salmi, A. Vuori, H. Haario, J. Lehtonen, A. Sundqvist & E. Tirronen (1997) Development of a kinetic model for the esterification of acetic acid with methanol in the presence of a homogeneous acid catalyst. *Chemical Engineering Science,* 52, 3369-3381,ISSN 0009-2509.

Salciccioli, M., M. Stamatakis, S. Caratzoulas & D. G. Vlachos (2011) A review of multiscale modeling of metal-catalyzed reactions: Mechanism development for complexity and emergent behavior. *Chemical Engineering Science,* 66, 4319-4355,ISSN 00092509.

Sanchez, N., A. Coteron, M. Martinez & J. Aracil (1992) Kinetic analysis and modeling of the esterification of oleic acid and oleyl alcohol using cobalt chloride as catalyst. *Industrial & Engineering Chemistry Research,* 31, 1985-1988,ISSN 0888-5885.

Santos Ph, D. (1996) Comparison study of lewis acid type catalysts on the esterification of octanoic acid and n octyl alcohol. *Chemical engineering & technology,* 19, 538-542 1521-4125.

Sanz, M., R. Murga, S. Beltran, J. Cabezas & J. Coca (2002) Autocatalyzed and ion-exchange-resin-catalyzed esterification kinetics of lactic acid with methanol. *Industrial & Engineering Chemistry Research,* 41, 512-517,ISSN 0888-5885.

Schmid, B., M. Döker & J. Gmehling (2008) Esterification of Ethylene Glycol with Acetic Acid Catalyzed by Amberlyst 36. *Industrial & Engineering Chemistry Research,* 47, 698-703,ISSN 0888-5885.

Schmitt, M. & H. Hasse (2006) Chemical equilibrium and reaction kinetics of heterogeneously catalyzed n-hexyl acetate esterification. *Industrial & Engineering Chemistry Research,* 45, 4123-4132 ,ISSN 0888-5885.

Schmitt, M., S. Blagov & H. Hasse (2008) Mastering the reaction is the key to successful design of heterogeneously catalyzed reactive distillation: A comprehensive case study of hexyl acetate synthesis. *Industrial & Engineering Chemistry Research,* 47, 6014-6024,ISSN 0888-5885.

Solomons, T. W. G. 1986. *Fundamentals of organic chemistry.* wiley New York etc, ,ISBN 047181184X.

Srilatha, K., C. Ramesh Kumar, B. L. A. Prabhavathi Devi, R. B. N. Prasad, P. S. Sai Prasad & N. Lingaiah (2011) Efficient solid acid catalysts for esterification of free fatty acids with methanol for the production of biodiesel. *Catalysis Science & Technology,* 1, 662,ISSN 2044-4753 2044-4761.

Streitwieser, A., C. H. Heathcock & E. M. Kosower. 1985. *Introduction to organic chemistry.* Macmillan NY; London, ,ISBN 0029467209.

Tesser, R., M. Di Serio, L. Casale, G. Carotenuto & E. Santacesaria (2010) Absorption of water/methanol binary system on ion-exchange resins. *The Canadian Journal of Chemical Engineering,* 88, 1044-1053,ISSN 00084034.

Tian, W. Y., Z. X. Zeng, W. L. Xue, Y. B. Li & T. Y. Zhang (2010) Kinetics of the Mono-esterification Between Terephthalic Acid and 1, 4-Butanediol. *Chinese Journal of Chemical Engineering,* 18, 391-396,ISSN 1004-9541.

Tiwari, N. & S. Sawant (2005) Kinetics of Esterification of Erucic Acid with Cetyl Alcohol and Oleyl Alcohol. *JOURNAL-OIL TECHNOLOGISTS ASSOCIATION OF INDIA,* 37, 14,ISSN 0970-4094.

Tiwari, N. J. & S. B. Sawant (2005) Behenic acid esters: kinetics and properties. *European Journal of Lipid Science and Technology,* 107, 30-35 ,ISSN 1438-7697 1438-9312.

Toor, A. P., M. Sharma, G. Kumar & R. K. Wanchoo (2011) Kinetic Study of Esterification of Acetic Acid with n-butanol and isobutanol Catalyzed by Ion Exchange Resin. *Bulletin of Chemical Reaction Engineering & Catalysis,* 6, 23-30,ISSN 1978-2993.

Toor, A. P., M. Sharma, S. Thakur & R. K. Wanchoo (2011) Ion-exchange Resin Catalyzed Esterification of Lactic Acid with Isopropanol: a Kinetic Study. *Bulletin of Chemical Reaction Engineering & Catalysis,* 6, 39-45 ,ISSN 1978-2993.

Tsai, Y.-T., H.-m. Lin & M.-J. Lee (2011) Kinetics of heterogeneous esterification of glutaric acid with methanol over Amberlyst 35. *Journal of the Taiwan Institute of Chemical Engineers,* 42, 271-277,ISSN 18761070.

Urteaga, L., N. Sánchez, M. Martinez & J. Aracil (1994) Kinetic study of the synthesis of n octyl octanoate using cobalt chloride as catalyst. *Chemical engineering & technology,* 17, 210-215 ,ISSN 1521-4125.

Vahteristo, K., A. Laari, H. Haario & A. Solonen (2008) Estimation of kinetic parameters in neopentyl glycol esterification with propionic acid. *Chemical Engineering Science,* 63, 587-598 ,ISSN 00092509.

Vahteristo, K., S. Maury, A. Laari, A. Solonen, H. Haario & S. Koskimies (2009) Kinetics of Neopentyl Glycol Esterification with Different Carboxylic Acids. *Industrial & Engineering Chemistry Research,* 48, 6237-6247 ,ISSN 0888-5885.

Xu, C. L., C. Y. Tao, H. P. Tu, M. S. Liu & X. H. Cao (2006) Study on the esterification. *Chemical Intermediates,* 1, 6-9

Yang, J. I., S. H. Cho, H. J. Kim, H. Joo, H. Jung & K. Y. Lee (2007) Production of 4 Hydroxybutyl Acrylate and Its Reaction Kinetics over Amberlyst 15 Catalyst. *The Canadian Journal of Chemical Engineering,* 85, 83-91 ,ISSN 1939-019X.

Yoshida, A., X. Hao, O. Yamazaki & J. Nishikido (2006) Development of Industrial Reaction Processes Using Fluorous Lewis Acid Catalysts. *QSAR & Combinatorial Science,* 25, 697-702,ISSN 1611-020X 1611-0218.

Zhang, H. L., G. Y. Feng & T. J. Wei (1995) New development and kinetics of esterification *Henan Chemical Industry,* 2, 5-8

Zubir, M. I. & S. Y. Chin (2010) Kinetics of Modified Zirconia-catalyzed Heterogeneous Esterification Reaction for Biodiesel Production. *Journal of Applied Sciences,* 10, 2584-2589,ISSN 1812-5654.

14

Progresses in Experimental Study of N_2 Plasma Diagnostics by Optical Emission Spectroscopy

Hiroshi Akatsuka
Tokyo Institute of Technology, Japan

1. Introduction

Nitrogen plasmas have been widely applied to material or electronic engineering, for example, metal-surface treatment for super-hard coating, preparation of innovative insulating layers, etc. For these processes, various plasma parameters are of great importance to control the characteristics of the prepared materials. From the engineering point of view, non-intrusive measurement method is desirable. Consequently, optical emission spectroscopy (OES) measurement is one of the best methods to examine various plasma parameters. In addition to applications, the nitrogen plasma plays an important role in many fundamental problems related to environmental issues. To understand the kinetics of radicals in the upper atmosphere or ionosphere including NOx generation or ozone destruction, we should study the kinetics of the electronic or vibrational excited states of nitrogen discharge (Fridman, 2008; d'Agostino et al., 2008; Guerra & Loureiro, 1997).

In most of industrial applications or geophysical phenomena, the nitrogen plasma is in a state of non-equilibrium. Consequently, the gas temperature is much lower than the electron temperature. In order to estimate approximate value to the gas temperature, rotational temperature measurement is being frequently applied in practical researches and industries (Hrachová et al., 2002). Particularly, the spectrum of the second positive system (2PS), emitted as transitions from C $^3\Pi_u$ state to B $^3\Pi_g$ state, is easy to obtain its vibrational and rotational temperatures owing to its simple transition scheme. These temperatures are determined as best theoretical fitting parameters for the spectrum observed experimentally. Observation of this band is also easy from the experimental point of view (Phillips, 1976; Koike et al., 2004; Kobori et al., 2004; Yuji et al, 2007).

In the meanwhile, the first positive system (1PS), another band in the visible wavelength region, was difficult to analyze because of the complicated selection rule of the corresponding transition from B $^3\Pi_g$ state to A $^3\Sigma_u^+$ state. In order to obtain many experimental parameters as well as to understand the characteristics of non-equilibrium of each electronically excited state, quantitative measurement of 1PS of several vibrational levels is also significant for the understanding of nitrogen plasma (Sakamoto et al., 2006).

Another important parameter for the practical applications or for fundamental discussion of the nitrogen plasma is the dissociation degree, which is considered to be the one of the most critical parameters for the processing. Many studies are being carried out both theoretically and experimentally on nitrogen dissociation in various discharge plasmas containing nitrogen gas. Experimentally, the most convenient method to measure the dissociation degree is the actinometry method based on optical emission spectroscopy (OES) measurement (Tatarova et al., 2005; Czerwiec et al., 2005). To deduce the dissociation degree of nitrogen molecules, we must know the ratio of the line intensity emitted from some excited states of atomic nitrogen to that from the excited actinometric molecule mixed into the plasma with its amount precisely controlled, for which argon has often been chosen. However, all of them severely overlap the 1PS band spectrum. Unless the dissociation degree is high enough to neglect the 1PS band intensity, precise evaluation of the dissociation degree seems almost impossible. If we calculate the 1PS band spectrum and subtract it from the observed emission spectrum, it is possible for us to extract the atomic nitrogen lines to apply the actinometry method by OES measurement.

Concerning the non-equilibrium of each band spectrum, it should be also remarked that the band spectra of molecular ions sometimes show their rotational temperatures different from those of neutral molecules. As for nitrogen ions, a number of papers reported that the first negative system (1NS), originated from B $^2\Sigma_u^+$ state of N_2^+ ion, shows higher rotational temperature than that from neutral molecules (e.g., Huang et al., 2008).

On the other hand, it is also quite important to study reaction kinetics in nitrogen plasmas to understand quantitative amount of various excited species including reactive radicals. Many theoretical models have been proposed to describe the number densities of excited states in the plasmas. Excellent models involve simultaneous solvers of the Boltzmann equation to determine the electron energy distribution function (EEDF) and the vibrational distribution function (VDF) of nitrogen molecules in the electronic ground state. Consequently, we have found noteworthy characteristics of the number densities of excited species including dissociated atoms in plasmas as functions of plasma parameters such as electron density, reduced electric field, and electron temperature (Guerra et al., 2004; Shakhatov & Lebedev, 2008).

From the viewpoints summarized above, we report our recent progress in spectroscopic analyses of 2PS, 1PS, and 1NS band spectra and actinometry measurement. We should also discuss a model to describe excitation kinetics in the nitrogen plasma. In section 2, the method to calculate the 2PS spectrum is described in detail. In section 3, a similar method to calculate 1PS spectrum is described. In section 4, we describe the similar fundamentals to analyze 1NS spectrum. In section 5, we concentrate on the actinometer measurement of dissociation degree of N_2 molecule by 1PS-subtraction, and discuss the dependence of the dissociation degree on the discharge conditions, particularly on the mixture ratio with rare gases. In section 6, we review a model to describe excitation kinetics in the nitrogen plasma. We also discuss dominant elementary processes to determine number densities of B $^3\Pi_g$ or C $^3\Pi_u$ states for the interpretation of spectroscopic data.

2. Spectrum of the N_2 Second Positive System (2PS)

The 2PS system corresponds to a transition between the electronic states C $^3\Pi_u$ and B $^3\Pi_g$. This band dominates the spectral region about 300 – 490 nm. We can find 2PS band in various nitrogen discharge or atmospheric gas discharge plasmas.

2.1 Theoretical background for spectral analysis of 2PS

First, let us consider the energy levels of upper and lower levels of the 2PS. Both states are the triplet system, which exhibits three sub-bands corresponding to the transitions $^3\Pi_0$ - $^3\Pi_0$, $^3\Pi_1$ - $^3\Pi_1$ and $^3\Pi_2$ - $^3\Pi_2$. Fortunately, the splitting is smaller than the separation of rotational lines. In the present study, we assume that the rotational lines remain unresolved, and consequently, we can justifiably neglect the spin splitting; the line strengths for the P, Q and R branches are combined (Phillips, 1976; Nunomura et al., 2006).

The energy of a N_2 molecule is given by a sum of its electronic E_e, vibrational $E_v(v)$ and rotational energies $E_r(v, J)$:

$$E(v,J) = E_e + E_v(v) + E_r(v,J), \tag{1}$$

where $E_v(v)$ and $E_r(v, J)$ are given by

$$E_v(v) = \omega_e\left(v+\frac{1}{2}\right) - \omega_e x_e\left(v+\frac{1}{2}\right)^2 + \ldots, \tag{2}$$

$$E_r(v,J) = B_v J(J+1) - D_v J^2(J+1)^2 + \ldots, \tag{3}$$

$$B_v = B_e - \alpha_e\left(v+\frac{1}{2}\right) + \cdots, \tag{4}$$

$$D_v = D_e - \beta_e\left(v+\frac{1}{2}\right) + \cdots. \tag{5}$$

Here, v and J are the vibrational and rotational quantum numbers, respectively. The coefficients in eqs. (2) – (5) are listed in Table 1. The energy of an emitted photon associated with an electronic transition from C $^3\Pi_u(v', J')$ to B $^3\Pi_g(v'', J'')$ is given by

$$E_{Bv'',J''}^{Cv',J'} = E_C(v',J') - E_B(v'',J''), \tag{6}$$

where $E_e(v, J)$ is the energy level of the electronic state e (e = B or C) with vibrational quantum number v and rotational quantum number J, and $E_{Bv'',J''}^{Cv',J'}$ is the energy of the emitted photon. The corresponding frequency and wavelength is given by

$$\nu_{Bv'',J''}^{Cv',J'} = E_{Bv'',J''}^{Cv',J'} / h, \quad \lambda_{Bv'',J''}^{Cv',J'} = hc / E_{Bv'',J''}^{Cv',J'}, \tag{7}$$

where h and c are the Planck constant and the speed of light in vacuum, respectively. Since 2PS is an electric dipole transition, we apply the following selection rule:

Electronic State	E_e [10^4 cm^{-1}]	ω_e [10^3 cm^{-1}]	$\omega_e x_e$ [10^1 cm^{-1}]	B_e [cm^{-1}]	α_e [10^{-2} cm^{-1}]
C $^3\Pi_u$	8.913 688	2.047 17	2.844 5	1.824 7	1.868
B $^3\Pi_g$	5.961 935	1.733 39	1.412 2	1.637 4	1.791

Table 1. Coefficients of the N_2 2PS.

$$\Delta J \equiv J' - J'' = 0, \pm 1, \tag{8}$$

except for $J' = 0 \rightarrow J'' = 0$. The values of ΔJ yield three branches: P, Q and R-branch, corresponding to $\Delta J = -1$, 0 and + 1, respectively.

Basically, the nitrogen plasmas in our low-pressure (~ 1 Torr) steady-state discharge can be considered to be optically thin, at least for the 2PS band. This is because the order of electron density is 10^{13} cm^{-3} at most, and the number density of the lower level is considered to be low enough for us to neglect reabsorption.[1] Under the optically thin condition, the intensity of the spectrum is proportional to the population density of the upper level $N_C(v', J')$ and the transition probability $A_{Bv'',J''}^{Cv',J'}$:

$$I_{Bv'',J''}^{Cv',J'} \propto A_{Bv'',J''}^{Cv',J'} \cdot N_C(v',J') \cdot \tag{9}$$

The population density of rotational levels is generally found to obey the Boltzmann distribution, at least for C $^3\Pi_u$ state, which we have confirmed for many 2PS spectra observed experimentally by theoretical fitting (Koike et al., 2004; Sakamoto et al., 2006; Yuji et al., 2007; Nunomura et al., 2006). On the other hand, the vibrational levels of N_2 C $^3\Pi_u$ state do not obey the Boltzmann distribution in general due to complicated kinetics to form vibrational levels, as later shown in section 6. We define the vibrational temperature T_V over several vibrational levels with the assumption that the levels are in the Boltzmann distribution. The population density is expressed as

$$N_C(v',J') = (2J'+1) N_C(0,0) \exp\left[-\frac{E_C(v',0) - E_C(0,0)}{kT_V}\right] \cdot \exp\left[-\frac{E_C(v',J') - E_C(v',0)}{kT_R}\right], \tag{10}$$

where k is the Boltzmann constant. The transition probability $A_{Bv'',J''}^{Cv',J'}$ is given by

$$A_{Bv'',J''}^{Cv',J'} = \frac{64\pi^4 \left(\nu_{Bv'',J''}^{Cv',J'}\right)^3}{3hc^3 g_C} \cdot \frac{1}{2J'+1} \sum_{j'j''} \left|R_{j'j''}\right|^2 \cdot q_{v'v''} S_{J'J''}, \tag{11}$$

where $\Sigma_{j'j''} |R_{j'j''}|^2$ is the transition moment and just a constant, g_C is the statistical weight of the C $^3\Pi_u$ state and also a constant, $q_{v'v''}$ is the Franck-Condon factor and $S_{J'J''}$ is the Hönl-London factor. Some of the Franck-Condon factors for small (v', v'') are listed in many textbooks, e.g., Ochkin, 2009. Meanwhile, we referred the Hönl-London factor $S_{J'J''}$ for P, Q, and R- branches to Phillips 1976, where the spin-splitting is neglected due to their smaller separation than the rotational lines, and the line strengths for the P, Q and R branches are combined. This approximation is allowed only when we treat the 2PS bands rotationally unresolved, which is exactly the case in the present analysis.

In actual spectrum measurement, the line spectrum is always broadened mainly due to a finite spectral resolution of an optical setup, where the line shape can be often approximated as Gaussian practically. When we introduce the spectral resolution as the full width of the half maximum (FWHM), the spectrum is finally written as follows:

---

[1] It should be noted that some pulse-discharge plasmas with high electron density can be optically thick even for 2PS transition.

$$I(\lambda) = \sum_{v',v'',J',J''} I_{Bv'',J''}^{Cv',J'} \exp\left[-\left(\frac{\lambda - \lambda_{Bv'',J''}^{Cv',J'}}{\Delta\lambda}\right)^2\right], \tag{12}$$

$$\Delta\lambda = \frac{\mathrm{FWHM}}{2\sqrt{\ln 2}}, \tag{13}$$

where λ is the wavelength of observed spectrum.

Figure 1 shows the spectrum of the N_2 2PS for $\Delta v = v' - v'' = -2$, calculated by eqs. (1) - (13). The 2PS spectrum has sharp band heads at the longer wavelength side and long tails at the shorter wavelength side. Since the 2PS spectrum has such a distinct feature, a fit of the observed spectrum to the calculated one yields T_V and T_R as best fitting parameters. Figure 2 is an example of comparisons between spectra calculated theoretically and measured experimentally for microwave discharge nitrogen plasma with its pressure 1 Torr.

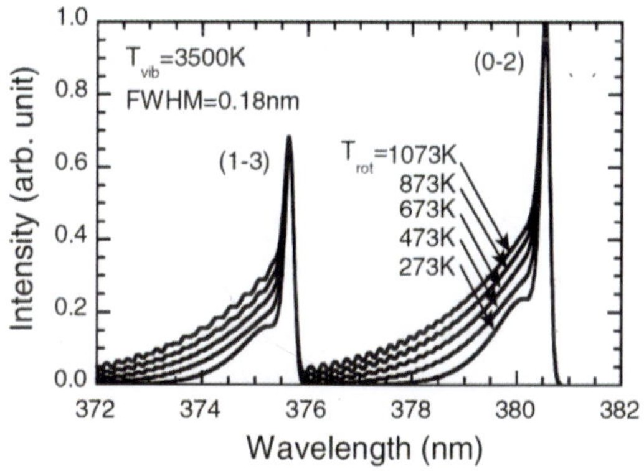

Fig. 1. Calculated spectrum of the N_2 2PS of $\Delta v = -2$, assuming T_V = 3500 K and FWHM = 0.18 nm (Nunomura et al., 2006).

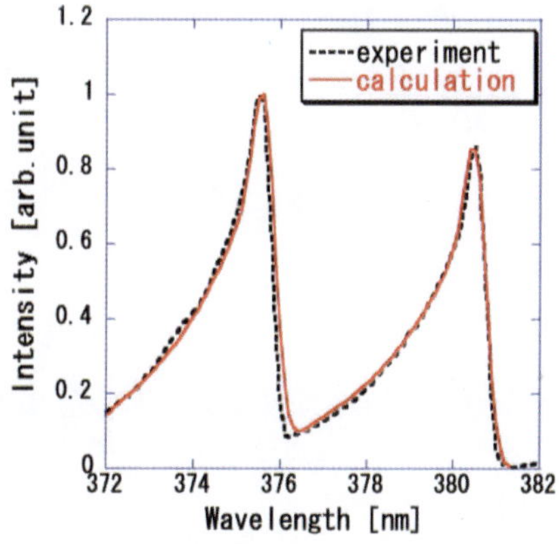

Fig. 2. Example of comparison between 2PS spectra calculated theoretically and measured experimentally, assuming T_V = 0.90 eV and T_R = 0.15 eV (Sakamoto et al., 2006, 2007).

2.2 Examples of 2PS spectra measured experimentally and discussion on the vibrational and rotational temperatures

In our laboratory, we have been examining spectroscopic characteristics of microwave discharge nitrogen plasma. Figure 3 shows the schematic diagram of our experimental setup. We generate a nitrogen plasma, using a rectangular waveguide with a cavity and a quartz tube, one end of which was inserted into a vacuum chamber. The quartz tube (i.d. 26 mm) was aligned in the direction of the electric field of the waveguide. The microwave frequency was 2.45 GHz and the output power was set at 600 W. The discharge pressure was 0.5 - 5.0 Torr. The gas feed rate was set at approximately 100 - 300 ml/min using a flow controller. Further details of the detection system are specified elsewhere (Sakamoto et al., 2006, 2007).

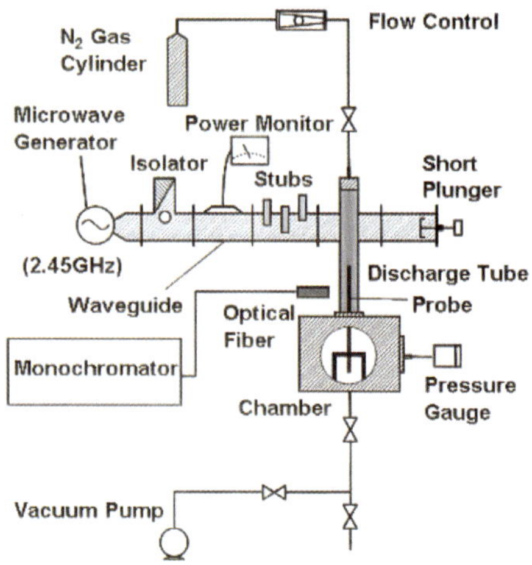

Fig. 3. Schematic diagram of microwave discharge apparatus and measurement system.

Figures 4 (a) and (b) shows T_R and T_V of the N_2 C $^3\Pi_u$ state, respectively. T_R decreased as the plasma flowed to the downstream direction, i.e., to larger z. It is considered that this result is

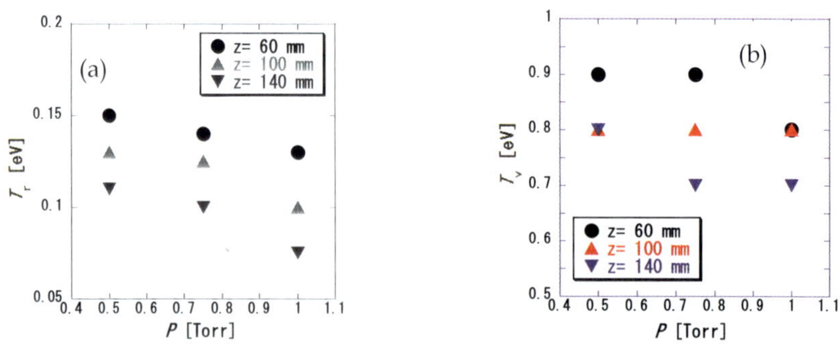

Fig. 4. (a) Rotational and (b) vibrational temperatures of C $^3\Pi_u$ state of N_2 plasma measured experimentally, generated in the apparatus schematically shown in Fig. 3 (Δv = - 2, v' = 0, 1) (Sakamoto et al., 2007).

obtained because of the cooling of neutral component of discharge species, since it is mostly heated at the discharge position $z = 0$. Consequently, the variation in the rotational temperature is considered to be useful for the analysis of macroscopic thermal structure of nitrogen plasma, which is mostly determined by the temperature of neutral particles (Nunomura et al., 2006; Yuji et al., 2007, 2008).

Concerning the vibrational temperature, there is some experimental error (± 0.05 eV) that is primarily caused by the fitting procedure. The vibrational temperature is much higher than the rotational temperature, since the vibrational kinetics is considerably determined by the electron impact excitation. The vibrational temperature decreased with increasing discharge pressure. It is considered that the collisional relaxation of molecules proceeds rapidly at higher discharge pressure (Sakamoto et al., 2006, 2007).

3. Spectrum of the N_2 First Positive System (1PS)

This transition appears between the electronic states B $^3\Pi_g$ and A $^3\Sigma_u^+$. Emission spectrum of 1PS is found in the wide wavelength region from 500 nm to 1100 nm.

3.1 Theoretical background for spectral analysis of 1PS

First, let us consider the energy levels of B $^3\Pi_g$ state, for which every rotational level K is subdivided into three sublevels with their quantum numbers J corresponding to $J = K + 1$, K, and $K - 1$. We must treat the energy level of the B $^3\Pi_g$ state more precisely for 1PS than for 2PS. We write subscript numbers 1, 2, and 3 corresponding to $J = K + 1$, K, and $K - 1$, respectively, in the following equations. The rotational term values are

$$F_1(J) = B_v\left[J(J+1) - \sqrt{Z_1} - 2Z_2\right] - D_v\left(J - \frac{1}{2}\right)^4, \tag{14}$$

$$F_2(J) = B_v\left[J(J+1) + 4Z_2\right] - D_v\left(J + \frac{1}{2}\right)^4, \tag{15}$$

$$F_3(J) = B_v\left[J(J+1) + \sqrt{Z_1} - 2Z_2\right] - D_v\left(J + \frac{3}{2}\right)^4, \tag{16}$$

with

$$Z_1 = Y(Y-4) + \frac{4}{3} + 4J(J+1), \tag{17}$$

$$Z_2 = \frac{1}{3Z_1}\left[Y(Y-1) - \frac{4}{9} - 2J(J+1)\right], \tag{18}$$

where

$$Y = A_v / B_v, \tag{19}$$

and A_v is the spin-orbit interaction parameter

$$A_v = 42.286 - 0.068\left(v + \frac{1}{2}\right) - 2.5 \times 10^{-3}\left(v + \frac{1}{2}\right)^2 - 2.6 \times 10^{-4}\left(v + \frac{1}{2}\right)^3 \text{ [cm}^{-1}\text{]}, \quad (20)$$

and B_v and D_v are defined by equations (4) and (5), respectively. For B $^3\Pi_g$ state, D_e = 5.52 x 10^{-6} cm^{-1}, and $\beta_e = 9 \times 10^{-8}$ cm^{-1}.
Next, for the electronic state A $^3\Sigma_u^+$, the rotational term values are

$$F_1(K) = B_v K(K+1) - D_v K^2 (K+1)^2 + \frac{6w(K+1)}{2K+3} - x(K+1), \quad (21)$$

$$F_2(K) = B_v K(K+1) - D_v K^2 (K+1)^2, \quad (22)$$

$$F_3(K) = B_v K(K+1) - D_v K^2 (K+1)^2 + \frac{6w(K+1)}{2K-1} - xK, \quad (23)$$

where w = 0.443 cm^{-1}, $x = 3 \times 10^{-3}$ cm^{-1}, B_e = 1.4539 cm^{-1}, α_e = 0.0175 cm^{-1}, $D_e = 5.46 \times 10^{-6}$ cm^{-1}, and $\beta_e = 1.1 \times 10^{-7}$ cm^{-1} (Sakamoto et al., 2006, 2007).

Since $^{14}N_2$ is a homonuclear molecule, we must consider the selection rule with respect to the symmetry (s) and anti-symmetry (a). Namely, the transitions s ↔ s and a ↔ a are allowed. We must keep the statistical weights for the symmetric and anti-symmetric levels are in the ratio 2 : 1 since $^{14}N_2$ is with nuclear spin I = 1 for each N. When we apply these regulations to 1PS transition, we have the selection rules as schematically shown in Fig. 5. For example, the transition P_{33} belongs to an a ↔ a transition and Q_{33} to an s ↔ s transition.

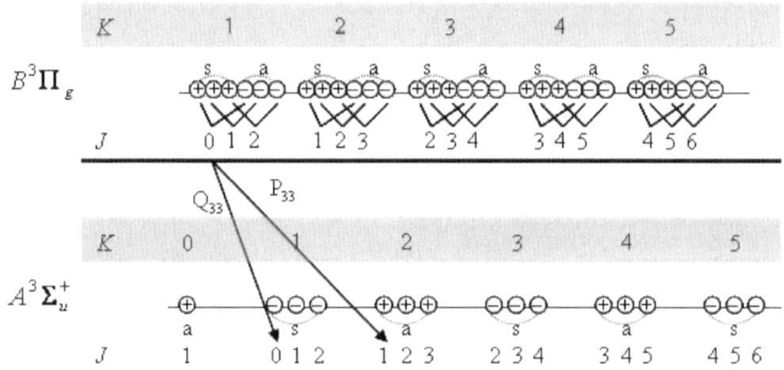

Fig. 5. Schematic diagram to illustrate the selection rule with respect to the symmetry (s) and anti-symmetry (a) of 1PS. The transitions s ↔ s and a ↔ a are allowed (Ichikawa et al., 2010).

During the course of our spectroscopic study of microwave discharge nitrogen plasma, we found that neither the Hund's coupling case (a) nor (b) holds for the 1PS transition for general discharge nitrogen plasmas with a high gas temperature owing to the large energy gap between highly excited rotational levels. We proposed the transition scheme in Fig. 6, where we consider 27 all the allowed transitions that satisfy the selection rule Δl = 0, ± 1 for variation in the rotational quantum number. The Franck-Condon and the Hönl-London factors used are specified elsewhere (Sakamoto et al., 2007).

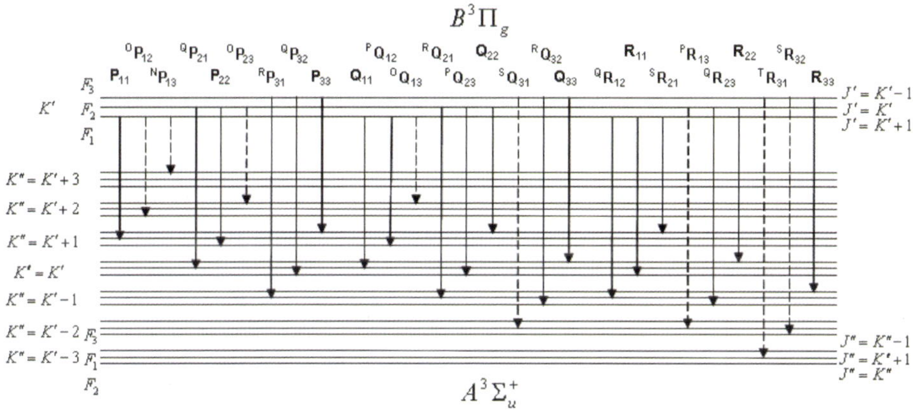

Fig. 6. Transition scheme of N_2 1PS. The filled lines denote the transitions given by Hund's coupling case (b), whereas the broken lines are those newly included in our study (Sakamoto et al., 2007; Ichikawa et al., 2010).

Figure 7 is an example of comparison between the 1PS spectrum calculated on the basis of the scheme indicated in Fig. 6 and the one measured experimentally from 635 nm to 655 nm. Obviously, the agreement is excellent. Small maxima around 641 and 648 nm are well reproduced theoretically and the agreement with the experimental results is satisfactory. In the meanwhile, we could not reproduce the maxima around 641 and 648 nm in Hund's (b) scheme, which did not agree with the experimental results well. These small maxima may be, in some sense, considered to be minor, and indeed, we can determine the rotational or vibrational temperatures as best fitting parameters. However, if we would like to reproduce the whole 1PS spectrum to find other line spectra overlapped in the wavelength region of 1PS, we should trace the shape of spectrum as precise as possible. Particularly, as shown in section 5, to extract lines of atomic nitrogen, we should calculate the spectra precisely. For this reason, the rigorous transition scheme should be reflected on the theoretical calculation of 1PS spectrum.

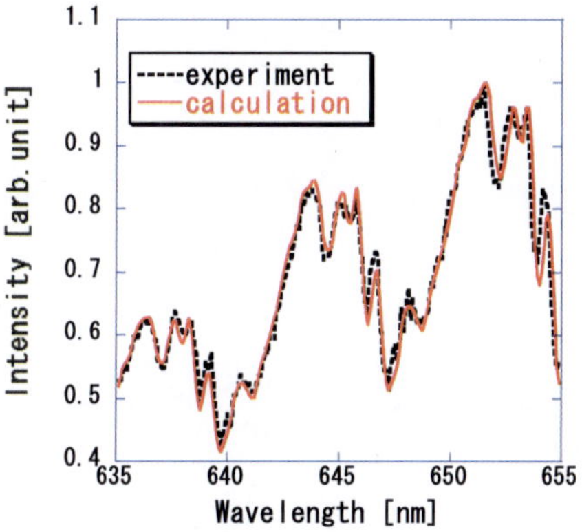

Fig. 7. Example of comparison between 1PS ($\Delta v = 3$) spectra calculated theoretically and measured experimentally, assuming $T_V = 0.65$ eV and $T_R = 0.15$ eV (Sakamoto et al., 2007).

3.2 Experimental results and discussion on vibrational and rotational temperatures determined from 1PS spectrum in comparison with those from 2PS spectrum

Figures 8(a) and 8(b) show the rotational and vibrational temperatures, respectively, determined from the 1PS spectrum observed in the same discharge apparatus that is schematically shown in Fig. 3 and under the same discharge conditions when we observed the temperatures shown in Figs. 4. Figures 8(a) and 4(a) indicate that the rotational temperatures of both 1PS and 2PS are not so different from each other for the discharge pressure 0.5 - 1.0 Torr, both of which can be considered as approximate value to the gas translational temperature. The rotational temperature of 1PS also becomes lower as the plasma flows toward the downstream direction, since the collisional relaxation becomes essential. Particularly, when the discharge pressure is 1.0 Torr, the rotational temperatures both of 1PS and of 2PS are almost the same throughout the observed domain over the microwave discharge. The pressure as high as 1 Torr can enhance the collisional relaxation, and in consequence, both rotational temperatures are considered to agree very well with each other. Basically, the rotational constant B_e of nitrogen molecules is very small not only for the ground state X $^1\Sigma_g^+$ but also for excited states B $^3\Pi_g$, C $^3\Pi_u$, etc. Therefore, the rotationally excited levels can frequently exchange kinetic energy with translational motion of neutral nitrogen molecules. Consequently, it is considered that the energy distribution of rotational levels is almost equilibrated with that of translational motion through a couple of collisions.

On the other hand, the vibrational temperature of 1PS is significantly lower than that of 2PS, as Figs. 8(b) and 4(b) indicate. However, the dependence on the discharge pressure is qualitatively similar, i.e., the vibrational temperature tends to decrease as the discharge pressure increases. This can also be attributed to the frequent collisional relaxation with neutral molecules. The discrepancy on vibrational temperatures between 1PS and 2PS can be explained by the dominant molecular processes for the excitation and de-excitation of the upper state of 1PS and 2PS, that is, B $^3\Pi_g$ and C $^3\Pi_u$. This will be discussed in section 6 in terms of elementary processes in the nitrogen plasma with low discharge pressure.

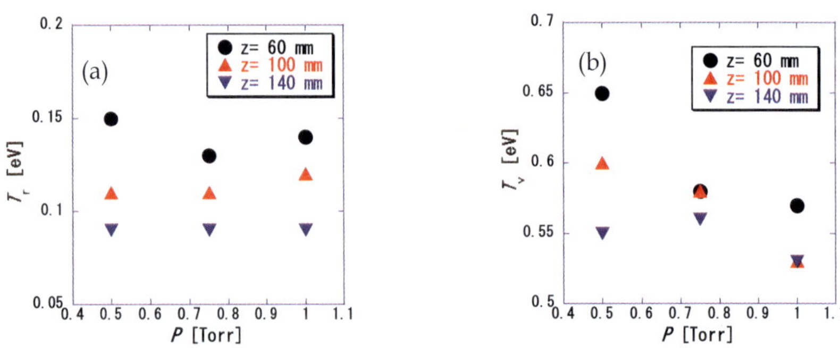

Fig. 8. (a) Rotational and (b) vibrational temperatures of B $^3\Pi_g$ state of N_2 plasma measured experimentally, generated in the apparatus schematically shown in Fig. 3 (Δv = 3, v' = 7, 8, 9) (Sakamoto et al., 2007).

4. Spectrum of the N_2^+ First Negative System (1NS)

1NS is originated from the transition between the excited sates of molecular ion N_2^+ B $^2\Sigma_u^+$ and the ground state of ion N_2^+ X $^2\Sigma_g^+$. It is found near UV through shorter visible wavelength range, from 320 to 450 nm, which almost overlaps the 2PS spectrum.

4.1 Theoretical background for spectral analysis of 1NS

Since 1NS is a $^2\Sigma_u^+ \rightarrow {}^2\Sigma_g^+$ transition, the coupling scheme is given by the Hund's (b) coupling case. Although 1NS can be basically approximated by a P- and an R-branches, this transition has a fine structure owing to spin multiplicity. However, the structure is sufficiently fine to be neglected in general. Then, the numbering of the branches should be dependent on *K* which appears in the Hund's (b), not on *J*. Consequently, the rotational energy should be described not with equation (3), but by the following equations:

$$E_1(K) = B_v K(K+1) + \frac{1}{2}\gamma K, \quad \left(J = K + \frac{1}{2}\right) \text{ (P}_1\text{, R}_1 \text{ branches)}, \tag{24}$$

$$E_2(K) = B_v K(K+1) - \frac{1}{2}\gamma (K+1), \quad \left(J = K - \frac{1}{2}\right) \text{(P}_2\text{, R}_2 \text{ branches)}, \tag{25}$$

where γ is the spin splitting constant. The rotational term is split into two components as eqs. (24) – (25) for two possible values of the quantum number *J*, where *J* is the absolute value of the vector ***J*** that is defined as the vector-like summation of ***J*** = ***K*** + ***S***. In the present scheme $S = |\boldsymbol{S}| = 1/2$. Each line is split into three components corresponding $\Delta J = J' - J'' =$ -1, 0, and + 1. This indicates that the essential transition structure of 1NS band spectrum is decomposed into the scheme as depicted in Fig. 9. However, the components with $\Delta J = 0$ (P_{Q12} and R_{Q21}) are weak enough to be neglected. In consequence, the 1NS spectrum can be satisfactorily reproduced by the summation of four components, P_1, P_2, R_1, and R_2, as shown in Fig. 9 (Bingel, 1967). Concerning Franck-Condon and Hönl-London factors of 1NS transition, we adopted Ochkin 2009, which is a practical and useful textbook published recently, and also briefly summarized other transition schemes (Ochkin, 2009).

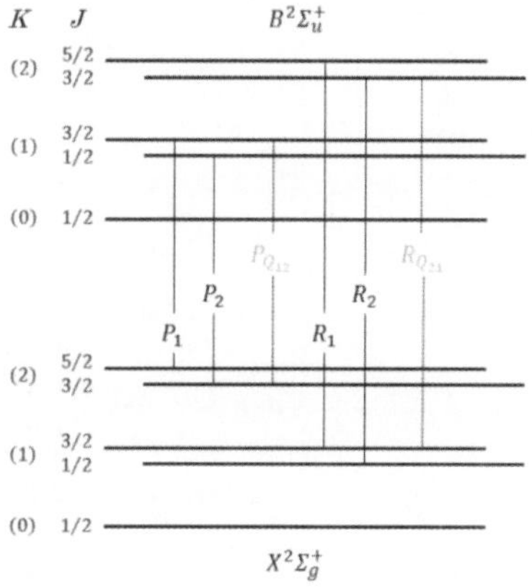

Fig. 9. Transition scheme of N_2^+ 1NS. Those indicated in thin lines are negligibly weak.

The band spectrum of 1NS $\Delta v = -1$, which has the strongest intensity in 1NS, is entirely overlapped with that of 2PS. Therefore, 1NS must be fitted simultaneously with 2PS. The intensity of 1NS in comparison with that of 2PS, of course, depends on the discharge conditions. In common low-temperature nitrogen discharge plasmas, the ionization degree is not so high, and consequently, the intensity of 1NS is weaker than that of 2PS. We chose the wavelength region from 410 to 430 nm ($\Delta v = -1$) where both intensities were almost comparable in the nitrogen plasma generated in our apparatus shown in Fig. 3. First, we determined the T_V and T_R of 2PS for $\Delta v = -2$ by the procedure in section 2 for the wavelength region from 372 to 382 nm. After that, we determine T_V and T_R of 1NS by fitting procedure for the spectrum from 410 to 430 nm with the previously fixed T_V(2PS) and T_R(2PS) for the band $\Delta v = -4$ of 2PS.

Figure 10 shows an example of comparison between the spectrum calculated theoretically and the one measured experimentally. We found a good agreement for the longer wavelength region in Fig. 10, i.e., from 421 to 428 nm, where there exist $(v', v'') = (0, 1), (1, 2)$ bands of 1NS and (1, 5) of 2PS. We found that the bands $\Delta v = -4$ of 2PS for the wavelength region shorter than 421 nm cannot be calculated precisely by the method described in section 2, particularly in the tail region where the R-branch becomes predominant. The spectrum of 2PS bands with (2, 6) or higher vibrational quantum numbers requires some modification. However, in the present analysis, the objective is to determine T_V and T_R of 1NS, which is practically carried out for the wavelength region from 421 to 428 nm precisely. The band heads of 1NS are much more sharp than that of 2PS, which allows us to determine T_V with satisfactory precision. On the other hand, (1, 2) band of 1NS is rather isolated, and in consequence, T_R can be determined satisfactorily (Kawano et al., 2011).

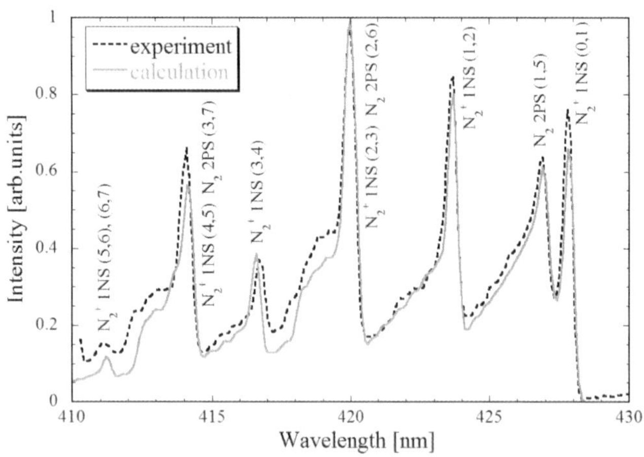

Fig. 10. Example of comparison between the spectrum of 1NS and 2PS calculated theoretically and the one observed experimentally (Kawano et al., 2011).

4.2 Results and discussion on difference in T_V and T_R between 1NS and 2PS

Figures 11(a) and 11(b) show the rotational and vibrational temperatures, respectively, determined from the 1NS spectrum observed in the same discharge apparatus schematically shown in Fig. 3 under the same discharge conditions as in Figs. 4 and 8, except the discharge pressure is fixed at 1 Torr. Figure 11(a) indicates that the rotational temperature of N_2^+ B $^2\Sigma_u^+$ ion ranges from 0.14 – 0.35 eV, which is about 1.5 times higher than that of neutral N_2 C $^3\Pi_u$ determined from the OES of 2PS, 0.08 – 0.18 eV. It is also found that T_R of N_2^+ B $^2\Sigma_u^+$ ion also decreases as the plasma flows to the downstream direction.

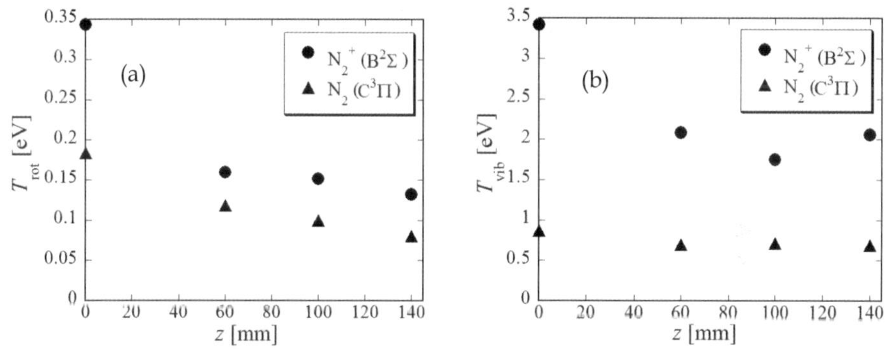

Fig. 11. (a) Rotational and (b) vibrational temperatures of N_2^+ B $^2\Sigma_u^+$ state of the plasma generated in the apparatus schematically shown in Fig. 3 (Kawano et al., 2011).

Basically, the rotational motion of the molecular species in the plasma is considered to be an approximate value to the gas translational temperature, which is the case for N_2 C $^3\Pi_u$ and B $^3\Pi_g$ states as already shown in sections 2 and 3. However, the rotational temperature of 1NS is higher than those of 1PS and 2PS, and consequently, it does not correspond to the translational temperature of neutral molecules. Similar results are reported on T_R of 1NS of low-pressure discharge nitrogen plasmas (Huang et al., 2008). These experimental results possibly indicate that the dominant population process of excited states B $^2\Sigma_u^+$ of N_2^+ is not the direct excitation from the ground state of neutral N_2 molecule, and not from excited states of neutral molecular state, either. Otherwise, the rotational energy distribution of N_2^+ B $^2\Sigma_u^+$ should become almost the same with the initial state of the molecule.

One possible reason for the higher T_R of 1NS is that the predominant population process of B $^2\Sigma_u^+$ of N_2^+ ion is the electron impact excitation from the ground state X $^2\Sigma_g^+$ of N_2^+ ion, not from any state of neutral molecules. Then, the rotational energy distribution of B $^2\Sigma_u^+$ of N_2^+ should be close to that of the ground state X $^2\Sigma_g^+$ of N_2^+ ion. It is also noteworthy that T_V of 1NS is also about twice as high as that of 2PS as in Fig. 11(b). Further discussion is necessary to conclude the reason for the higher rotational temperature of 1NS.

5. Measurement of dissociation degree of N_2 molecule in the nitrogen plasma by actinometry method with the help of 1PS subtraction

As we described in the introduction, one of the most important parameters to control the nitrogen plasma processes in industrial applications is the density of nitrogen atoms, or the dissociation degree of the nitrogen molecules in the discharge plasma. The most convenient and practical method of its measurement is the actinometry method. To do so, however, we must extract emission lines of atomic nitrogen, by the subtraction of 1PS band spectrum. In this section, we describe the actinometry method with the help of 1PS subtraction to measure the dissociation degree of nitrogen (Ichikawa et al., 2010). We also experimentally examined the effect on the nitrogen dissociation degree of admixture of rare gases.

5.1 Basic principle of actinometry measurement for about 1 Torr discharge

In the general actinometer measurement of density of nitrogen atoms in the nitrogen plasma, we almost always choose argon as an actinometer. As actinometric signals, we generally choose the line intensities of λ = 746.83 nm for N I [3p $^4S^o$ (12.00 eV) $\rightarrow$ 3s $^4P_{5/2}$], and λ = 811.53 nm for Ar I [2p$_9$ (i.e., 4p[5/2], 13.07 eV) $\rightarrow$ 1s$_5$ (i.e., 4s[3/2]^o)]. In our study, we treat the N_2-rare gas mixture plasmas to examine the dissociation degree that must depend on the gas mixture ratio. In this subsection, we describe the basic principle of actinometry including atomic and molecular processes of the N_2-gas mixture discharge plasmas, which was applied to N_2-O_2 mixed discharge (Ichikawa et al., 2010). Regarding the population and depopulation of these states, we must consider the following reactions due to collisional relaxation by the ground-state molecules of N_2 for about a 1-Torr discharge to deduce the number density of nitrogen atoms.

$$\mathrm{N} + \mathrm{e}^- \longrightarrow \mathrm{N}^* + \mathrm{e}^- \quad (\text{rate coefficient } k_{\mathrm{N+e}}^{\mathrm{dir}}), \tag{26}$$

$$\mathrm{N}_2 + \mathrm{e}^- \longrightarrow \mathrm{N}^* + \mathrm{N} + \mathrm{e}^- \quad (\text{rate coefficient } k_{\mathrm{N}}^{\mathrm{diss}}), \tag{27}$$

$$\mathrm{N}^* \longrightarrow \mathrm{N}^{**} + h\nu \quad (\text{transition probability } A_{\mathrm{N}}), \tag{28}$$

$$\mathrm{N}^* + \mathrm{N}_2 \longrightarrow \mathrm{N} + \mathrm{N}_2 \quad (\text{rate coefficient } k_{\mathrm{N+N_2}}^{\mathrm{Q}}), \tag{29}$$

$$\mathrm{Ar} + \mathrm{e}^- \longrightarrow \mathrm{Ar}^* + \mathrm{e} \quad (\text{rate coefficient } k_{\mathrm{Ar}}^{\mathrm{exc}}), \tag{30}$$

$$\mathrm{Ar}^* \longrightarrow \mathrm{Ar}^{**} + h\nu \quad (\text{transition probability } A_{\mathrm{Ar}}), \tag{31}$$

$$\mathrm{Ar}^* + \mathrm{N}_2 \longrightarrow \mathrm{Ar}^{**} + \mathrm{N}_2 \quad (\text{rate coefficient } k_{\mathrm{Ar+N_2}}^{\mathrm{Q}}). \tag{32}$$

For these transitions in the present discharge pressure range, the spectrum intensity ratio becomes

$$\frac{I_{\mathrm{N}}}{I_{\mathrm{Ar}}} = \frac{A_{\mathrm{N}}}{A_{\mathrm{Ar}}} \cdot \frac{\sum A_{\mathrm{Ar}} + k_{\mathrm{Ar+N_2}}^{\mathrm{Q}}[\mathrm{N_2}]}{\sum A_{\mathrm{N}} + k_{\mathrm{N+N_2}}^{\mathrm{Q}}[\mathrm{N_2}]} \cdot \frac{k_{\mathrm{M+e}}^{\mathrm{dir}}[\mathrm{N}]}{k_{\mathrm{Ar}}^{\mathrm{exc}}[\mathrm{Ar}]} \cdot \frac{\lambda_{\mathrm{Ar}}}{\lambda_{\mathrm{N}}} \cdot \frac{C(\lambda_{\mathrm{N}})}{C(\lambda_{\mathrm{Ar}})}, \tag{33}$$

where [M] is the number density of species M, k^{Q} is the rate coefficient of the quenching reaction of the excited states at the line emission of the present OES measurement with their subscripts denoting the reactions [eqs. (29) and (32)], k^{dir} is that of direct electron impact excitation from the atomic ground state of N to produce the corresponding OES level [eq. (26)], k^{exc} is that for Ar [eq. (30)], λ is the wavelength of the transitions given by eqs. (28) and (31), A is the atomic transition probability of the corresponding transition, and C(λ) is the detection coefficient of the spectrometric system for the wavelength λ. If we add oxygen, rare gas or other dilution gas into nitrogen, we must consider the quenching effect of excited species by the admixture gas and modify eq. (33). We summarized the transition probabilities and rate coefficients required to eqs. (26) – (33) elsewhere in Ichikawa et al., 2010.

In the present analysis, the EEDF is determined by solving the Boltzmann equation as a function of the reduced electric field E/N so that the electron mean energy equals 3/2 times the electron temperature experimentally measured by the probe. The Boltzmann equation is simultaneously solved with the master equations for the vibrational distribution function (VDF) of the N_2 X $^1\Sigma_g^+$ state, since the EEDF of N_2-based plasma is strongly affected by the VDF of N_2 molecules owing to superelastic collisions with vibrationally excited N_2 molecules. A more detailed account of obtaining the EEDF is given in the next section.

Strictly speaking, the actinometry levels are also generated by the radiative decay of their upper levels, in addition to eq. (26), which is referred to as cascade processes. These processes are generally negligible for actinometry measurement in the present microwave discharge plasmas, which are categorized into ionizing plasmas. Further discussion was described elsewhere (Ichikawa et al., 2010).

5.2 Subtraction of 1PS-band spectrum as background signal to extract atomic nitrogen lines, and the lower limit of number density of nitrogen atoms

As we already showed in Fig. 7, we demonstrated theoretical fitting of 1PS as functions of vibrational and rotational temperatures for the transition series $\Delta v = v' - v'' = 3$. In order to extract the lines emitted from excited nitrogen atoms, we must calculate the 1PS spectrum with $\Delta v = v' - v'' = 2$, which can be done by the same procedure. After we experimentally measure the 1PS spectrum of the vibrational quantum numbers $\Delta v = v' - v'' = 2$ in the wavelength region of 730 – 760 nm, we determine T_v and T_r by the numerical fitting method. We consider that an argon line with a large peak appears at 750.4 nm. Consequently, we fit the spectrum excluding the wavelength region of 750 – 752 nm. Then, after we subtract the overall 1PS spectrum calculated as a background signal from the observed spectrum, we obtain the line of the excited nitrogen atom at 746.83 nm.

Figure 12(a) shows an example of fitting the 1PS band spectrum experimentally observed in the wavelength region of 730 – 760 nm with the one calculated theoretically, and Fig. 12(b) shows the result of subtraction, which indicates the successful extraction of atomic nitrogen line spectra, not only at 746.83 nm but also at 744.23 and 742.36 nm, which corresponds to the transitions 3p $^4S^o_{3/2} \rightarrow$ 3s $^4P_{5/2,\,3/2,\,1/2}$, respectively. The simultaneous extraction of these three lines indicates that the present method is reliable and that the contamination by other lines can be neglected with respect to other excited states of nitrogen and argon species. The line at 746.83 nm has the largest intensity among the three lines, and we chose it for the actinometry measurement. Here, we discuss the lower limit of the number density of nitrogen atoms that measured by the present method. Figure 12(b) is a typical example, which corresponds to a density of nitrogen atoms of 1.4×10^{12} cm^{-3}, whereas the fluctuation of the baseline is about 1/20 times the peak height of the actinometry signal. The subtracted baseline illustrated in Fig. 12(b) is common to almost all the discharge conditions throughout the present experiments. As a result, the lower limit of the number density of nitrogen atoms is considered to be about $< 7 \times 10^{10}$ cm^{-3} (Ichikawa et al., 2010).

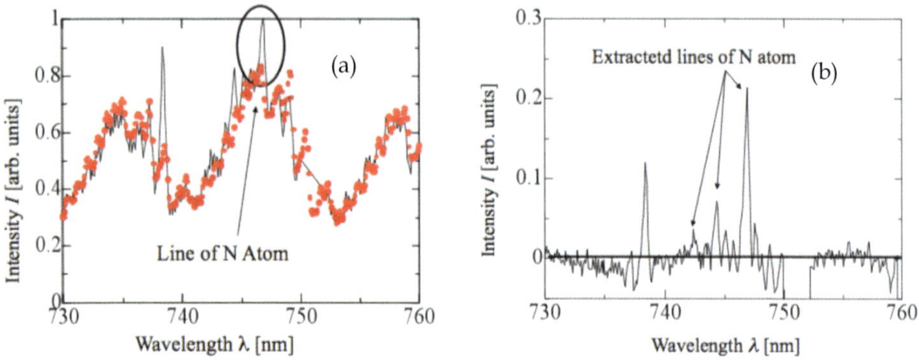

Fig. 12. (a) Schematic diagram of the spectrum fitting of N_2-1PS band spectrum and (b) the extracted lines of nitrogen atom. (a) Line - experimentally measured spectrum, dots - calculated spectrum by our method. We did not plot the experimental results in the wavelength region 750 - 752 nm since an Ar atomic line appears in this position with a large intensity (Ichikawa et al., 2010).

5.3 Results and discussion of actinometry measurement of dissociation degree of nitrogen molecule in N_2-rare gas mixed microwave discharge plasma

In this study, we define the dissociation degree D(N) of nitrogen as follows:

$$D(\mathrm{N}) = [\mathrm{N}]/(2[\mathrm{N}_2]), \tag{34}$$

where [X] is the number density of species X. The density [N_2] is calculated from the discharge partial pressure and gas temperature, with the assumption that the number densities of any excited species are negligibly smaller than that of the ground state.

We experimentally examined the dependence of the dissociation degree of nitrogen on the mixture ratio of O_2 (Ichikawa et al., 2010) and various rare gas species (Kuwano et al., 2009). Here, we concentrate on rare-gas admixture. First, we examined the electron temperature and density by a Langmuir Double probe, as function of the gas mixture ratio. The admixture of lighter rare-gas species increases the electron temperature, since the lighter rare-gas species have higher ionization potential. On the other hand, the heavier rare-gas species have lower ionization potential, and consequently, the electron temperature can become lower and the electron density increases with increasing the volumetric ratio of heavier rare-gas species.

Figure 13 shows the measured dissociation degree plotted against the rare gas mixture ratio for the microwave discharge N_2-rare gas plasma. When helium is mixed into the nitrogen plasma, we found a small increase in the nitrogen dissociation degree. This can be explained by an increase in the electron temperature by the helium admixture. On the other hand, when the argon or krypton with low-ionization energy was mixed into the nitrogen plasma, we found lowering of electron temperature and resultant reduction in the nitrogen dissociation degree. For these three kinds of rare gases, the variation in their dissociation degree is reasonable since it corresponds to the variation in the electron temperature (Kuwano et al., 2009).

Figure 13, however, shows that the neon admixture markedly enhances the nitrogen dissociation degree. This tendency was found even at considerable downstream positions like z = 140 mm. We now consider that the spectroscopic contamination of Ne I 747.24 nm into N I 746.83 nm is negligible owing to sufficient resolution of experimental setup. Some nitrogen plasma process may be conducted several hundred times faster than the conventional processes with neon admixture. We now consider that one of the possible mechanisms is that the energy-transfer collision between the metastable neon (16.62 or 16.72 eV) and nitrogen molecules, which makes it excited to the dissociation curve. Further discussion and cross-examination by other experimental methods are necessary to understand the dissociation of nitrogen molecules by neon admixture (Akatsuka et al., 2010).

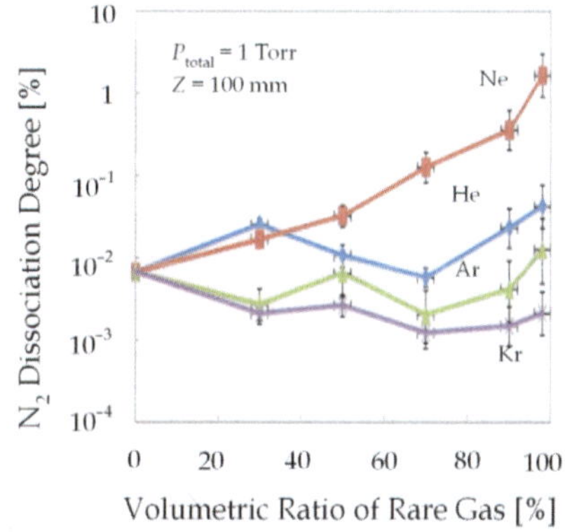

Fig. 13. Dissociation degree of nitrogen molecule plotted against N_2 : rare-gas mixture ratio.

6. Numerical modelling of excitation kinetics in the N_2 plasma

Numerical studies on number densities of various excited states in the N_2 plasma have eagerly been carried out all over the world (Guerra et al., 2004; Shakhatov & Lebedev, 2008). We also make a numerical code to calculate number densities as functions of the following parameters: gas temperature T_g, electron density N_e, total discharge pressure P, and reduced electric field E/N as a rather simplified model (Akatsuka et al., 2008; Ichikawa et al., 2010).

First, we assume that the geometry is axially symmetric and neglect the z-dependence. Concerning the density [A] of species A, we have the following partial differential equation:

$$\frac{\partial[\mathrm{A}]}{\partial t} = -\nu_{\mathrm{W}} \cdot [\mathrm{A}] + G, \qquad (35)$$

where ν_w is the particle loss frequency due to wall collision or diffusion, and G is the net particle generation or loss due to volumetric reactions. We discuss the number densities of $N_2(X\,^1\Sigma_g^+)$, $N_2(A\,^3\Sigma_u^+)$, $N_2(B\,^3\Pi_g)$, $N_2(C\,^3\Pi_u)$, $N_2(a\,^1\Pi_g)$, $N_2(a'\,^1\Sigma_u^-)$, N_2^+, N_4^+, $N(2p\,^4S^o)$, and e^-. The cross sections, rate coefficients, or any required atomic and molecular data required in this section are summarized elsewhere in Ichikawa et al., 2010.

6.1 The Boltzmann equation

In order to calculate the various rate coefficients to solve eq. (35) as well as to evaluate the actinometry signal in the present experiments using eq. (33), we need the electron energy probabilistic function (EEPF) in the discharge plasma, and consequently, we must solve the Boltzmann equation to describe the EEPF. To analyze cw discharge, the EEPF may be treated by a two-term approximation owing to the sufficiently small anisotropy. Consequently, the Boltzmann equation for the isotropic component of the EEPF $f_0(\varepsilon)$ is formulated as follows (Sakamoto et al., 2007; Mizuochi et al, 2010):

$$-\frac{\mathrm{d}}{\mathrm{d}\varepsilon}\left\{\frac{1}{3}\left(\frac{E}{N}\right)^2\frac{\varepsilon}{\sigma_c(\varepsilon)}\frac{\mathrm{d}f_0(\varepsilon)}{\mathrm{d}\varepsilon}+\frac{2m_e}{M}\varepsilon^2\sigma_c(\varepsilon)\left[f_0(\varepsilon)+\frac{kT_g}{e}\frac{\mathrm{d}f_0(\varepsilon)}{\mathrm{d}\varepsilon}\right]\right\}$$

$$+\sum_l \varepsilon\frac{N_l}{N}\sigma_l^{si}(\varepsilon)f_0(\varepsilon)-\sum_l\left(\varepsilon+\varepsilon_l^{si}\right)\frac{N_l}{N}\sigma_l^{si}\left(\varepsilon+\varepsilon_l^{si}\right)f_0\left(\varepsilon+\varepsilon_l^{si}\right)=0\,, \tag{36}$$

where e is the elementary charge, ε is the electron energy, σ_c is the momentum transfer cross section, σ_l^{si} is the lth inelastic collision cross section with the energy change of ε_l^{si}, m_e is the electron mass, M denotes the molecular mass of the elastic collision partner of the electron, and N_l is the number density of the lth inelastic collision partner. Table 2 summarizes the inelastic collisions included in eq. (36), where the EEPF $f_0(\varepsilon)$ is normalized as follows:

$$\int_0^\infty f_0(\varepsilon)\varepsilon^{1/2}\mathrm{d}\varepsilon=1\,. \tag{37}$$

Inelastic Collisions		
$e^- + N_2(X)$	$\rightarrow e^- + N_2(Y)$	($Y = A^3\Sigma_u^+$, $B\ ^3\Pi_g$, $C\ ^3\Pi_u$, $a'\ ^1\Sigma_u^-$, $a\ ^1\Pi_g$, $w\ ^1\Delta_u$, $B'\ ^3\Sigma_u^-$, $W\ ^3\Delta_u$)
$e^- + N_2(X)$	$\rightarrow e^- + e^- + N_2^+$	
$e^- + N_2(X, v)$	$\leftrightarrow e^- + N_2(X, w)$	($v, w = 0 - 8$)

Table 2. List of inelastic collisions included in the collision term in eq. (36).

6.2 Vibrational distribution function (VDF) of $N_2\ X\ ^1\Sigma_g^+$ state

We must solve the Boltzmann equation [eq. (36)] simultaneously with the master equations to describe the VDF of the ground state of the nitrogen molecule. We consider the elementary processes shown in Table 3. We treat N plasmas with a very low dissociation degree of its order about 10^{-3}, and consequently, we neglect the V-T relaxation by nitrogen atoms. We also neglect the vibrational wall-relaxation, since we treat plasmas where the V-V and V-T processes dominate the wall relaxation. In the V-V and V-T processes, we consider only single-quantum transition processes. We assume that the total density of nitrogen molecules is constant owing to their small dissociation degree. As a result, the dissociated nitrogen atoms are assumed to associate into the vth vibrational level with probability R_v immediately after dissociation, which is assumed to be constant over v. Hence, we have the following master equation for the VDF of $N_2\ X\ ^1\Sigma_g^+$ state:

$$\frac{\mathrm{d}N_v}{\mathrm{d}t}=N_e\sum_{w=0,\neq v}^{M}N_wC_{wv}-N_eN_v\sum_{w=0,\neq v}^{M}C_{vw}+N_{v-1}\sum_{w=0,\neq v}^{M-1}N_{w+1}Q_{v-1,v}^{w,w+1}$$

$$+N_{v+1}\sum_{w=0,\neq v}^{M-1}N_wQ_{v+1,v}^{w,w+1}-N_v\left(\sum_{w=0,\neq v}^{M-1}N_{w+1}Q_{v,v+1}^{w+1,w}+\sum_{w=0,\neq v}^{M-1}N_wQ_{v,v-1}^{w,w+1}\right)$$

Reactions		Process
N_2 (X; v = 0 – 8) + e^-	↔ N_2 (X; w = 0 – 8 ≠ v) + e^-	e-V
N_2 (X; v) + N_2 (X; w)	↔ N_2 (X; v + 1) + N_2 (X; w – 1)	V-V
N_2 (X; M) + N_2 (X; w)	→ 2N (2p $^4S^o$) + N_2 (X; w – 1)	V-Diss
N_2 (X; v) + N_2 (X)	↔ N_2 (X; v – 1) + N_2 (X)	V-T

Table 3. List of collisions included in the master equation of VDF, eq. (38).

$$+[\mathrm{N}_2]\left(N_{v-1}P_{v-1,v}+N_{v+1}P_{v+1,v}\right)-N_v[\mathrm{N}_2]\left(P_{v,v-1}+P_{v,v+1}\right)+R_v\,, \tag{38}$$

where N_v is the number density of the N_2 X state at the vth vibrationally excited level, C_{wv} is the rate coefficient of the electron impact vibrational excitation ($w < v$) or deexcitation ($w > v$) from level w to v, Q and P are the rate coefficients of V-V transfer and V-T relaxation, respectively, between the levels given by the following suffixes for N_2–N_2 collisions, and R_v is the rate of atomic nitrogen recombination into the vth level. The upper limit of the summation M is set at v = 45, which is considered to be the dissociation level of the nitrogen molecule, considered to be followed by instantaneous association into level v, which corresponds to the term R_v in eq. (38).

6.3 Reactions relevant to formation of excited species in the model

We include the electron-impact processes as in Table 4, and some of their reverse processes. To obtain the cross section of the reverse process, we apply the principle of detailed balance, which is known as the Klein-Rosseland equation formulated below:

$$\frac{\sigma_{pq}(\varepsilon')}{\sigma_{qp}(\varepsilon'')}=\frac{g_q}{g_p}\cdot\frac{\varepsilon''}{\varepsilon'}\,, \tag{39}$$

Electron Impact Excitation		
e^- + $N_2(X\,^1\Sigma_g^+)$	↔	e^- + $N_2(A^3\Sigma_u^+)$
e^- + $N_2(X\,^1\Sigma_g^+)$	↔	e^- + $N_2(B\,^3\Pi_g)$
e^- + $N_2(X\,^1\Sigma_g^+)$	↔	e^- + $N_2(C\,^3\Pi_u)$
e^- + $N_2(X\,^1\Sigma_g^+)$	↔	e^- + $N_2(a'\,^1\Sigma_u^-)$
e^- + $N_2(X\,^1\Sigma_g^+)$	↔	e^- + $N_2(a\,^1\Pi_g)$
Electron Impact Ionization		
e^- + $N_2(X\,^1\Sigma_g^+)$	→	e^- + e^- + N_2^+
Electron Impact Dissociation		
e^- + $N_2(X\,^1\Sigma_g^+)$	→	e^- + 2N(2p $^4S^o$)
Dissociative Recombination		
e^- + N_2^+	→	2N($^4S^o$)
e^- + N_4^+	→	2 $N_2(X\,^1\Sigma_g^+)$

Table 4. List of electron collision processes included in term G in eq. (35).

where $\sigma_{pq}(\varepsilon')$ is the cross section for the electron impact reaction from level p to q with energy difference $\varepsilon_{pq} > 0$ for electron energy ε', $\sigma_{qp}(\varepsilon'')$ is that of the reverse reaction with electron energy $\varepsilon'' = \varepsilon' + \varepsilon_{pq}$, and g_p is the statistical weight of state p.

We also take the atomic and molecular collision processes into account listed in Table 5. We also include one of their reverse processes, whose rate coefficient k_r is obtained from that of the forward reaction k_f and the equilibrium constant K_{eq} as

$$k_f/k_r = K_{eq}. \tag{40}$$

We calculate the equilibrium constant using the partition functions involved in the reactions.

Chemical Reactions included in term G of eq. (35)		
$N_2(a'\ ^1\Sigma_u^-) + N_2(X\ ^1\Sigma_g^+)$	$\rightarrow$	$N_2(B\ ^3\Pi_g) + N_2(X\ ^1\Sigma_g^+)$
$N_2(C\ ^3\Pi_u) + N_2(X\ ^1\Sigma_g^+)$	$\rightarrow$	$N_2(a'\ ^1\Sigma_u^-) + N_2(X\ ^1\Sigma_g^+)$
$N_2(a\ ^1\Pi_g) + N_2(X\ ^1\Sigma_g^+)$	$\leftrightarrow$	$N_2(a'\ ^1\Sigma_u^-) + N_2(X\ ^1\Sigma_g^+)$
$N_2(B\ ^3\Pi_g) + N_2(X\ ^1\Sigma_g^+)$	$\rightarrow$	$2N_2(X\ ^1\Sigma_g^+)$
$N_2(A\ ^3\Sigma_u^+) + N_2(X\ ^1\Sigma_g^+)$	$\rightarrow$	$2\ N_2(X\ ^1\Sigma_g^+)$
$N_2(A\ ^3\Sigma_u^+) + N(2p\ ^4S^o)$	$\rightarrow$	$N_2(X\ ^1\Sigma_g^+) + N(2p\ ^4S^o)$
$N_2(A\ ^3\Sigma_u^+) + N_2(A\ ^3\Sigma_u^+)$	$\rightarrow$	$N_2(B\ ^3\Pi_g) + N_2(X\ ^1\Sigma_g^+)$
$N_2(A\ ^3\Sigma_u^+) + N_2(A\ ^3\Sigma_u^+)$	$\rightarrow$	$N_2(C\ ^3\Pi_u) + N_2(X\ ^1\Sigma_g^+)$
$N_2(a'\ ^1\Sigma_u^-) + N_2(X\ ^1\Sigma_g^+)$	$\rightarrow$	$N_2^+ + N_2(X\ ^1\Sigma_g^+) + e^-$
$N_2(a'\ ^1\Sigma_u^-) + N_2(a'\ ^1\Sigma_u^-)$	$\rightarrow$	$2N_2^+ + 2e^-$
$N_2(X\ ^1\Sigma_g^+, v \geq 6) + N_2(A\ ^3\Sigma_u^+)$	$\rightarrow$	$N_2(B\ ^3\Pi_g) + N_2(X\ ^1\Sigma_g^+)$
$N_2(B\ ^3\Pi_g) + N_2(X\ ^1\Sigma_g^+)$	$\rightarrow$	$N_2(A\ ^3\Sigma_u^+) + N_2(X\ ^1\Sigma_g^+)$
$2N(2p\ ^4S^o) + N(2p\ ^4S^o)$	$\rightarrow$	$N_2(B\ ^3\Pi_g) + N(2p\ ^4S^o)$
$N_2(a'\ ^1\Sigma_u^-) + N_2(A\ ^3\Sigma_u^+)$	$\rightarrow$	$N_4^+ + e^-$
$N_2(a'\ ^1\Sigma_u^-) + N_2(a'\ ^1\Sigma_u^-)$	$\rightarrow$	$N_4^+ + e^-$

Table 5. List of atomic and molecular processes included in term G in eq. (35).

Some radiative decay processes of excited species are essential for the population kinetics due to large absolute value, which are summarized in Table 6. We must also include wall loss processes due to diffusion or thermal motion for several excited species, particularly for metastable states and ions. From the wall loss probability γ, we can calculate the wall loss frequency ν_W as follows:

$$\nu_W = \frac{\gamma v_{th}}{2R} \quad \text{for } \gamma << 1, \tag{41}$$

$$\nu_W = \left(\frac{2.405}{R}\right)^2 D \quad \text{for } \gamma \sim 1, \tag{42}$$

where R is the discharge tube radius, v_{th} is the thermal velocity of the particle considered, and D denotes the diffusion coefficient. For ionic species, we apply ambipolar diffusion coefficient. Table 7 shows the wall loss processes considered in the present model.

Radiative transitions			Name of Transition
$N_2(B\ ^3\Pi_g)$	$\rightarrow$	$N_2(A\ ^3\Sigma_u^+) + h\nu$	1st Positive System
$N_2(C\ ^3\Pi_u)$	$\rightarrow$	$N_2(B\ ^3\Pi_g) + h\nu$	2nd Positive System
$N_2(a\ ^1\Pi_g)$	$\rightarrow$	$N_2(a'\ ^1\Sigma_u^-) + h\nu$	Farlane Infrared System
$N_2(a\ ^1\Pi_g)$	$\rightarrow$	$N_2(X\ ^1\Sigma_g^+) + h\nu$	Lyman-Birge-Hopfield System
$N_2(a'\ ^1\Sigma_u^-)$	$\rightarrow$	$N_2(X\ ^1\Sigma_g^+) + h\nu$	Ogawa-Tanaka-Wilkinson-Mulliken System

Table 6. List of radiative transitions included in term *G* in eq. (35).

Wall loss processes included in term G of eq. (35)			
$\gamma << 1$ [eq.(41)]			
$2N\ (2p\ ^4S^o)$ + wall	$\rightarrow$	$N_2(X\ ^1\Sigma_g^+)$	$\gamma = 1.0 \times 10^{-4}$
$N_2(a'\ ^1\Sigma_u^-)$ + wall	$\rightarrow$	$N_2(X\ ^1\Sigma_g^+)$	$\gamma = 1.0 \times 10^{-2}$
$\gamma \sim 1$ [eq.(42)]			
$N_2(A\ ^3\Sigma_u^+)$ + wall	$\rightarrow$	$N_2(X\ ^1\Sigma_g^+)$	$\gamma = 1.0$
$N_2(a\ ^1\Pi_g)$ + wall	$\rightarrow$	$N_2(X\ ^1\Sigma_g^+)$	$\gamma = 1.0$
N_2^+ + wall	$\rightarrow$	$N_2(X\ ^1\Sigma_g^+)$	$\gamma = 1.0$

Table 7. List of wall loss processes included in term *G* of eq. (35).

6.4 Numerical procedure

We calculate the number densities of the excited species depicted in Fig. 14. We solve eq. (35) for each species until we find that a steady state is accomplished for every state. The input parameters are the reduced electric field E/N, electron number density N_e, gas temperature T_g, and discharge pressure P. It should be remarked that the electron density is chosen as an input parameter, and consequently, the resultant ion density does not necessarily equal N_e. In order to maintain quasi-neutrality in the present calculation, we modify the value of P or T_g and repeat the algorithm in Fig. 14 until the quasi-neutral condition is fulfilled (Akatsuka et al., 2008; Ichikawa et al., 2010).

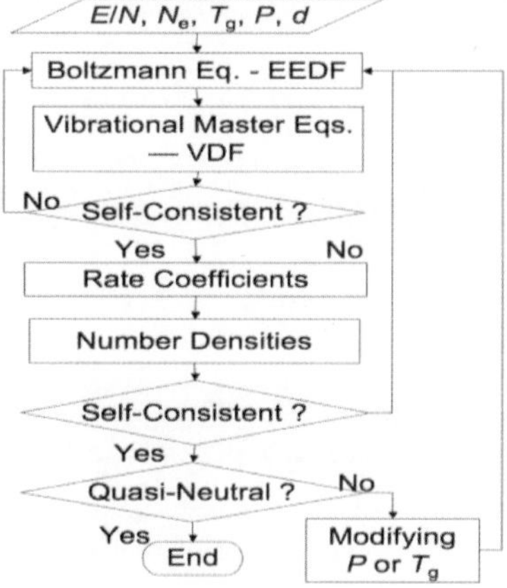

Fig. 14. Flow chart of the numerical procedure (Akatsuka et al., 2008; Ichikawa et al., 2010).

6.5 Numerical results and discussion

Figures 15(a) and 15(b) show the calculation results of EEPF and VDF of N_2 X, respectively. The calculations were run at T_g = 1200 K, N_e = 5.0 × 10^{11} cm^{-3} and T_e = 2.5 - 4.5 eV. These parameters were chosen to correspond to our experimental results at P = 1.0 Torr and z = 60 mm obtained in the experimental apparatus shown in Fig. 3. It should be repeated that we choose a reduced electric field so that the electron mean energy $\langle\varepsilon\rangle$ equals $(3/2)kT_e$ when we compare the numerical calculation with the number densities obtained experimentally by OES measurement. Obviously, the EEPF is not like Maxwellian. It has a dip in the range from 2 to 3 eV owing to frequent consumption of electrons with this energy range due to inelastic collisions to make vibrationally excited molecules. Meanwhile, Fig. 15(b) shows that the VDF is also quite far from the Maxwellian distribution. The number density of the vibrational levels shows rapid decrease first, then moderate decrease, and rapid decrease again as the vibrational quantum number increases. This behaviour of the VDF of N_2 X state has been frequently reported, and consequently, our model is also considered to be appropriate. If we can assume corona equilibrium of some excited states of N_2 molecule, for example, N_2 C state, we can calculate the number density of the vibrational levels of the excited state that can be experimentally observed. This indicates that we can verify the appropriateness of the calculated VDF of the N_2 X state as shown in Fig. 15(b).

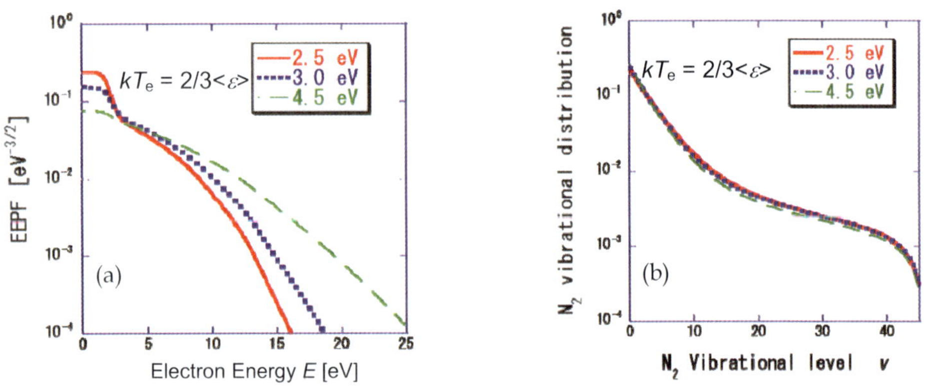

Fig. 15. (a) EEPF and (b) VDF of nitrogen plasma calculated numerically by the present scheme with pressure P = 1 Torr, T_g = 1200 K and N_e = 5.0 × 10^{11} cm^{-3}.

Another interesting result of this modelling is the identification of essential kinetic processes of population and depopulation of each excited state of N_2 molecule. Table 8 shows reaction rates of dominant population and depopulation processes for B and C state of nitrogen molecule, calculated for T_e = 3.0 eV, N_e = 4.0 × 10^{11} cm^{-3}, and P = 1.0 Torr (Akatsuka et al., 2008). When we examined the essential processes to populate and depopulate N_2 B state and N_2 C state, we found a marked difference between them. That is, the C state populates mainly by electron impact excitation from the N_2 X state, the ground state of molecule, and depopulates mainly by radiative decay to the B state, i.e., by 2PS emission. It indicates that the C state is almost in the state of corona equilibrium. In the meanwhile, the B state populates mainly by intermolecular collision between N_2 X ($v \geq 6$) and N_2 A states, and depopulates by collisional quenching to N_2 A state by the ground state molecule.

Consequently, the B state is quite far from the corona equilibrium. We should notice that the vibrational states of N_2 X is, indeed, essential to calculate the populations of excited states like B state, where the excitation through the intermolecular collisions plays an important role. Therefore, we must calculate the VDF together with the excitation kinetics of electronically excited states of N_2 molecule.

	Population Reaction	Rate [$cm^{-3} s^{-1}$]
C	$N_2(X) + e^- \rightarrow N_2(C) + e^-$	6.8×10^{17}
	$N_2(A) + N_2(A) \rightarrow N_2(C) + N_2(X)$	1.2×10^{17}
	Depopulation Reaction	Rate [$cm^{-3} s^{-1}$]
	$N_2(C) \rightarrow N_2(B) + h\nu$	8.0×10^{17}
	Population Reaction	Rate [$cm^{-3} s^{-1}$]
B	$N_2(X, v \geq 6) + N_2(A) \rightarrow N_2(B) + N_2(X)$	1.84×10^{18}
	$N_2(X) + e^- \rightarrow N_2(B) + e^-$	1.23×10^{18}
	$N_2(C) \rightarrow N_2(B) + h\nu$	0.80×10^{18}
	$N_2(A) + N_2(A) \rightarrow N_2(B) + N_2(X)$	0.24×10^{18}
	$N_2(a') + N_2(X) \rightarrow N_2(B) + N_2(X)$	0.01×10^{18}
	Depopulation Reaction	Rate [$cm^{-3} s^{-1}$]
	$N_2(B) + N_2(X) \rightarrow N_2(A) + N_2(X)$	2.09×10^{18}
	$N_2(B) \rightarrow N_2(A) + h\nu$	1.89×10^{18}
	$N_2(B) + N_2(X) \rightarrow N_2(X) + N_2(X)$	0.14×10^{18}

Table 8. Reaction rates of essential population and depopulation processes for B and C states of nitrogen molecule, calculated for $T_e = 3.0$ eV, $N_e = 4.0 \times 10^{11}$ cm^{-3}, and $P = 1.0$ Torr.

This is also experimentally confirmed by the spectroscopic observation of vibrational levels of N_2 B and C states. If we assume the corona equilibrium of the excited states, we can calculate the vibrational distribution of the states from that of N_2 X state with the application of the Franck-Condon principle. Figures 16(a) and 16(b) show the comparison between the calculated and measured vibrational number densities of B $^3\Pi_g$ (v = 7, 8, 9) state and those of C $^3\Pi_u$ (v = 0 – 4) state, respectively, at P = 1.0 Torr and z = 60 mm measured with the

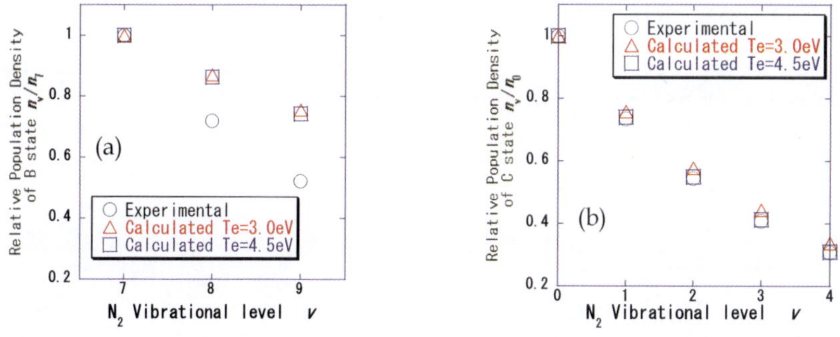

Fig. 16. Measured and calculated number densities of vibrational levels of N_2. (a) B $^3\Pi_g$ v = 7, 8, and 9 and (b) C $^3\Pi_u$ v = 0 – 4 (Sakamoto et al., 2007).

apparatus shown in Fig. 3. The agreement in the number densities observed by OES measurement with those calculated theoretically is excellent in C $^3\Pi_u$ (v = 0 – 4) state. On the other hand, it is found that of B $^3\Pi_g$ (v = 7, 8, 9) state does not agree with each other at all. One of the essential reasons for these findings lies in the respect that C state is in the corona equilibrium, while B state is not. Anyway, when we discuss the number densities of electronically excited states of N_2 in discharge plasmas, we should include the kinetics of vibrational levels as well as of population-depopulation mechanisms.

7. Conclusion

There still remain innovative and challenging applications about OES measurement of nitrogen plasma relevant to atomic and molecular processes. Following the introduction, section 2 introduced how to analyze 2PS spectrum with unresolved rotational structures, by which we can understand thermal structure of plasma processes.

Next in section 3, we introduced analysis of the 1PS spectrum. Although the procedure to analyze 1PS bands becomes far more complicated than 2PS bands, the basic strategy is the same as that of 2PS. We also demonstrated the resultant rotational temperature of 1PS is almost the same with that of 2PS for our microwave discharge nitrogen plasma. We should further examine its characteristics of vibrational non-equilibrium.

In chapter 4, we reviewed analysis of 1NS spectrum from N_2^+ ions. We also found that the rotational temperature of 1NS bands is much higher than that of 1PS or 2PS. We must further examine the reason why the 1NS bands of nitrogen show higher rotational temperature through atomic and molecular processes in the gas discharge.

In section 5, we demonstrated actinometry measurement of density of nitrogen atoms by subtracting the calculated 1PS spectrum from the one observed experimentally. Since lines from excited nitrogen atoms in the near-visible wavelength region severely overlap the 1PS band spectrum, it has been considered to be difficult to apply to nitrogen plasmas with low-dissociation degree. We overcame the problem and created another method to measure the number density of nitrogen atoms with inexpensive equipment with low-resolution.

In section 6, we introduced our simple modelling to analyze the excitation kinetics in the nitrogen plasma, which have been widely studied all over the world. This kind of modelling is essential to understand the spectroscopic characteristics of nitrogen plasmas, particularly the nonequilibrium kinetics of the vibrational levels.

We should not consider that nitrogen plasma is a commonplace industrial tool, but must scientifically respect its complicated excitation kinetics. Spectroscopic observation is one of the best experimental methods to understand it, simple and inexpensive. However, to do so, we must study its chemical kinetics after due consideration. We hope many researchers will become interested and take part in the study of this field.

8. Acknowledgment

The author thanks Mr. S. Koike, Mr. H. Kobori, Mr. R. Toyoyoshi, Mr. K. Naoi, Mr. N. Kitamura, Mr. T. Ichiki, Mr. S. Kakizaka, Mr. Y. Ohno, Mr. Y. Ichikawa, Mr. J. Mizuochi, Mr. Y. Shimizu, Mr. Y. Kittaka, Mr. T. Shibata, Mr. W. Takai, Mr. K. Kuwano, Mr. H. Kawano and, particularly, Dr. T. Sakamoto for their cooperation in spectroscopic study or atomic-molecular processes of plasmas. The author also thanks Prof. T. Yuji of University of Miyazaki, Prof. H. Matsuura, Dr. M. Matsuzaki and Mr. A. Nezu of Tokyo Institute of Technology for their helpful discussion. This study was partly supported by Grant-in-Aids for Scientific Research from the Japan Society for the Promotion of Science.

9. References

Akatsuka, H.; Ichikawa, Y.; Sakamoto, T.; Shibata, T. & Matsuura, H. (2008). Population Kinetics and Number Densities of Excited Species in Low-Pressure Discharge Nitrogen Plasma, *Proceedings of The 6th EU-Japan Joint Symposium on Plasma Processing (EU-Japan JSPP)*, pp. 13-14, Okinawa Convention Centre, Okinawa, Japan, April 2008

Akatsuka, H.; Kuwano, K.; Nezu, A. & Matsuura, H. (2010). Measurement of Nitrogen Dissociation Degree of Nitrogen Discharge Plasma by Actinometry Method with Subtraction of First Positive Band Spectrum; *Proceedings of the 63rd Gaseous Electronics Conference 2010 & 7th International Conference on Reactive Plasmas (GEC10/ ICRP7)*, pp. 59-60, ISBN 978-4-86348-101-5, Paris, France, October 2010

Bingel, W. A. (1967). Theorie der Molekülspektren, In: *Chemische Taschenbücher No. 2*, W. Foerst & H. Grünewald (Eds.) Verlag Chemie, ISBN 978-3-527-25017-2 Weinheim/ Bergstr Germany [in German]

Czerwiec, T.; Greer, F. & Graves, D. B. (2005). Nitrogen Dissociation in a Low Pressure Cylindrical ICP Discharge Studied by Actinometry and Mass Spectrometry. *J. Phys. D : Appl. Phys.*, Vol. 38, No. 24, (December 2005), pp. 4278-4289, ISSN 0022-3727

D'Agostino, R.; Favia, P.; Kawai, Y.; Ikegami, H.; Sato, N & Arefi-Khonsari, F. (Eds.). (2008). *Advanced Plasma Technology*, Wiley-VCH, ISBN 978-3-527-40591-6, Weinheim, Germany

Fridman, A. (2008). *Plasma Chemistry*, Cambridge University Press, ISBN-13 978-0-521-84735-3, New York, USA

Guerra, V. & Loureiro J. (1997). Self-Consistent Electron and Heavy-Particle Kinetics in a Low-Pressure N_2-O_2 Glow Discharge. *Plasma Sources Sci. Technol.*, Vol. 6, No. 3, (August 1997), pp. 373-385, ISSN 0963-0252

Guerra V.; Sá, P. A. & Loureiro J. (2004). Kinetic Modeling of Low-Pressure Nitrogen Discharges and Post-Discharges. *Eur. Phys. J. Appl. Phys.*, Vol. 28, No. 2, (November 2004), pp. 125-152, ISSN 1286-0042

Hrachová, V.; Diamy, A.-M.; Kylián, O.; Kaňka A. & Legrand, J.-C. (2002). Behaviour of Glow and Microwave Discharges of Oxygen, In: *Advances in Plasma Physics Research*, F. Gerard, (Ed.), pp. 33-54, Nova Science Publishers, ISBN 1-59033-329-2, New York, USA

Huang, X.-J.; Xin Y.; Yang, L.; Yuang, Q.-H. & Ning, Z.-U. (2008). Spectroscopic Study on Rotational and Vibrational Temperature of N_2 and N_2^+ in Dual-Frequency Capacitively Coupled Plasma. *Phys. Plasmas*, Vol. 15, No. 11, (November 2008), pp. 113504-1–113504-6, ISSN 1070-664X

Ichikawa, Y.; Sakamoto, T.; Nezu, A.; Matsuura, H. & Akatsuka, H. (2010). Actinometry Measurement of Dissociation Degrees of Nitrogen and Oxygen in N_2-O_2 Microwave Discharge Plasma. *Jpn. J. Appl. Phys.*, Vol. 49, No. 10, (October 2010), pp. 106101-1–106101-16, ISSN 1347-4065

Kawano, H.; Nezu, A.; Matsuura, H. & Akatsuka, H. (2011). Estimation of Vibrational and Rotational Temperatures of N_2^+ of Microwave Discharge Nitrogen Plasma by

Optical Emission Spectroscopy Measurement. *The Papers of Technical Meeting on "Plasma Science and Technology", IEE Japan,* Vol. PST-11, No. 2, pp. 15-18, [in Japanese]

Kobori, S; Koike, S.; Watanabe, S.; Matsuzaki M.; Matsuura, H. & Akatsuka, H. (2004). Dependence of Nitriding Degree of Ti Surface by Non-LTE Nitrogen Plasma on Various Plasma Parameters. *Thin Solid Films,* Vol. 457, No. 1, (June 2004), pp. 69-77, ISSN 0040-6090

Koike, S.; Sakamoto, T.; Kobori, H.; Matsuura, H. & Akatsuka, H. (2004). Spectroscopic Study on Vibrational Nonequilibrium of a Microwave Discharge Nitrogen Plasma. *Jpn. J. Appl. Phys.,* Vol. 43, No. 8A, (August 2004), pp. 5550-5557, ISSN 1347-4065

Kuwano, K.; Nezu, A.; Matsuura, H. & Akatsuka, H. (2009). Fundamental Study on Discharge Characteristics of Nitrogen-Rare Gas Microwave Plasma; *Proceedings of 6th Asia-Pacific International Symposium on the Basic and Application of Plasma Technology (APSPT 6),* Minghsin University of Science and Technology, Hsinchu, ROC, December 2009 pp. 207-210

Mizuochi, J.; Sakamoto, T.; Matsuura, H. & Akatsuka, H. (2010). Evaluation of Electron Energy Distribution Function in Microwave Discharge Plasmas by Spectroscopic Diagnostics with Collisional Radiative Model. *Jpn. J. Appl. Phys.,* Vol. 49, No. 3, (March 2010), pp. 036001-1–036001-14, ISSN 1347-4065

Nunomura, S.; Kondo, M. & Akatsuka, H. (2006). Gas Temperature and Surface Heating in Plasma Enhanced Chemical-Vapour-Deposition. *Plasma Sources Sci. Technol.,* Vol. 15, No. 4, (November 2006), pp. 783-789, ISSN 0963-0252

Ochkin, V. N. (2009). *Spectroscopy of Low Temperature Plasma,* WILEY-VCH, ISBN 978-3-527-40778-1, Weinheim, Germany

Phillips, D. M. (1976). Determination of Gas Temperature from Unresolved Bands in the Spectrum from a Nitrogen Discharge. *J. Phys. D: Appl. Phys.,* Vol. 9, No. 3, (March 1976), pp. 507-521, ISSN 0022-3727

Sakamoto, T; Matsuura, H. & Akatsuka, H. (2006). Spectroscopic Study on Vibrational Distribution of N_2 C $^3\Pi$ and B $^3\Pi$ States in Microwave Nitrogen Discharge. *Jpn. J. Appl. Phys.,* Vol. 45, No. 10A, (October 2006), pp. 7905-7910, ISSN 1347-4065

Sakamoto, T; Matsuura, H. & Akatsuka, H. (2007). Spectroscopic Study on the Vibrational Populations of N_2 C $^3\Pi$ and B $^3\Pi$ States in a Microwave Nitrogen Discharge. *J. Appl. Phys.,* Vol. 101, No. 2, (February 2007), pp. 023307-1–023307-7, ISSN 0021-8979

Shakhatov, V. A. & Lebedev, Yu. A. (2008). Kinetics of Excitation of N_2 (A $^3\Sigma_u^+$, v_A), N_2 (C $^3\Pi_u$, v_C), and N_2 (B $^3\Pi_g$, v_B) in Nitrogen Discharge Plasmas as Studied by Means of Emission Spectroscopy and Computer Simulation, *High Energy Chemistry,* Vol. 42, No. 3, (May 2008), pp. 170-204, ISSN 0018-1439

Tatarova, E.; Dias, F. M.; Gordiets, B. & Ferreira, C. M. (2005). Molecular Dissociation in N_2–H_2 Microwave Discharges. *Plasma Sources Sci. Technol.,* Vol. 14, No. 1, (February 2005), pp. 19-31, ISSN 0963-0252

Yuji, T.; Suzaki, Y.; Yamawaki, T.; Sakaue, H. & Akatsuka, H. (2007). Experimental Study of Temperatures of Atmospheric-Pressure Nonequilibrium Ar/N_2 Plasma Jets and Poly(ethylene terephtalate)-Surface Processing. *Jpn. J. Appl. Phys.,* Vol. 46, No. 2, (February 2007), pp. 795-798, ISSN 1347-4065

Yuji, T.; Urayama, T.; Fujii, S.; Mungkung, N. & Akatsuka, H. (2008), Temperature Behavior of Atmospheric-Pressure Non-Equilibrium Microwave Discharge Plasma Jets for Poly(ethylene naptharate)-Surface Processing. *Surface & Coatings Technology,* Vol. 202, No. 22-23, (August 2008), pp. 5289-5292, ISSN 0257-8972

Part 5

Application of Chemical Kinetics

15

Application of Catalysts to Metal Microreactor Systems

Pfeifer Peter
Institute for Micro Process Engineering, Karlsruhe Institute of Technology, Germany

1. Introduction

Applying microsystems for heterogeneously catalyzed processes means that the surface of tiny channels or structures has to be functionalized. Considering the surface-to-volume ratio of microchannels, volume specific surfaces of microchannels in the order of 10^5 up to 10^6 m^2/m^3 can be obtained. However, when combining the channels to reactors the entire fabrication technique and the necessary connection to conventional equipment lowers the overall surface-to-volume ratio to roughly $2*10^3$ up to $2*10^4$ m^2/m^3 and thus increases costs for materials and manufacture. Taking into account the demand of catalysis, i.e. the necessary "edges and corners" of the active species and the surface area of conventional catalyst support materials of 10^7 up to 10^9 m^2/m^3, the surface-to-volume ratio of the microsystems is not necessarily sufficient. Reviewing the literature only few cases are reported, where the geometric surface of the microsystem, e.g. channels made in copper or silver metal, is high enough ensuring cost competitive micro process engineering equipment. The reaction rates per surface site need to be very high, so that the volume specific heat flux is in a range that the advantage of microsystems, i.e. the high heat transfer rates, can be utilized for improving chemical processes in terms of process intensification.

Two approaches are often applied for increasing the geometric surface, the application of a micro fixed bed, also often called "packed bed microreactors", or the surface coating with support material and catalytically active species. Regarding the process requirements it is obvious that both approaches have Pros and Cons. So for example, commercial catalyst can directly be applied for the packed bed system while catalyst coating may take a serious time for its development. Catalysts can be removed in packed bed arrangements whereas the coating may only be removed with the whole microreactor. On the other hand coating technology provides new insights into catalysis due to quasi isothermal conditions so that much higher activity of the catalysts can be applied or obtained.

This book chapter will give information on interplay between reaction engineering aspects, material science and microfabrication which have to be considered when developing a specific heterogeneously catalysed microreactor process. A brief introduction in the individual coating approaches and exemplarily in new coating developments will be given.

2. Reaction engineering, materials and fabrication interplay

A whole set of parameters listed in Table 1 has to be considered for every kind of application and there is no easy decision for a specific catalyst integration technique. For decision making, the issues which have to be considered can be divided into three sets of categories, a) the reaction engineering, i.e. the catalyst and reaction dependent, b) the materials linked with preparation methods and c) the implications from microstructure fabrication and process.

Catalyst and reaction dependent issues	Method and material dependent issues	Implications of micro-fabrication and process
Volume specific catalyst loading	Homogeneous distribution of catalyst	Deactivation rate versus regeneration / removal
Mass specific activity of catalyst	Thermal expansion	Reactor joining method
Heat of reaction and heat transport/transfer	Adhesion (stationary / transient operation)	Stacking schemes and modular approaches
Catalyst and reactor costs	Chemical compatibility	Migration effects
Mass transport/transfer	Development effort	Reactor size implications T/p-requirements

Table 1. Categories for decision on packed bed microreactor versus various options of catalyst wall coatings in microreactors for heterogeneous catalysis

2.1 Reaction engineering aspects

From reaction engineering point of view it is not only the single parameter, i.e. the ratio of catalyst amount to mass of the reactor or the mass specific activity of the catalyst which determines the choice. It is often a combination such as the product flow per reactor mass which is a major parameter since it combines the activity of the catalyst with the occupied volume ratio of the catalyst inside the microreactor. In the following subsections the headings refer basically to the items in Table 1 - except for the latter issue – and details the individual aspects.

2.1.1 Product flow per reactor mass

Klemm et al. (2007) pointed out by a simple geometric analysis that, in comparison to a normal packed bed multi-tubular reactor, microchannel reactors suffer from small volume specific catalyst loading unless the coating layer occupies almost half the volume of the microchannels. For their comparison they assumed the same catalyst working in microchannel and the standard fixed bed under microkinetic regime, i.e. that the pore effectiveness (η) is unity. Their analysis was slightly more favourable for the microreactor in a comparison to a core-shell catalyst or at an effectiveness factor of 0.3 in conventional equipment. However, they did not explicitly mention that other possibilities of catalyst integration such as the packed bed microreactor or the use of non-standard catalysts with higher mass specific activity is feasible under excellent temperature control.

In Pfeifer et al. (2011) this comparison was extended for the packed bed microreactor approach, showing that, with different catalyst systems for the oxidation reaction of SO_2 to SO_3, both approaches can be competitive with conventional tubular reactors (Table 2).

System	V_{cat}/V_{react} or %	$m_{Stainless}/V_{cat}$ t/m³	$m_{Stainless}/m_{cat}$-	Cat.-Activity kg/kgh	$m_{Stainless}/(m_{Product}$*t) kgh/kg
Packed bed (bundle) η=1	12-15*	10*	4.2*	2	2.1
Packed bed (bundle) η=0.3	4-5*	30*	12.6*	2	6.3
Micro packed bed (commercial V_2O_5/SiO_2 catalyst)	52.7	5.4	2.3	1.8	1.3
Coated channel (Pt/TiO_2 catalyst)	1.3	251.5	105.3	30.1	3.5

Table 2. Comparison of catalyst volume fraction and influence of catalyst productivity in the oxidation of SO_2 to SO_3 on product flow per reactor mass (* data from Klemm et al. (2007)).

2.1.2 Heat of reaction and heat transport/transfer

The catalyst loading and the catalyst implementation route are strongly linked with the heat of reaction. Since the intention for the use of a microreactor is a good temperature control in the reaction fluid and the catalyst, a severe temperature gradient should be avoided. Regarding the criteria for evaluation of temperature gradients in a packed bed microreactor design it is possible to reduce the complexity of calculation to a 2-D geometrical similar tubular design or a 2-D slit design. Then it is possible to calculate temperature gradients in the micro packed bed with simplified heat balance. Knochen et al. (2010) have analysed the microreactor performance under the aspect of microchannel slit height for the Fischer-Tropsch synthesis reaction and came to the conclusion that even at 1.5 mm slit height the system works nearly isothermal.

For a possible heat transfer limitation particle-to-fluid the equation from Mears (1971) can be applied to the packed bed microreactor (Eq. 1). The same is true for a possible heat transport limitation within the catalyst particle (Anderson (1963), Eq. 2).

$$\frac{(-\Delta H_R) r_{v,eff} r_p^2}{(1-\varepsilon)\lambda_{cat}^{eff} T_s} \frac{E_A}{RT_s} < 1 \qquad 0.95 \le \eta \le 1.05 \tag{1}$$

$$\frac{(-\Delta H_R) r_{v,eff} r_p}{(1-\varepsilon)\alpha_{p,g} T_g} \frac{E_A}{RT_g} < 0.15 \qquad 0.95 \le \eta \le 1.05 \tag{2}$$

For the negligible heat transport limitations in the case of the wall-coated microreactor the equations have to be different due to the geometric changes for derivation of the criteria. Looking at Fig. 1 it becomes clear that two cases have to be distinguished with regard to the microreactor stacking scheme: A) the strictly cooled case and B) the monolithic system, where most of the channels with reaction are located next to each other.

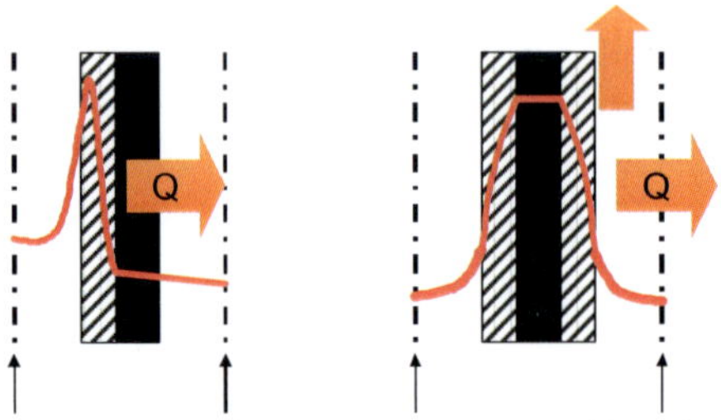

Fig. 1. Two cases which have to be distinguished for heat transfer limitation: a strictly cooled system (left) and a monolithic system (right). The different directions of heat flux and the temperature profiles are indicated (porous catalyst = shaded, microreactor wall = black).

Due to the fact that the microsystem usually operates in the region of laminar flow (small Reynolds numbers) the following order of heat resistances can be applied:

$$\alpha_g = \frac{\lambda_g}{\delta_g} \approx \frac{\lambda_g}{r_{channel}} << \frac{\lambda_{cat}^{eff}}{\delta_{cat}} << \frac{\lambda_{wall}}{s_{wall}} \tag{3}$$

That means that the maximum temperature in case A is near to the gas phase and almost all heat flux is transferred to the cooling fluid, when the cooling is effective. By approximation of the temperature profile in the catalyst as almost linearly falling instead of the real un-symmetric parabolic profile, one can derive a modified Anderson criteria like Eq. 4, which was published in Görke et al. (2009). The heat transport to the gas mixture is not relevant in case A.

$$\frac{(-\Delta H_R) r_{v,eff} \left(\frac{V_{cat}}{O_{cat,\,geo}}\right)^2}{\lambda_{cat}^{eff} T_R} \frac{E_A}{RT_R} < 0.1 \tag{4}$$

For case B the monolithic system, the heat transport to the reaction fluid has to be considered instead. Eq. 5 has been published in Görke et al. (2009).

$$\frac{(-\Delta H_R) r_{v,eff} \frac{V_{cat}}{O_{cat,geo}}}{\alpha_g T_R} \frac{E_A}{RT_R} < 0.05 \tag{5}$$

The missing porosity factor in Eqs. 4,5 compared to 1,2 is due to different assumptions for the reaction rate, i.e. the change in volume due to wall coating is assumed to be negligible.

The heat conduction along the walls of the microreactor is difficult to describe by one criterion. So a pseudo-homogenous approach for the description is necessary (see section 2.3.5).

Taking into account the maximum possible slit height of the reactor or the maximum coating thickness from reaction aspects, influence on the material aspects is obvious.

2.1.3 Catalyst and reactor costs

Catalyst costs and reactor costs may significantly change with respect to the issues which have been raised above. Higher catalyst loadings and higher allowed temperature gradients will decrease the cost of investment but temperature gradients might also increase the costs for catalyst removal due to faster deactivation. With regard to the choice of the catalyst implementation technique the costs for the catalyst might differ due to different species, i.e. when noble metals are needed for high activity in the coated system and lower specific costs can be obtained with the micro packed bed, the deactivation rate might influence the decision for the catalyst implementation method. In both cases a cost competitive system should be obtained in comparison to tubular reactors or other techniques like the fluidized bed apparatus.

Approaches for mass production of catalyst layers, i.e. reducing the coating cost are rarely reported. A cheap possibility has been demonstrated by O'Connell et al. (2011) by screen printing in the application of micro-engineered fuel reformers for hydrogen production. Such a coating is shown in Fig. 2.

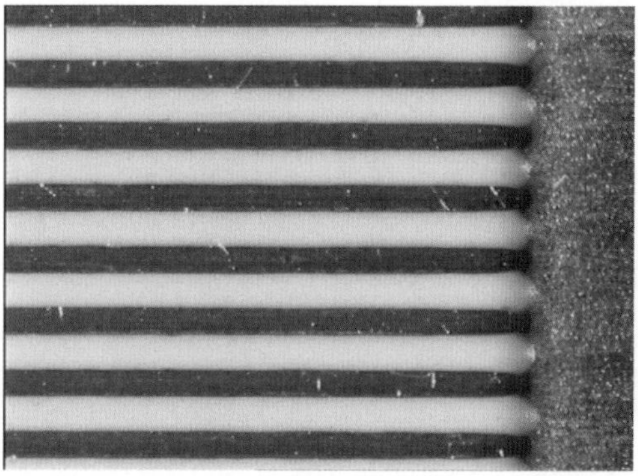

Fig. 2. Picture of an individual microchannel plate after screen printing, taken from O'Connell et al. (2011).

2.1.4 Mass transport or transfer

Due to short diffusion pathways in the microsystem, the overall mass transport in the phases or the transfer via phase boundaries is often magnitudes higher than in conventional reactor systems. However, with regard to the desired high loadings with catalyst and low cost for fluid compression or pumping, the mass transfer to the catalyst and the mass transport within porous catalyst still has to be effective. As for the heat transport the differentiation between packed bed and wall-coated microreactor is necessary for mass transport considerations. The mass transport in packed bed microreactors is not significantly different to normal tubular packed bed reactors, so that equations like the Mears criteria (Eq. 6) can be used.

$$\frac{r_{v,eff} r_p}{(1-\varepsilon) k_g c_{i,bulk}} < \frac{0.15}{n} \tag{6}$$

The assumption of laminar flow can be used to substitute the gas transport coefficient by the ratio of the diffusion coefficient of the reaction species in the mixture and half of the mean distance between the particles. Diffusion limitation in the pores of the catalyst particles can be excluded by the Weisz-Prater criteria (Eq. 7).

$$\frac{r_{v,eff} r_p^2}{(1-\varepsilon) D_i^{eff} c_{i,g}} < 1 \qquad \eta > 0.95 \qquad n \neq 0 \tag{7}$$

In the case of the wall-coated microchannel system Eq. 6 rewrites in the form of Eq. 8 (Görke et al. (2009)) due to the accessible geometric surface of the catalyst is different and the mass balance between transport to the surface and the reaction in the catalyst has to be fulfilled.

$$\frac{r_{v,eff} \frac{V_{cat}}{O_{cat,geo}}}{k_g c_{i,bulk}} < \frac{0.05}{n} \tag{8}$$

Again, the mass transport coefficient can be substituted by the ratio of the diffusion coefficient in the gas phase with the diffusion pathway, which is the radius of the free cross section or the radius of the microchannel minus the catalyst coating thickness (Eq. 9).

$$\frac{r_{v,eff} (r_{channel} - \delta_{cat}) \frac{V_{cat}}{O_{cat,geo}}}{D_i c_{i,bulk}} < \frac{0.05}{n} \tag{9}$$

This approach has been proven to be valid in simulation work by Lopes et al.(2011). For catalyst coating internal mass transport limitation the Eq. 7 can be transformed to Eq. 10.

$$\frac{r_{v,eff} (\frac{V_{cat}}{O_{cat,geo}})^2}{D_i^{eff} c_{i,g}} < 0{,}1 \qquad \eta > 0.95 \qquad n \neq 0 \tag{10}$$

The validation of negligible heat transport limitation is only possible via control of observable temperature gradients, e.g. in the cooling fluid or across the reactor walls. A sensor influence is predictable on the temperature measurement due to the small inner structures of the microreactor. In terms of mass transport resistances, some experimental approaches can be used to validate their absence.

Taking into account laminar flow occurring in microstructures, conventional tests like changing the reaction gas velocity at constant weight-hourly space velocity (WHSV) will not result in significant change of the mass transfer to the catalyst as Walter (2003) pointed out. This is due to the fact that in conventional equipment turbulent flow in the conventional packed bed is usually assumed and that the increase in velocity changes the thickness of the laminar boundary layer around the catalyst particle. In both cases, the packed bed microreactor and the wall coated system, this is not valid due to laminar flow. An experimental procedure for wall coated systems was applied by Kölbl et al. (2004). A reduction of total pressure or change of inert gas in the reaction fluid, both at constant reactant pressure, was tested on basis of the calculated change of the diffusion coefficient of the reactant in the reactant mixture. Such procedure has effect on the mass transport to the catalyst and the inner pore diffusion if Knudsen diffusion contributes to mass transport. The same kind of approach was then transferred by Bakhtiary (2010) to the micro packed bed system in which laminar flow is also dominating. Working at high pressure of 5-8 MPa under conditions of methanol synthesis reaction, he tested for a change of the conversion by changing the total pressure and the carrier gas while leaving the reactant pressure constant. In both experimental studies it was shown that no mass transport limitation in the gas phase occurred.

Experimental investigations on the mass transport limitations in catalyst layers are much more difficult as discussed by Walter (2003). Only when the change of catalyst layer thickness does not significantly change the free cross section of some microchannel arrangement, an interpretation is possible without changing the channel size either. However, when Knudsen diffusion significantly contributes to the mass transport in the catalyst, a change in the reactant diffusion coefficient could also identify a mass transport resistance in the catalyst. In packed bed microreactors the conventional method of changing the catalyst particle size is applicable for test of catalyst internal mass transport limitation (Bakhtiary (2010)).

A practical approach to overcome a possible problem of diffusion limitation in the catalyst and increasing the catalyst layer thickness is a hierarchical layer structure, which can be obtained in different ways. One way is the use of material which is microporous, i.e. possesses mainly pore diameters in the range of less than 2 nm, and which is brought onto the wall of the microsystem in shape of particles with binders. Materials such as TS1 can be sprayed as particles with diameter of roughly 5 μm onto the microchannel substrate and by using adjusted suspensions large pores can be provided (Schirrmeister et al. (2006)). The same result can be obtained by combining so-gel methods and nanoparticles. Görke & Pfeifer (2011) prepared a catalyst layer from cerium-based sol and α-alumina particles with mean particle size of 60 nm which was impregnated with platinum. This yielded a composition of 13 wt.% CeO_2 on alumina with a surface enlargement E of 3052 m^2/m^3. E is defined according to

$$E = \frac{O_{cat,BET}}{O_{wall,geo}} \tag{11}$$

Advantage of this procedure is the high catalyst amount of 17 mg/cm^2 of microchannel surface. A pure ceria layer based on sol-gel technology would only yield 0.3 mg/cm^2 and a surface enlargement of 200 m^2/m^3. The nanoparticles provide a thickness increase by factor of higher than 10 but large pores in the range of the particle size. The particle surrounding layer of cerium oxide produces then a large surface area for the introduction of the catalytically active species. A micrograph of the layer in one microchannel is shown in Figure 3.

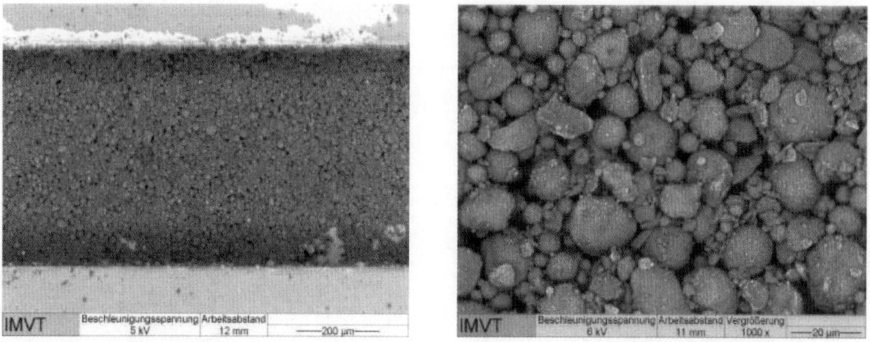

Fig. 3. SEM of a coating with 5 wt.% Pt on 13 wt.% CeO_2 on alumina nanoparticles; left: in one microchannel; right: increased magnification.

2.2 Materials and methods

From a material point of view the chemistry of the interfaces between the microstructure and the catalyst is an important issue. Influence on the catalyst distribution and the adhesion are to be considered and the effort for developing a catalyst coating is essential for its application.

2.2.1 Homogeneous distribution of catalyst

Metallic surfaces and small dimensions turn out to be critical issues, when trying to apply catalyst coatings to the microchannel walls. One critical issue is a well-defined residence time. Every microchannel may be taken as a small single reactor. Obviously, different diameters resulting, e.g. from non-uniformity of catalyst layer thickness would lead to different residence times. A simple approach can be used to show the importance for flow distributions. From calculations the pressure drop difference and therefore the mass flow difference between an 80 and a 90 μm rectangular channel is approximately 27% (assuming constant gas velocity). For heterogeneously catalysed reactions the consequences of different hydrodynamic diameters are quite difficult to elucidate, as performance loss is dependent on kinetics of the reactions occurring on the catalyst. However, if the inner diameters of 80 and 90 μm are result from a 10 or 5 μm thick coating on the channel walls in 100 μm channels, respectively, half the catalyst mass and the 27% flow increase occur in the greater channel. Thus the overall catalyst load, i.e. the flow per catalyst mass increases by 154% compared to the 10 μm thick coating, and totally different conversion or selectivity for the reaction application could be expected in the individual channels.

Important parameters for the homogeneous distribution are the methods and parameters during the preparation of the catalyst layer. An automated spraying technology, reported for example by Schirrmeister et al. (2006), can result in very homogeneous layers. Also drying rate is an important parameter for washcoating, as demonstrated in Pfeifer et al. (2004). However, the most important parameter is the order of manufacturing steps. Catalyst layers can be applied onto open microstructures (pre-coating) or into completely fabricated microdevices (post-coating) as schematically explained in Fig. 4.

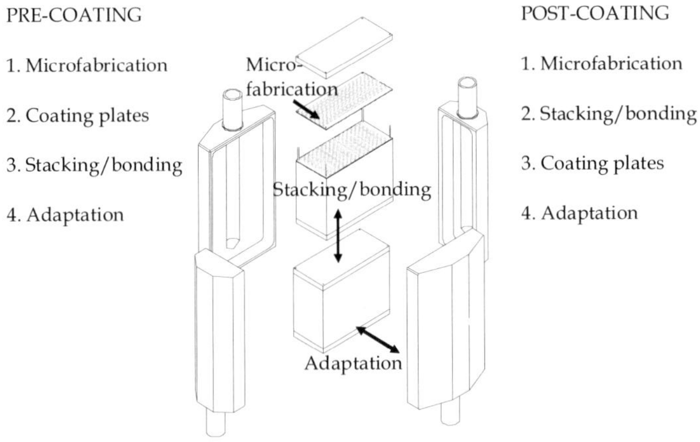

Fig. 4. Fabrication steps of microreactors including two possible routes in the consecutive order of fabrication steps (pre- and post-coating) having influence on the introduction of catalyst; the corresponding microreactor hardware is described in Pfeifer et al. (2009).

When pre-coating is applied, the subsequent bonding steps must not harm the catalyst system, i.e. no sintering or poisoning may occur. And the bonding step should not be influenced by the sintering process (see section 2.3.2). Otherwise post-coating should be applied. In that case it becomes clear that several of the coating methods can not be used, such as sputtering, spraying, ink-jet or screen printing as they require a direct accessible surface.

SEM pictures of the coatings or cutting the microstructured foils and analysing the distribution of the layer thickness can only give a qualitative impression about coating uniformity. In addition, these methods can only be applied before the microstructured foils are assembled to a complete reactor. Flow distribution has been made more uniform by introduction of regions with high pressure drop, like shown in the review of Rebrov et al. (2011). A practical approach for investigating the uniformity of catalyst layers was developed by help of hot wire anemometry of the gas velocity at the exit of the microchannel array by Pfeifer et al. (2004) and was further developed for 3-D arrangements (Pfeifer & Schubert (2008)). Work on the flow distribution in micro packed bed systems is currently under progress.

2.2.2 Thermal expansion

Due to the fact that most of the applied microreactors are made from metal and that the catalyst support layers are of ceramic nature, the thermal expansion creates large mechanical stress. During preparation of the layers often temperatures of several hundred degrees Celsius are necessary to remove binders or the precursor anion either for the support or the catalytically active species. For reactions on the catalyst, seldom lower temperatures than 100°C are sufficient and a start-up of the microreactor to operation temperature is necessary. The factors influencing the thermal shock resistance are the layer thickness, the microchannel shape, and the porosity of the support. Large continuously coated area, increasing thickness, and low porosity reduce the resistance. A high roughness of the microchannel surface can increase the stability and the thermal expansion coefficients can be adjusted in a certain extent to the ceramic material. Materials such as Crofer 22 APU® or alloy 800, which are adjusted to the properties of the membrane cermets in solid oxide fuel cells, can also be a good choice for catalyst coatings.

2.2.3 Adhesion

Adhesion and thermal expansion are very strongly linked, as the sticking properties at low temperature have certainly an effect on the ability of the catalyst layer to stick at higher temperature. Cracks in the surface, however, can still occur while heating the microsystem to the application temperature. The factors improving the adhesion are basically the same as for the thermal resistance. Often intermediate layers are used to adjust the chemical compatibility between the metal surface and the ceramic catalyst support.

The influence of the microfabrication method on the adhesion is clearly visible from the comparison of etched stainless steel versus mechanically fabricated rectangular microchannels in Figure 5. A sol-gel coating of the different microstructures was performed by Kreuder et al. (2011) yielding alumina layers with a thickness of roughly 2 μm.

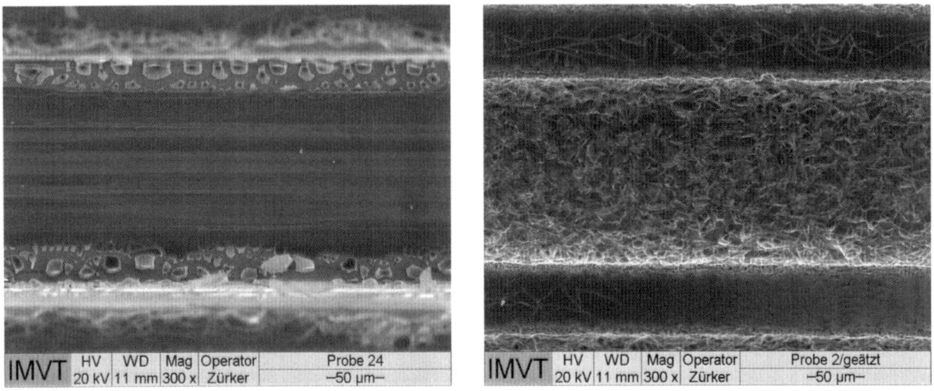

Fig. 5. Alumina layers on 316 L (1.4404) stainless steel; left: coating on mechanically fabricated rectangular microchannel; right: coating on chemically etched microchannel.

The methods to test the adhesion properties are dependent on the type of application, if it is a stationary application or if the microreactor is operated in transient mode. Mobile applications like reformer for fuel cell applications have special demand for vibration resistance of the coating. A procedure for the testing can be the determination of the weight difference after putting an adhesive tape on top of the catalyst layer and its removal or slight bending of the metallic microstructure. Some kind of standardized tests is proposed in Schwarz et al. (2010) - the loss of catalyst layer according to DIN EN ISO 4624 (bending test).

2.2.4 Chemical compatibility

Chemical compatibility can be discussed in three different ways: the compatibility with regard to the adhesion (discussed before), the compatibility with regard to the reaction gases and the diffusion of species from the catalyst into the metallic microchannel wall or vice versa (see section 2.3.4). Special attention should also be paid on the interaction between catalytically active species and the metal microstructure, since the electronic properties of e.g. noble metals can be influenced by the metal substrate and selectivities can be shifted. This effect has been recognized very early in Pfeifer et al. (2004b), where the influence of the steel or aluminum microstructured substrate was observed for a PdZn alloy catalyst. While under the conditions of methanol steam reforming on this catalyst the main route is directly to CO_2 and hydrogen, the CO byproduct formation increased by the contact of the PdZn with the substrate. This effect could also occur in the case of the micro packed bed approach. However, no literature addressed this issue so far. Activity of the microstructure wall with regard to conversion of reactants may very prohibitive as discussed by several authors, e.g. severe byproduct formation was found by Walter (2003) for the selective oxidation of isoprene to citraconic anhydride due to the large surface area provided in microstructured reactors. On the other hand, appropriate choice of the metal can lead to significant potential for process intensification. Myrstad et al. (2009) showed that the microstructured reactor wall made from stainless steel does not influence the product distribution or the catalyst deactivation in the Fischer-Tropsch synthesis reaction.

2.2.5 Development effort

The more complex the catalyst system the longer is the time needed for formulation of a well-known powder catalyst as a coating. Using conventional catalyst, some studies have demonstrated that the use dissolved or colloidal binders like pseudo-boehmite or sodium silicate (waterglass) is not recommended. Active sites can be covered and surface area of the support can be lost, as stated by Nijhuis et al. (2001) or Groppi et al. (2000). On the other hand, some studies exist where such approach was successful. E.g. a mixture of $CuO/ZnO/Al_2O_3$ catalyst was deposited with alumina sol on stainless steel sheets by Park et al. (2004). For approaches where new precursors are needed to prepare the catalytic coating, the development time might increase by orders of magnitude. So, rapid screening of coatings on microstructured supports would be desired. These approaches have been started by Claus et al. (2001). However, the time needed for preparation of the layers and the different layer thickness from different chemical precursors are critical issues as pointed out in section 2.2.1.

2.3 Implications of microfabrication and process

The microfabrication and the applied processes, e.g. for bonding, as well as the application conditions can have influence on the discussion of catalyst incorporation into the microsystem. The following subsections will detail these issues further.

2.3.1 Deactivation rate versus catalyst regeneration / removal

One of the most critical issues for applying catalyst layers is, that strong adhesion is the demand during operation of the microreactor, but when deactivation occurs the removal of the catalyst layer may then become a challenging task. Reactor costs must be low, so that the reactor can be removed as low cost assembly, but in most cases the life cycle analysis and the life cycle costing may not allow such approach. Microchannel catalyst coating reviews by Meille (2006) or Renken & Kiwi-Minsker (2010) give no information on catalyst removal topics.

Investigations at IMVT at KIT show that a certain potential for multiple coating with sol-gel approach is possible since the coating thickness is seldom larger than 2-3 μm. For alumina support the removal of the support including the catalytically active species is possible on stainless steel supports by the use of NaOH solutions. Cerium oxide layers and silica layers are hardly to remove but their tolerance to poisoning or deactivation is often lower than for other supports. Cerium oxide is proven to stabilize catalysts for soot tolerance in steam reforming of diesel type fuels as demonstrated by Thormann et al. (2008) and (2011). Regeneration under air atmosphere and reaction temperature led to a full recovery of the initial catalyst activity.

In first consideration on removal of catalyst from packed bed microreactors one could easily forget the phenomena of catalyst morphology changes during in-situ activation or reaction operation, sintering or densification of the catalyst bed and possible residues from reaction. Catalyst morphology changes often occur on copper catalysts due to continuous change between Cu^+ and Cu(0) species in methanol synthesis or methanol steam reforming to hydrogen. However, no issue was observed in the work of Bakhtiary et al. (2011) and Hayer et al. (2011). The aspect of residues from reaction can be much more challenging in the case of Fischer-Tropsch synthesis like in the work from Myrstad et al. (2009). Here a wax fraction from the catalysis remains on the catalyst and a purge flow of solvent to remove the catalyst is necessary. A purge flow of ethanol was also proven to work for charcoal catalyst removal in microstructures of the type shown in Figure 6.

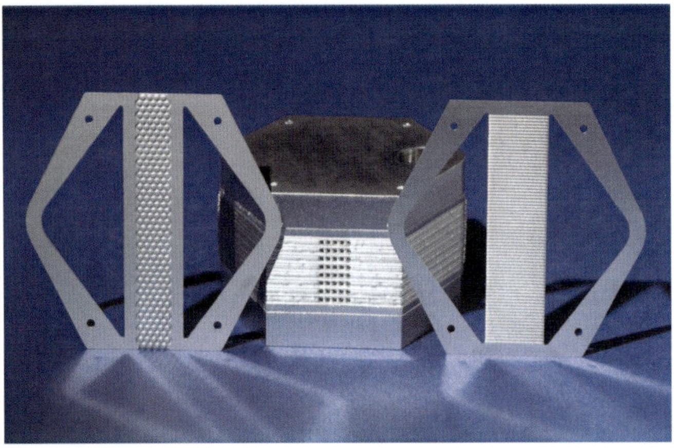

Fig. 6. Pillar type microstructures (left) and heat exchange microstructure (right) used at IMVT at KIT for the implementation of a packed bed into microreactor assemblies (middle) for several applications and catalysts, such as charcoal and alumina based catalysts.

2.3.2 Reactor joining method

As stated in section 2.2.1 the joining of the microstructures to a form an assembled microreactor system can be before or after the coating, suggested denotation post-coating or pre-coating respectively. Due to non-accessible walls of the microstructure in the inner part of assembled microreactors only a flow coating method can be applied, either in the liquid phase (see Fig. 7) or from the gas phase. Procedures which can apply to the flow coating are

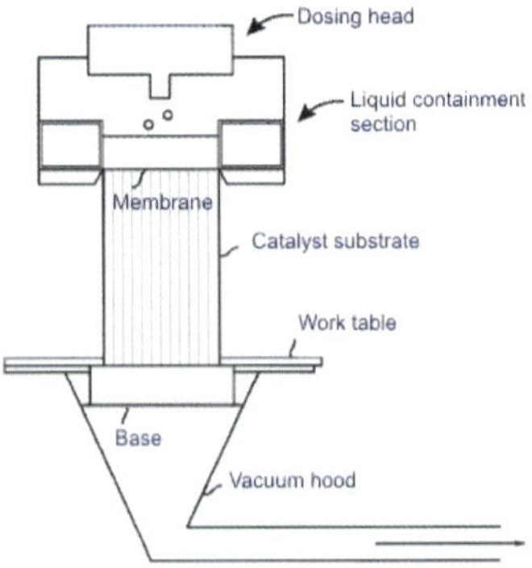

Fig. 7. Schematic of a catalyst coating apparatus used for monoliths as well as microreactors, adapted from Aderhold et al. (2003).

liquid or suspension methods such as sol-gel technology and washcoating. However, viscosities of the fluids or suspensions and precursor loading have to be thoroughly adjusted. Too thin layers or blocking can result from inadequate composition. Rebrov & Schouten (2011), for example, have carried out a study on the necessary viscosity for titania sols for dip-coating which could also apply for flow coating procedures.

From the gas phase only Chemical Vapour Deposition [CVD] can be applied in certain circumstances for a post-coating with catalyst. The deposition rate which is influencing the gas phase content of the support or active species precursor will determine the homogeneity of the catalyst along the microchannels. The deposition rate is mainly influenced by the parameters: microstructure wall temperature, microchannel diameter and the flow velocity in the microchannels at constant pressure. These parameters relate to the diffusivity of the precursor. Appropriateness of CVD methods for coating with Al_2O_3 has been shown very early by Janicke et al. (2000).

For the electro-assisted methods, like electrophoretic deposition and anodic oxidation of aluminum/titanium alloys as material of the microstructure have also limitations in length and shape of the microchannels. The schematic of the apparatus, unpublished so far, for such coating is shown in Figure 8. Flow of the suspension or the electrolyte is established through the microreactor assembly and the microreactor metal represents the anode. Cathodes are located in front of inlet and outlet of the microreactor. The flow rate of the suspension or the electrolyte should be high enough to avoid reduction of the particle load in the liquid or of the electrolyte ions, respectively. Bends are not allowed in the channel shape as they prevent a continuous electric field. The accessible channel length is linked with the channel size, as a decrease in channel size will reduce the strength of the electric field. Coatings produced by these methods are presented in Wunsch et al. (2002) and Pfeifer et al. (2002).

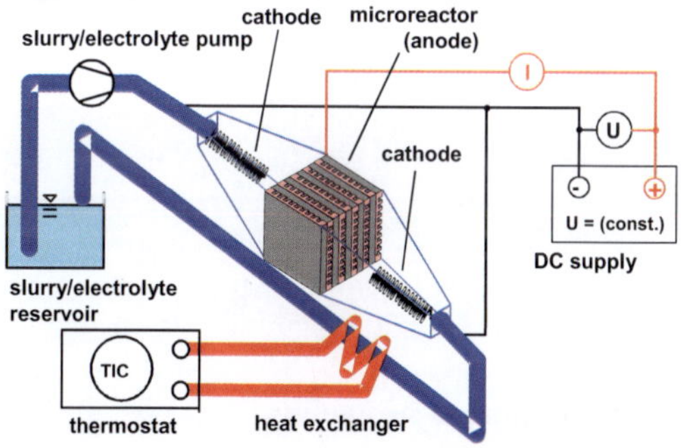

Fig. 8. Schematic of a catalyst coating apparatus for electrophoretic deposition or anodic oxidation inside assembled microreactors.

The joining methods for microstructures which end up in the necessity for flow coating are usually soldering/brazing or diffusion bonding. Temperature for these joining processes are ranging from 400 to 1400°C and start usually with melting of copper brazes and end up with roughly 2/3 of the melting temperature of the material from which the microstructures are built for diffusion bonding. No catalyst material should be located on the bonding planes. Procedures which apply to coated microstructures are laser or electron beam welding. In the latter case some temperature influence on the catalyst system may be feasible near the location of the weld seam.

2.3.3 Reactor size implications

In practical pre-coating most of the methods known are nearly unlimited concerning the size of the plates to coat. Even for Physical Vapour Deposition [PVD] and sputtering one could imagine a very large chamber for the coating procedure. For the post-coating some size and shape limit exists as pointed out in the previous section. For CVD, anodic oxidation and electrophoretic deposition the highest limitations exist. Larger catalyst bed heights are not necessarily a problem regarding the pressure drop due to low particle sizes (50 - 150 μm) in the micro packed bed approach, as reported by Myrstad et al. (2009).

The joining methods may have additional limitations regarding the materials and by that possibly on the outer size of the reactor. Materials, like aluminum and titanium, which tend to segregate oxygen-rich surface species, are hardly to join by diffusion bonding. The same is true for material with temperature sensitive segregation of phases. Since the material implies again some limitations in the catalyst coating procedure and by this on the total reactor size.

The microstructure size, e.g. microchannel width and height, which belongs to the reactor size attributes, is influenced by the microfabrication method. The individual microfabrication methods imply different surface roughness and shape, and impact on the catalyst incorporation technique is obvious.

2.3.4 Migration effects

Migration effects can occur between the metal microstructure and the catalyst due to soldering/brazing materials or in course of operation in reaction medium. Copper and silver as brazing components have high diffusivity and can mix up with e.g. noble metals like palladium or platinum. The migration effects occurring under reaction conditions were investigated by Enger at el. (2008). They found that, under conditions of methane partial oxidation to synthesis gas, the alumina layers created from annealing aluminum-rich FeCrAlloy® steel prevents chromium enrichment in the support and the rhodium catalytically active species. Support layers of alumina prepared by sol-gel route did not prevent a contamination of rhodium with chromium from Alloy 800 steel (Fig. 9). New investigations at IMVT show that cerium oxide is a much better inhibitor for migration.

2.3.5 Stacking schemes and modular approaches

Since costs for microfabrication may hinder the industrial competitiveness of microreactors, the use of optimum stacking schemes and modular approaches can be an approach to reduce the costs of the overall assembly. Reducing the number of microstructured plates for cooling/heating of catalytically modified microstructured plates will automatically reduce the costs. This changes also the stacking scheme. In the ideal temperature controlled situation each plate with integrated catalyst is adjacent to a microstructure for heating/cooling (alternating stacking scheme 1:1). Under reduced costs several plates with catalyst will be adjacent to each other. With regard to the catalyst temperature control, the heat conduction in the walls of the microreactor has to be described. A pseudo-homogenous approach for the description was developed therefore in Pfeifer et al. (2003). Based on a

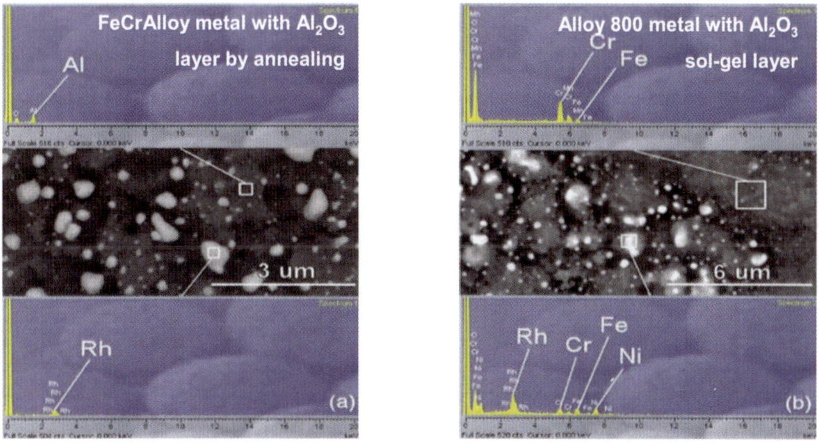

Fig. 9. Energy Dispersive X-ray Analysis and SEM of the rhodium containing alumina catalyst layer on top of the steel microstructure; a) catalyst prepared by segregation of alumina during annealing on FeCrAlloy® with subsequent incipient wetness impregnation with rhodium precursor, b) sol-gel alumina layer with rhodium by incipient wetness impregnation on alloy 800.

volumetric heat production rate due to reaction the stack temperature gradient can be calculated.

$$\Delta T = \frac{|\dot{q}_V| s_{max}^2}{2\lambda_{wall}} \quad (12)$$

The volume basis for this simple model is the material of the fins or pillars between the channels or in the slits, respectively. This specific volume is responsible for transport through a stack of several catalytically modified microstructured plates without intermediate cooling or heating. Assumption for this simple solution of the heat transport equation is a temperature constant heat production rate, so that only small predicted gradients fit the experiment. The stack height without intermediate cooling/heating is $2{*}s_{max}$.

Modular approaches, meaning that several stacks of microstructures are operated in parallel or series, can help to reduce the reactor size implications but a maintenance and fluid distributions strategy amongst the modules has to be developed for process control. Also the costs reduction for fabrication will not necessarily be significant by increasing the number of modules. This might then lead to low economies of scale in chemicals production with the microreactor system.

2.3.6 T/p-requirements

The temperature and pressure requirements of the chemical process which should be conducted on the catalyst integrated in the microreactor are influencing the method of catalyst implementation with regard to the material choice. High temperatures of more than 600°C imply the use of materials like alloy 800 or FeCrAlloy®, whereas stainless steel is sufficient below that temperature under moderate pressure conditions. Above 950°C the thin walls between the microchannels or microstructures get attacked by high temperature corrosion and the problem of metal choice is not sufficiently solved there.

With regard to the pressure resistance, diffusion bonding and soldering presumably are the methods of choice for the joining procedure, which limits the materials for the microstructure and thus the catalyst integration technique.

3. Conclusion

The individual parameters which influence the choice of the catalyst with regard to reaction engineering, material science and fabrication issues are discussed. The crosslink between the individual parameters is shown on basis of some reaction engineering examples and relevant literature is cited. Indications for the design of microreactors are given by criteria, which allow for judgement of necessary efforts for miniaturisation.

However, it becomes obvious that there is no clear overall indication which way of catalyst integration is the best for obtaining the highest degree of process intensification with minimum investment and lowest operation costs. Every chemical process has to be judged on its own, before the choice for the approach is done.

4. Acknowledgment

I would like to thank all the colleagues, co-workers and PhD students for contributing to this book chapter in experimental and theoretical background. My special thanks also go to Hilde, Hamid, Fatemeh, Xuyen, Ingrid, Björn, Rune and Anders in Norway for the long lasting nice collaboration.

5. List of symbols

α_g	Heat transfer coefficient at catalyst layer
$\alpha_{p,g}$	Heat transfer coefficient at catalyst particle
$c_{i,bulk}$	Concentration of species i in the gas (fluid) bulk phase
$c_{i,g}$	Concentration species i in the gas (fluid) phase at catalyst surface
δ_{cat}	Catalyst layer thickness
δ_g	Thickness of laminar heat transfer layer
D_i^{eff}	Effective diffusion coefficient species i in the solid catalyst
E	Surface enhancement factor
E_A	Activation energy
ε	Porosity
η	Pore efficiency
ΔH_R	Reaction enthalpy
k_g	Mass transport coefficient
λ_{cat}^{eff}	Effective catalyst heat conduction coefficient
λ_g	Heat conduction coefficient gas (fluid)

λ_{wall} Heat conduction coefficient microchannel wall
n Reaction order
$O_{cat,BET}$ Catalyst inner surface, measured by BET method
$O_{cat,\,geo}$ Catalyst geometric surface
$O_{wall,geo}$ Geometric surface of the microchannel
$\dot{q}_V$ Volumetric heat production rate due to reaction
R Gas constant
$r_{channel}$ Radius of the microchannel
r_p Mean catalyst particle radius
$r_{v,eff}$ Observed volumetric reaction rate
s_{max} Half of the microchannels stack height
s_{wall} Thickness microchannel wall
T_g Gas (fluid) temperature
T_R Reaction temperature
T_s Solid (catalyst) temperature
ΔT Temperature gradient in the microchannel stack
V_{cat} Catalyst volume

6. References

Aderhold, D., Haynes, A.G., Spencer, M.L.W. & Winterborn D.J.W. (2003). Monolith coating apparatus and method therefore, *US Patent 6,599,570* (Johnson Matthey).

Anderson, J.B. (1963). A criterion for isothermal behaviour of a catalyst pellet. *Chemical Engineering Science*, Vol. 18, 147-148.

Bakhtiary, H.D. (2010). Performance assessment of a packed bed microstructured reactor – heat exchanger for methanol synthesis from syngas. *PhD Thesis, NTNU*, Norway, 2010:205.

Bakhtiary, H.D., Hayer, F., Phan, X.K., Myrstad, R., Venvik, H.J., Pfeifer, P. & Holmen, A. (2011), Characteristics of an Integrated Micro Packed Bed Reactor-Heat Exchanger for methanol synthesis from syngas. *Chemical Engineering Journal*, Vol. 167, 496–503.

Claus, P., Hönicke, D. & Zech, T. (2001). Miniaturization of screening devices for the combinatorial development of heterogeneous catalysts. *Catalysis Today*, Vol. 67, Iss. 4, 319-339.

Enger, B.C., Walmsley, J., Bjoergum, E., Loedeng, R., Pfeifer, P., Schubert, K., Holmen, A. & Venvik, H.J. (2008). Performance and SEM characterization of Rh impregnated microchannel reactors in the catalytic partial oxidation of methane and propane. *Chemical Engineering Journal*, Vol. 144, 489-501.

Görke, O. & Pfeifer, P. (2011). Preferential CO oxidation over a platinum ceria aluminia in a microchannel reactor with distributed gas feeding. *International Journal of Hydrogen Energy*, Vol. 36, 4673-4681.

Görke, O., Pfeifer, P. & Schubert, K. (2009). Kinetic study of ethanol reforming in a microreactor. *Applied Catalysis A: General*, Vol. 360, 232–241.

Groppi, G., Cristiani, C., Valentini, M. & Tronconi, E. (2000). Development of novel structured reactors for highly exothermic reactions. *Proceedings of the 12th*

International Congress on Catalysis, Studies in Surface Science and Catalysis, Vol. 130, 2747–2752.

Hayer, F, Bakhtiary, H.D., Myrstad, R., Venvik, H., Pfeifer, P. & Holmen, A. (2011), Synthesis of Dimethyl Ether from Syngas in a Microchannel Reactor - Simulation and Experimental Study. *Chemical Engineering Journal*, Vol. 167, Iss. 2-3, 610-615.

Janicke, M.T., Kestenbaum, H., Hagendorf, U., Schüth, F., Fichtner, M. & Schubert, K. (2000). The Controlled Oxidation of Hydrogen from an Explosive Mixture of Gases Using a Microstructured Reactor/Heat Exchanger and Pt/Al_2O_3 Catalyst. *Journal of Catalysis*, Vol. 191, 282–293.

Klemm, E., Döring, H., Geißelmann, A. & Schirrmeister, S. (2007). Mikrostrukturreaktoren für die heterogene Katalyse. *Chemie Ingenieur Technik*, Vol. 79, No. 6, p. 697-706.

Knochen, J., Güttel, R., Knobloch, C. & Turek, T. (2010). Fischer–Tropsch synthesis in milli-structured fixed-bed reactors: Experimental study and scale-up considerations, *Chemical Engineering and Processing*. Vol. 49, 958-964.

Kölbl, A., Pfeifer, P., Kraut, M., Schubert, K., Fichtner, M., Liauw, M.A. & Emig, G. (2004). Characterization of Flow Distribution in Microchannel Reactors. *Chemical Engineering and Technology*, Vol. 27, Iss. 6, 671-675.

Kreuder, H., Pfeifer, P. & Dittmeyer, R. (2011). Catalyst preparation for dehydrogenation of cycloalkanes in a microreactor. *1st International Symposium on Chemistry of Energy Conversion and Storage [ChemEner]*, February 27th to March 2nd 2011, Berlin – Germany, Poster No. 20.

Lopes, J.P., Cardoso, S.S.S. & Rodrigues, A.E. (2011). Criteria for kinetic and mass transfer control in a microchannel reactor with an isothermal first-order wall reaction. *Chemical Engineering Journal*, doi:10.1016/j.cej.2011.05.088.

Mears, D.E. (1971). Tests for Transport Limitations in Experimental Catalytic Reactors. *Industrial Engineering Chemistry Process Design and Development*, Vol. 10, 541-547.

Meille, V. (2006). Review on methods to deposit catalysts on structured surfaces. *Applied Catalysis A – General*, Vol. 315, 1-17.

Myrstad, R., Eri, S., Pfeifer, P., Rytter, E. & Holmen, A. (2009). Fischer-Tropsch synthesis in a microstructured reactor. *Catalysis Today*, Vol. 147, Suppl. 1, 301-304.

Nijhuis, T.A., Beers, A.E.W., Vergunst, T., Hoek, I., Kapteijn, F. & Moulijn, J.A. (2001). *Catalysis Reviews, Science and Engineering*, Vol. 43, 345–380.

O'Connell, M., Kolb, G., Schelhaas, K.-P., Wichert, M., Tiemann, D., Pennemann H. & Zapf R. (2011). Towards mass production of microstructured fuel processors for application in future distributed energy generation systems: A review of recent progress at IMM. *Chemical Engineering Research and Design*, doi:10.1016 /j.cherd.2011.08.002

Park, G.-G., Seo, D.J., Park, S.-H., Yoon, Y.-G., Kim, C.-S. & Yoon W.-L. (2004). Development of microchannel methanol steam reformer. *Chemical Engineering Jorunal*, Vol. 101, 87–92.

Pfeifer, P. & Schubert K. (2008). Hot wire anemometry for experimental determination of flow distribution in multilayer microreactors. *Chemical Engineering Journal*, Vol. 135, Supplement 1, S173-S178

Pfeifer, P., Görke, O. & Schubert, K. (2002). Waschcoats and electrophoresis with coated and uncoated nanoparticles on microstructured metal foils and microstructured reactors. Proceedings of IMRET 6, *AIChE Spring Meeting Pub. 164*, 281–287.

Pfeifer, P., Haas-Santo, K. & Görke, O. (2009). Application and Operation of Microreactors for Fuel Conversion, *in Handbook of Micro Process Engineering*, Eds. V. Hessel, A. Renken, J.C. Schouten, and J. Yoshida, Vol. 2: Devices, Reactions, Applications, Wiley, 405-420.

Pfeifer, P., Schubert, K., Liauw, M.A. & Emig G. (2004). Characterization of flow distribution in microchannel reactors. *AIChE Journal*, Vol. 50, Iss. 2, 418-425.

Pfeifer, P., Schubert, K., Liauw, M.A. & Emig G. (2004b). PdZn-Catalysts prepared by washcoating microstructured reactors. *Applied Catalysis A - General*, Vol. 270, 165-175.

Pfeifer, P., Schubert, K., Liauw, M.A. & Emig, G. (2003). Electrically heated microreactors for methanol steam reforming. *Chemical Engineering Research and Design*, Vol. 81, A7, 711-720.

Pfeifer, P., Zscherpe, T., Haas-Santo, K. & Dittmeyer, R. (2011). Investigations on a Pt/TiO_2 catalyst coating for oxidation of SO_2 in a microstructured reactor for operation with forced decreasing temperature profile. *Applied Catalysis A: General*, Vol. 391, 289–296.

Rebrov, E.V. & Schouten J.C. (2011). Limiting withdrawal rate and maximum film thickness during dip-coating of titania sols onto a Si substrate. *Chemical Engineering and Processing: Process Intensification*, doi:10.1016/j.cep.2011.05.025.

Rebrov, E.V., Schouten, J.C. & de Croon M.H.J.M. (2011). Single-Phase Fluid Flow Distribution and Heat Transfer in Microstructured Reactors. *Chemical Engineering Science*, Vol. 66, Iss. 7, 1374-1393.

Renken, A. & Kiwi-Minsker, L. (2010), Microstructured Catalytic Reactors, *Advances in Catalysis*, Vol. 53, 47-122.

Schirrmeister, S., Büker, K., Schmitz-Niederau, M., Langanke, B., Geißelmann, A., Becker, F., Machnik, R., Markowz, G., Schwarz, T. & Klemm, E. (2006). Katalytisch beschichtete Träger, Verfahren zu dessen Herstellung und damit ausgestatteter Reaktor sowie dessen Verwendung. *EP 10 2005 019 000 A1*, 26.10.2006.

Schwarz, T., Schirrmeister, S., Döring, H. & Klemm, E. (2010). Herstellung von Wandkatalysatoren für Mikrostrukturreaktoren mittels Niederdruckspritz-technologie, *Chemie Ingenieur Technik*, Vol. 82, 921-928.

Thormann, J., Pfeifer, P. & Kunz U. (2011). Dynamic Performance of Hexadecane Steam Reforming in a Microstructured Reactor. *Chemical Engineering Journal*, doi:10.1016/j.cej.2011.08.011.

Thormann, J., Pfeifer, P., Schubert, K. & Kunz U. (2008). Reforming of diesel fuel in a micro reactor for APU systems. *Chemical Engineering Journal*, Vol. 135, Suppl. 1, S74-S81.

Walter, S. (2003). Mikrostrukturreaktoren für selektive Oxidationsreaktionen: Isopren zu Citraconsäureanhydrid. *PhD Thesis, Shaker*, Aachen, 2003.

Wunsch, R., Fichtner, M., Görke, O., Haas-Santo, K. & Schubert, K. (2002), Process of applying Al_2O_3 coatings in microchannels of completely manufactured reactors. *Chemcal Engineering and Technology*, Vol. 25, 700–703.

Permissions

The contributors of this book come from diverse backgrounds, making this book a truly international effort. This book will bring forth new frontiers with its revolutionizing research information and detailed analysis of the nascent developments around the world.

We would like to thank Dr. Vivek Patel, for lending his expertise to make the book truly unique. He has played a crucial role in the development of this book. Without his invaluable contribution this book wouldn't have been possible. He has made vital efforts to compile up to date information on the varied aspects of this subject to make this book a valuable addition to the collection of many professionals and students.

This book was conceptualized with the vision of imparting up-to-date information and advanced data in this field. To ensure the same, a matchless editorial board was set up. Every individual on the board went through rigorous rounds of assessment to prove their worth. After which they invested a large part of their time researching and compiling the most relevant data for our readers. Conferences and sessions were held from time to time between the editorial board and the contributing authors to present the data in the most comprehensible form. The editorial team has worked tirelessly to provide valuable and valid information to help people across the globe.

Every chapter published in this book has been scrutinized by our experts. Their significance has been extensively debated. The topics covered herein carry significant findings which will fuel the growth of the discipline. They may even be implemented as practical applications or may be referred to as a beginning point for another development. Chapters in this book were first published by InTech; hereby published with permission under the Creative Commons Attribution License or equivalent.

The editorial board has been involved in producing this book since its inception. They have spent rigorous hours researching and exploring the diverse topics which have resulted in the successful publishing of this book. They have passed on their knowledge of decades through this book. To expedite this challenging task, the publisher supported the team at every step. A small team of assistant editors was also appointed to further simplify the editing procedure and attain best results for the readers.

Our editorial team has been hand-picked from every corner of the world. Their multi-ethnicity adds dynamic inputs to the discussions which result in innovative outcomes. These outcomes are then further discussed with the researchers and contributors who give their valuable feedback and opinion regarding the same. The feedback is then collaborated with the researches and they are edited in a comprehensive manner to aid the understanding of the subject.

Apart from the editorial board, the designing team has also invested a significant amount of their time in understanding the subject and creating the most relevant covers. They scrutinized every image to scout for the most suitable representation of the subject and create an appropriate cover for the book.

The publishing team has been involved in this book since its early stages. They were actively engaged in every process, be it collecting the data, connecting with the contributors or procuring relevant information. The team has been an ardent support to the editorial, designing and production team. Their endless efforts to recruit the best for this project, has resulted in the accomplishment of this book. They are a veteran in the field of academics and their pool of knowledge is as vast as their experience in printing. Their expertise and guidance has proved useful at every step. Their uncompromising quality standards have made this book an exceptional effort. Their encouragement from time to time has been an inspiration for everyone.

The publisher and the editorial board hope that this book will prove to be a valuable piece of knowledge for researchers, students, practitioners and scholars across the globe.

List of Contributors

Stefano Zambelli
University of Padova, Italy

Victor Martinez-Luaces
Electrochemistry Engineering Multidisciplinary Research Group, University of the Republic of Uruguay, Montevideo, Uruguay

Boris M. Kaganovich, Alexandre V. Keiko, Vitaly A. Shamansky and Maxim S. Zarodnyuk
Melentiev Energy Systems Institute, Russia

E.V. Kustova and E.A. Nagnibeda
Saint Petersburg State University, Russia

Terese Løvås
Department of Energy and Process Engineering, Norwegian University of Science and Technology, Norway

Hiroshi Kawanabe
Graduate School of Energy Science, Kyoto University, Japan

Ock Taeck Lim
University of Ulsan, Republic of Korea

Norimasa Iida
Keio University, Japan

David M. Holloway
Mathematics Department, British Columbia Institute of Technology, Canada

Ruggero Barni and Claudia Riccardi
Department of Physics G. Occhialini, University of Milano-Bicocca, Milan, Italy

Ramasamy Pothiraja, Nikita Bibinov and Peter Awakowicz
Institute for Electrical Engineering and Plasma Technology, Ruhr-University Bochum, Germany

Boris A. Mosienko
Siberian Research Institute of Geology, Geophysics and Mineral Resources, Novosibirsk, Russia

Zuoxiang Zeng, Li Cui, Weilan Xue, Jing Chen and Yu Che
Institute of Chemical Engineering, East China University of Science and Technology, P.R.China

Hiroshi Akatsuka
Tokyo Institute of Technology, Japan

Pfeifer Peter
Institute for Micro Process Engineering, Karlsruhe Institute of Technology, Germany